The Physical Principles of Diagnostic Radiology

The Physical Principles of Diagnostic Radiology

by

Perry Sprawls, Jr., Ph.D.
Professor of Radiology
Emory University School of Medicine

University Park Press
Baltimore • London • Tokyo

UNIVERSITY PARK PRESS
International Publishers in Science and Medicine
Chamber of Commerce Building
Baltimore, Maryland 21202

Typeset by The Composing Room of Michigan, Inc.
Manufactured in the United States of America by Universal Lithographers, Inc., and The Optic Bindery Incorporated

Library of Congress Cataloging in Publication Data

Sprawls, Perry.
The physical principles of diagnostic radiology.

Includes index.
1. Diagnosis, Radioscopic. 2. Radiation. I. Title.
[DNLM: 1. Radiography. 2. Health physics.
WN110 S767p]
RC78S683 616.07′572 77-8531
ISBN 0-8391-0968-7

Contents

Preface

This book is designed to be used by persons studying for a career in diagnostic radiology. It is based on material that has been presented in the training programs of the Department of Radiology of the Emory University School of Medicine.

Training in the physical principles of radiology, or radiological physics, as it is commonly known, is undergoing a significant change in many institutions. For many years most radiologists trained in both the diagnostic and therapeutic applications of radiation. Traditionally, the physics training was heavily oriented toward the therapeutic applications. However, in recent years there has been a major emphasis placed on the physics of diagnostic radiology, because most radiologists are entering that field and also because the diagnostic x-ray systems are increasingly sophisticated. It is these changes that have produced a need for a book of this type.

The book assumes that the reader has no background in physics. It begins by introducing the basic physical principles necessary to the understanding of x-ray machine function and image formation. The intent of the book is to present the various principles and concepts in a specific sequence, introducing new concepts only after the underlying principles have been thoroughly discussed.

Most persons embarking on the study of radiological physics are apprehensive about the mathematics required. Any reader who feels this way is strongly urged to begin his study with the materials covered in the appendix. After reviewing the various mathematical concepts that apply to radiology and working the exercises, he should find that mathematics has become an aid, rather than a hindrance, to his understanding of the physics concepts.

Acknowledgments

The preparation of this book has been aided by the significant contribution of many individuals, who are gratefully acknowledged.

The illustrations were prepared by Jake D. Paulk.

Judith Lolkema typed and edited the text material. Christine Weinberg also participated in the manuscript preparation. The editorial assistance of my wife Charlotte is gratefully acknowledged.

Jack E. Peterson has graciously read and contributed many suggestions during the preparation of this text. Other physicists who assisted with selected sections are Robert H. Rohrer and Gary T. Barnes.

Many of the hours that have gone into the preparation of this book were possible only because of the generosity of others. The understanding and support of my son Charles in this respect is gratefully acknowledged.

I wish to express my sincere appreciation to Dr. H. S. Weens, Chairman, Department of Radiology, for his many years of encouragement and support in the development of diagnostic radiological physics at Emory University. It is his interest and high standards in training future radiologists that have made this book possible.

The Physical Principles of Diagnostic Radiology

Chapter 1

Introduction to X-ray Imaging

The development of pathological conditions and trauma often produces changes in the physical structure of the human body. The early practitioners of the healing arts were able to observe only those gross physical changes that modified the body's exterior appearance. The vast majority of physical manifestations were undetectable, either because they were small in size, i.e., at the cellular level, or because they were hidden within the body. The development of the microscope and associated techniques permitted visualization of the minute tissue changes, and the discovery of x-rays opened up all points within the body to direct observation.

Diagnostic medical radiology began in 1896, only a few months after a German physicist, Wilhelm Konrad Roentgen, discovered a form of penetrating radiation, to which he gave the name x-rays.

Modern radiology is built on the same basic concepts and techniques that were demonstrated by Roentgen. However, technological evolution has moved the realm of medical x-ray from the simple table-top apparatus of Roentgen's day to complex systems that use the latest developments in electronics and computers.

The purpose of this book is to explore the physical principles upon which modern x-ray imaging systems are based.

ROENTGEN'S DISCOVERY

The forerunners of x-rays were cathode rays, which were later identified as electrons. In the last half of the nineteenth century, several scientists were studying the characteristics of cathode rays, which were being produced in partially evacuated glass tubes, energized by high voltage electrical sources. On November 8, 1895, Wilhelm Roentgen was conducting experiments with this type of apparatus. It had been discovered that the so-called cathode rays could penetrate several centimeters of air, expose photographic plates (film), and also cause certain fluorescent materials to glow in the dark. On this particular afternoon, Roentgen was setting up an experiment, with apparatus similar to that shown in Figure 1, that was designed to determine whether the cathode rays could penetrate the walls of a tube not equipped with a special thin window. While energizing the tube in the darkened laboratory, he noticed a weak light coming from something located on a nearby bench. He quickly discovered that the light occurred only when an electrical current was passing through the tube. He lit a match to locate the source of the light and discovered that it was a barium platinocyanide screen, which had been placed on the bench. These fluorescent screens could be caused to glow by cathode ray bombardment, but in this case the distance between the tube and screen was much greater than the penetrating range of cathode ray electrons.

This initial discovery was followed by days of excited experimentation in which Roentgen studied the characteristics of this new penetrating radiation. In late December he submitted a paper for publication to the Wurzburg Physical Medical Society entitled: "On a New Kind of Rays, a Preliminary Communication."

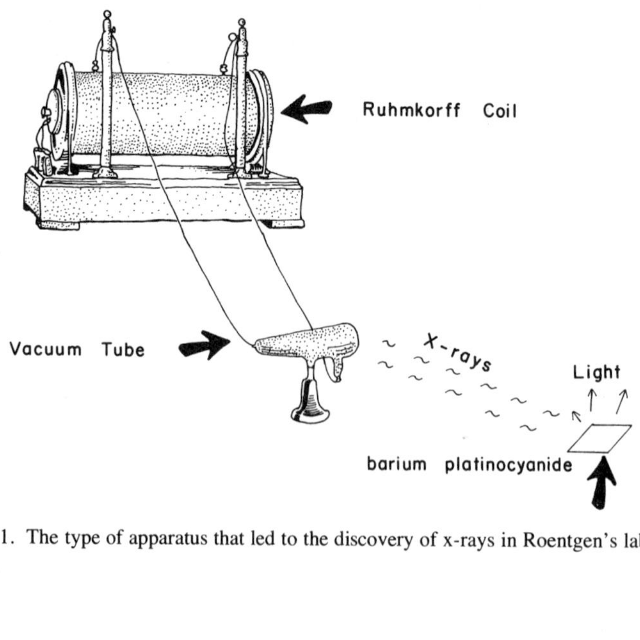

Figure 1. The type of apparatus that led to the discovery of x-rays in Roentgen's laboratory.

This classic scientific paper of approximately 10 printed pages begins with the following description of Roentgen's discovery.

> If one passes the discharges of a fairly large Ruhmkorff induction coil through a Hittorf vacuum tube, a sufficiently evacuated Lenard or Crookes tube, or a similar apparatus, and if one covers the tube with a rather closely fitting envelope of thin black cardboard, one observes in the completely darkened room that a piece of paper painted with barium platinocyanide lying near the apparatus glows brightly or becomes fluorescent with each discharge, regardless of whether the coated surface or the other side faces the discharge apparatus. The fluorescence is still visible at a distance of 2 m from the apparatus.

In this publication, Roentgen, after just a few weeks of intense work, described most of the important physical characteristics of x-radiation known even today. He described how x-rays could be detected or observed by allowing them to fall on fluorescent materials or expose photographic plates and films. He quickly discovered that a unique characteristic of the new radiation was its ability to penetrate many solid objects. He felt, however, that the penetration depended on properties of the object, such as thickness and density. He reported how the x-rays would cast a shadow of his hand, but one in which the bones were visible. His clever experiments soon confirmed that his discovery was not just another type of light, or cathode rays (electrons), but was indeed a new type of radiation, which he designated as x-rays.

In 1901 Wilhelm Konrad Roentgen was awarded the first Nobel Prize in Physics for his discovery of x-rays.

PROPERTIES OF X-RAYS

X-rays, a form of radiation energy, have several important properties that make them useful in both diagnostic and therapeutic applications. Five of these properties are illustrated in Figure 2. X-radiation is not necessarily unique with respect to any individual property, but gets its importance from the specific combination of properties shown. It is helpful to introduce diagnostic radiology with a brief look at these effects of x-radiation.

Penetration

Perhaps the characteristic of x-radiation that caused Roentgen to realize that it was something new was its penetrating ability. This gives x-radiation the ability to image structures within the human body. With respect to penetration, a significant fact is that all materials are not penetrated equally, as Roentgen discovered. This allows certain objects, such as the

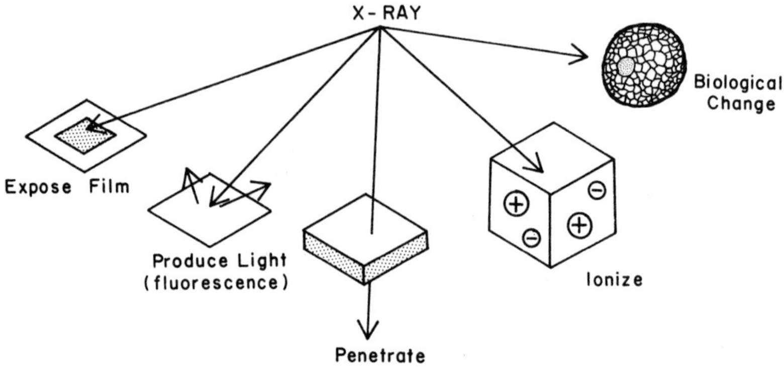

Figure 2. The five important properties and effects produced by x-radiation.

bones, to form shadow-type images because they permit less penetration than the surrounding soft tissue.

Fluorescence

X-rays are a form of radiation that is invisible to the human eye. In fact, Roentgen and other scientists had been producing x-rays long before their discovery but were unaware of their presence. It was only when the invisible x-rays fell upon a piece of barium platinocyanide and produced light that their presence was noticed. The production of light by bombarding certain materials, such as barium platinocyanide, with other forms of radiation is known as fluorescence. This property is used in most x-ray imaging systems to convert the invisible x-ray image into a light image that can be observed directly, recorded on film, or processed electronically.

Film Exposure

X-radiation, like light, will expose photographic-type film. Although this provides a possible means for recording x-ray images, it is seldom used in modern radiology. Today most x-ray images are formed by first producing a light image by fluorescence and allowing the light to expose the film.

Ionization

Because of the relatively high amount of energy carried by each individual x-ray unit (photon), it has the ability to disrupt atoms within material through which it passes. This disruption is in the form of electron removal or ionization. Since ionization in gases, such as air, is relatively easy to measure, this provides a means for detecting and measuring quantities of x-radiation. Because of this property, x-rays are often referred to as ionizing radiation.

Biological Effects

As x-radiation passes through living matter, a portion of the energy will be absorbed and can produce changes at the cellular level. The ultimate results of these interactions depend on many factors, which form the science of radiation biology. In diagnostic applications of x-rays, the biological effects constitute an undesirable factor that should be minimized as much as possible. However, the entire field of therapeutic radiology is based on this particular radiation property.

X-RAY IMAGING

This new type of radiation, later to be designated as Roentgen rays, had two crucial properties that would cause it to be the medium for an entirely new approach to medical diagnosis. These properties, illustrated in Figure 3, are the ability 1) to produce a visible image by causing certain materials

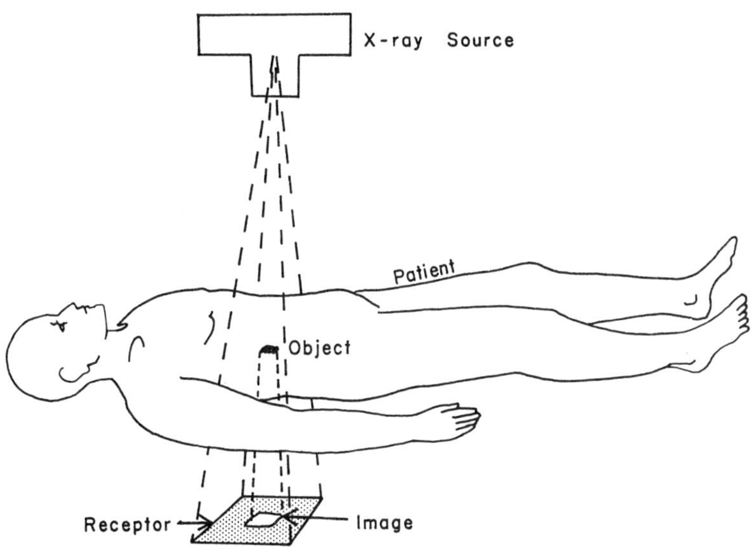

Figure 3. The basic principle of producing an x-ray image of an object within the human body.

to fluoresce (emit light) or photographic emulsions to be exposed, and 2) to be selectively absorbed by various materials which causes shadow images to be formed. Casting shadows of internal body structures was to be the underlying principle of all x-ray examinations for approximately eighty years. No other method of x-ray image formation was used until the mid-1970s, with the introduction of computed tomography imaging systems.

X-RAY SYSTEM

Perhaps it is best to introduce the x-ray machine not as a single device, but as a system comprised of several components, each with its own specific function. The basic components of the general diagnostic x-ray machine are shown in Figure 4.

Components

The heart of the system is the x-ray tube itself. Its function is simply to convert electrical energy into x-ray energy. Although the design of modern x-ray tubes has little in common with those of Roentgen's day, the operating principle is essentially the same.

X-rays can be produced only if the tube is energized by a very high electrical voltage. The relatively low voltage from power lines is not adequate for this purpose. Therefore, it is necessary to include a power

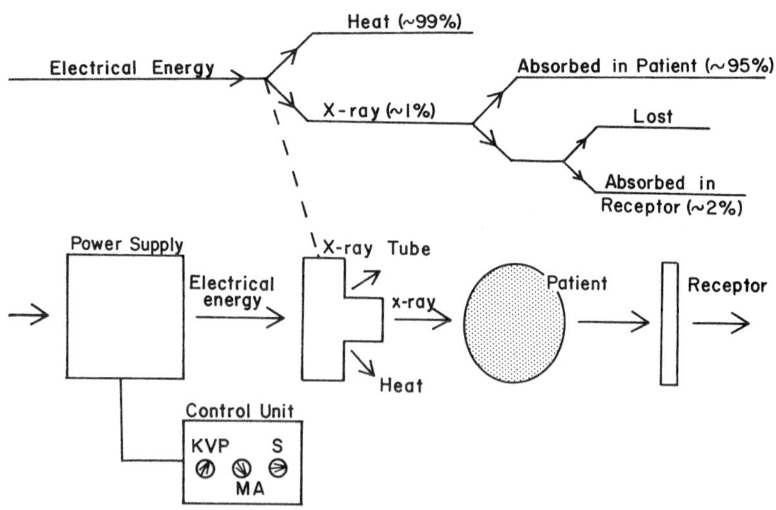

Figure 4. The basic components of the x-ray imaging system and the associated flow of energy. KVP, peak kilovoltage; MA, tube current; S, seconds.

supply in the system. Actually, this is not the source of energy or power as the name would imply, but is an energy converter. It converts electrical energy from the power distribution system to a voltage and form that can be used for x-ray production.

Closely associated with the power supply is a control unit, which is used to select the quantity and characteristics of the electrical energy applied to the x-ray tube. This, in turn, determines the quantity and characteristics of the x-rays produced. The final component in the system is the image receptor. Its purpose is to convert the invisible x-ray image into one that can be viewed by the physician. Receptors are of two basic types. Those that produce an immediate image are used in the fluoroscopic system. The name fluoroscope comes from the fluorescent screens that were used as receptors for many years. X-ray systems that produce a permanent image on film operate in the radiographic mode.

From the technical standpoint, the patient's body becomes part of the x-ray system. The formation of a quality image depends heavily on the proper selection of correct system operating parameters in accordance with the characteristics of the body section being examined. Within the patient's body, the x-ray beam does two things: it forms the image and deposits most of its energy.

Energy Flow

It should always be remembered that an x-ray system is an information-gathering system that utilizes a flow of energy between its components. There are two points within the system at which the desired energy transfer is very inefficient. Most of the electrical energy applied to the x-ray tube is converted into potentially damaging heat. Usually, less than 1% of the energy leaves the tube in the form of useful x-radiation. Most of the x-ray energy that enters the patient is absorbed by the body and only a small fraction passes through and carries the image to the receptor.

The basic purpose of a diagnostic x-ray system is to obtain information from within the body concerning its physical structure. In all forms of communication or movement of information, a carrier of some form must be used. In the case of x-ray examinations, the information is moved by a flow of energy. Energy, i.e., x-radiation, flows from the x-ray tube, through the patient, and on to the receptor where the visible image is formed. Unfortunately, most of the energy is absorbed within the patient's body. It is not that the quantity of energy in one examination is so great, but it is the ability of x-radiation to produce chemical and biological changes in living tissue that is the cause for concern. X-ray diagnosis, like many other medical procedures, is not without risk. Perhaps the ultimate goal in the design of x-ray systems is to obtain a maximum of information with the smallest possible quantity of energy deposited in the patient. Continued technological advancement has both dramatically increased the information obtained and reduced the amount of energy required. It is probably safe to say that the ratio of information, a quantity that is extremely difficult to measure, to patient exposure has been increased by a factor of several hundred during the "lifetime" of radiology.

The user of x-ray equipment must also be aware of another aspect of the information-radiation relationship. In a very general sense, the amount of information obtained in an examination is related to patient radiation exposure, perhaps somewhat like the graph shown in Figure 5. Although the actual shape of the curve is pure conjecture, it allows some very pertinent points to be made.

One consideration in "designing" an examination is the following. How much information is actually required in order to make the diagnosis? Using a system that might provide more, but unnecessary, information (image detail) subjects the patient to unnecessary radiation exposure. And, conversely, using a system that might deliver less patient exposure might also fall short with respect to the information content of the image. Unfortunately, there are no infallible rules that one can use to select the "perfect" system for a given type of examination. Hopefully, the user who has a thorough understanding of the x-ray system components and characteristics can make these judgments with some degree of confidence.

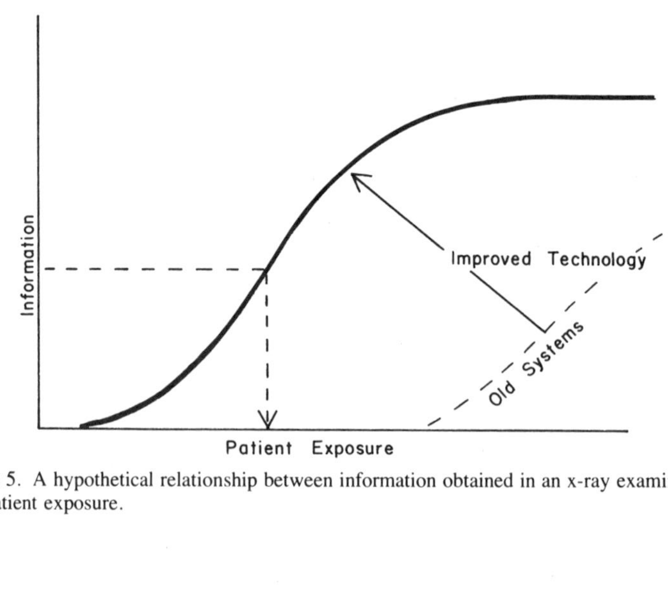

Figure 5. A hypothetical relationship between information obtained in an x-ray examination and patient exposure.

Both the lower and upper portions of the curve deserve comment. There is a lower radiation limit below which very little useful information can be gathered. This is primarily because of the random nature of x-rays, which will be discussed thoroughly in a later chapter. The upper end carries the message that increasing exposure above the "necessary" level not only produces unnecessary information, but at some point might not produce any additional information at all.

REFERENCES

Donizetti, P. 1967. Shadow and Substance—The Story of Medical Radiography. Pergamon Press, Long Island City, New York. 213 pp.

Glasser, O. 1939. What kind of tube did Roentgen use when he discovered the x-rays? Radiology 27:138.

Glasser, O. 1958. Dr. W. C. Roentgen. Charles C, Thomas, Publisher, Springfield, Ill. 169 pp.

Chapter II Energy and Radiation

A point of emphasis in the last chapter was that there is a general flow of energy between most of the components in the x-ray system. In most instances the energy is either transmitted in the form of radiation or is carried by electrons. Both forms of energy transport will be considered in detail, but first a discussion of the units used to quantitate energy is necessary.

Energy is often defined simply as the ability to do work. Although this definition is technically correct, it gives very little insight into energy as it relates to radiology. Perhaps a more appropriate description is that energy is essentially the ability to produce a physical change in matter or, in some situations, produce a stimulus to the human body. In our daily routines, we observe many forms of energy. A very common form is heat, which can raise the temperature of an object, cause water to boil, and can produce a reaction when applied to the human body. The wind is but one type of mechanical energy and its effect on trees and sailboats is easily observed. The chemical energy of gasoline is converted into another form—mechanical—by the engine and it moves the automobile down the street. Electrical energy flows into our homes to be used, in many instances, as a substitute for energy from the human body.

UNITS OF ENERGY

Energy is a measurable quantity. Throughout the years, many different units have been used to specify quantities of energy. A great variety of energy units occurs because different countries have developed their own systems of physical quantities, such as the British system and the metric system, and because different units are needed for large and small quantities of energy. Another trend has been to ''invent'' special energy units for the different forms of energy. For example, the British thermal unit (Btu) is an energy unit used almost exclusively for one form of energy, heat. In some fields, heat energy is specified in calories, and radiology has its own special unit for heat, the heat unit.

Obviously, all possible energy units are not used in radiology, but there is a sufficient number to benefit from some attempt at organization. Figure 1 shows the relationship among three of the basic general purpose energy units. These are the electron volt (eV), the erg, and the joule (J), which is also called the watt-second. All of these are units for specifying quantities of the same thing, energy. The major difference is in their size.

The smallest energy unit is the electron volt. The light emitted by a single atom would generally have an energy of several electron volts. This

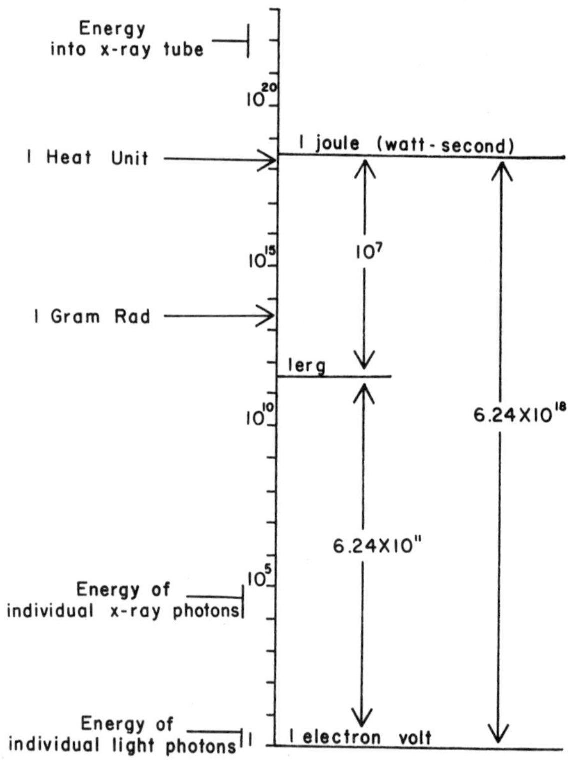

Figure 1. A scale showing the relationship of different energy units. The numerical values on the scale represent energy in electron volts.

quantity of energy is much too small to be seen or felt by humans. A somewhat larger unit, by a factor of 6.24×10^{11}, is the erg. When a photograph is made, the amount of light energy that passes through the lens during the exposure is typically in the order of several ergs. An even larger energy unit is the joule. If a 100-watt light bulb is turned on for 10 sec, the amount of energy dissipated (light and heat) would be 1,000 J, or watt-seconds. Even for the same form of energy, such as light, different energy units are needed. It depends on whether we are specifying the energy from a single atom or from a floodlight.

It should be noticed that the scale in Figure 1 is logarithmic (see Appendix I) and covers a very large range of values. This wide range of energy quantities is encountered in radiology. For example, the total energy transferred to an x-ray tube during a single exposure is perhaps 10^{22} times more than the energy of one of the light photons that exposes the radiographic film.

Two other energy units that are more or less unique to radiology are the heat unit (HU) and the gram-rad. The relationship between these units and the general purpose units shown in Figure 1 is:

$$1 \text{ heat unit (HU)} = 0.71 \text{ J}$$

$$1 \text{ gram-rad} = 100 \text{ ergs}$$

POWER

In many situations, the significant quantity is the rate at which energy is being transferred. This quantity is power. The most common power unit is the watt. One watt is 1 J per sec. Since power is a rate, the total amount of energy transferred is the product of power and time. Going back to the earlier example of the light bulb, the bulb that transfers at a rate of 100 watts continuously for 10 sec transfers a total energy of 1,000 J or watt-seconds. A 10-watt light bulb can transfer the same total amount of energy, but only if it is turned on for 100 sec.

INTENSITY

Whereas power describes energy transfer with respect to time, intensity is the relationship between power and the area through which the energy passes. Intensity is generally defined as the rate of energy transfer per square centimeter of beam cross-sectional area. It can be considered as the concentration of power in a given area.

Table 1. Unit multiples and prefixes encountered in radiology

Multiple	Prefix	Symbol	Example
10^6	mega-	M	megahertz (Mhz)
10^3	kilo-	k	kilovolt (kV)
10^{-2}	centi-	c	centimeter (cm)
10^{-3}	milli-	m	milliroentgen (mR)
10^{-6}	micro-	μ	microsecond (μsec)
10^{-9}	nano-	n	nanometer (nm)

UNIT MULTIPLES

Even when there is a variety of units available for expressing physical quantities, such as energy, it is often desirable to use additional units that are either factor of 10 multiples or submultiples of basic units. The name of the derived unit is established by an appropriate prefix, which indicates the multiple value. Table 1 contains most of the multiple units encountered in radiology.

ELECTROMAGNETIC RADIATION

Radiation is the movement of energy through space. There are two basic types of radiation. One type consists of small particles traveling at very high velocities and carrying energy. Typical examples are alpha and beta particles emitted from radioactive materials. The other type of radiation, which includes x-radiation, consists of pure energy. Radiation of this type, which has no particles or mass associated with it, is classified as electromagnetic radiation. Figure 2 illustrates the flow of electromagnetic radi-

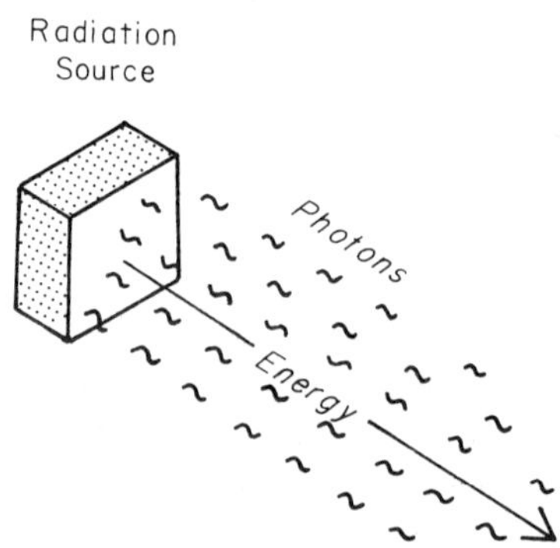

Figure 2. The quantum concept of radiation.

ation from a source. One of the most significant characteristics of electromagnetic radiation is that it is emitted by the source as a shower of small individual units of energy, called photons. Each photon is a certain quantity of energy. A photon is often said to be a quantum of energy.

There are many different types of electromagnetic radiation, such as light, radio, and television signals, and, of course, x-ray. What distinguishes one type of electromagnetic radiation from another are characteristics of the individual photons. Several of the physical characteristics of photons are discussed below, but it will be shown that they are all related. For example, if you know the energy of a photon, you can easily determine its other physical characteristics and classify it according to type of electromagnetic radiation.

Photon Energy

Since a photon is simply a unit of energy, one of its important characteristics is the quantity of energy that it contains. Photon energies are usually specified in the units of electron volts or appropriate multiples.

If all of the various types of electromagnetic radiation were analyzed with respect to the photon energies, and then arranged on a scale, as shown in Figure 3, the results would be the so-called electromagnetic spectrum. It should be emphasized that it is the energy of the individual photons which determines the type of electromagnetic radiation, i.e., light, x-ray, or radio signals. X-radiation produced by machines for diagnostic purposes is made up of photons with energies ranging from about 10 keV (10,000 eV) to slightly above 100 keV. X-ray machines do not produce photons of all the same energy, nor do they produce the same number of photons at each energy. The expanded segment in Figure 3 shows a typical x-ray energy spectrum that might be encountered in diagnostic work. The spectrum of photon energies coming from an x-ray machine can be changed by altering the operating parameters. This will be discussed in detail later.

It will soon be shown that there is a significant difference, even among the x-ray photons, as to how they interact with matter. The lower energy x-ray photons are often referred to as soft radiation, whereas the higher energy end of the spectrum would be so-called hard radiation. One important aspect of photon energy is that it generally determines the penetrating ability of the radiation. High energy (hard) x-radiation is, in most situations, more penetrating than the softer portion of the spectrum.

Photon Velocity

All electromagnetic radiation travels with the same velocity through space. Because light is one of the most common forms of electromagnetic radia-

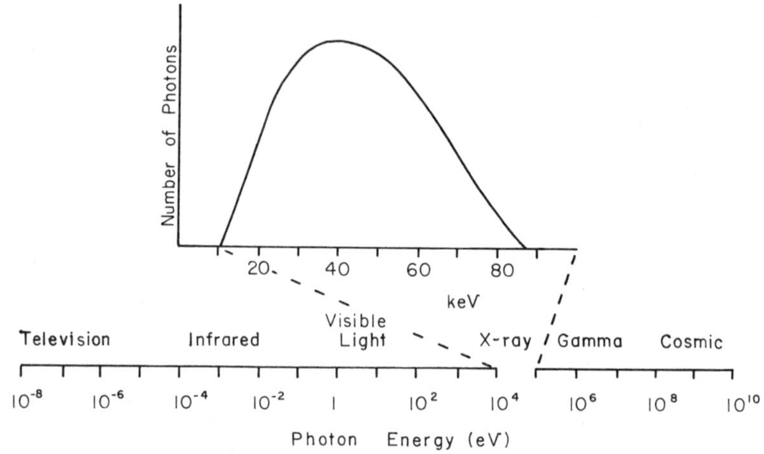

Figure 3. The electromagnetic radiation spectrum with an expanded view of the x-ray segment.

tion and its velocity is known, it is often said that x-rays and other electromagnetic radiations travel with the "speed of light." In free space, this is a velocity of 3×10^8 meters per sec. If it is assumed that the average x-ray photon travels a distance of 1 m between the time it is created and absorbed, the average lifetime of a photon would be 3.3×10^{-9} sec. Photons cannot be stored or suspended in space. Once a photon is created and emitted by a source, it travels with this very high velocity until it interacts with and is absorbed by some material, as shown in Figure 4. In

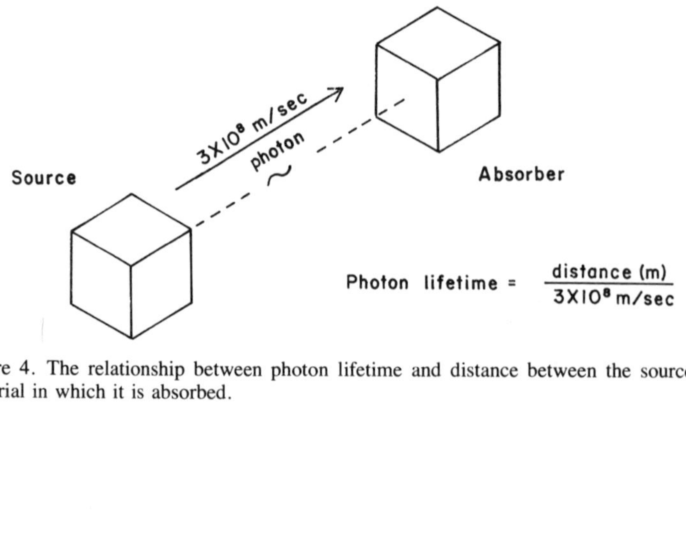

Figure 4. The relationship between photon lifetime and distance between the source and material in which it is absorbed.

its very short lifetime, the x-ray photon moves a small amount of energy from the source to the absorbing material.

Frequency

Another characteristic of all types of electromagnetic radiation is its frequency. Frequency denotes a rate of vibration or oscillation. One of the laws of physics which applies to electromagnetic radiation is that a photon's energy (E) and frequency (f) are directly proportional, with the relationship being:

$$E = hf$$

In this relationship, h is Planck's constant, which has a value of 6.625×10^{-27} erg-sec, and f is frequency in hertz (Hz, cycles per second). Although, theoretically, x-radiation has a frequency associated with it, the concept is never used. However, for other types of electromagnetic radiation, such as radio and television signals, frequency is the characteristic most used in describing radiation. For example, radio station WSB in Atlanta emits radiation that has a frequency of 760,000 Hz. Radio receivers are tuned to receive a desired signal according to frequency.

Wavelength

Various physical phenomena observed with electromagnetic radiation suggest that the radiation has certain wavelike properties. A characteristic of any type of wave is the distance between two successive peaks, which is the wavelengh (λ). This is also the distance the radiation moves forward during the period of one oscillation.

Wavelength can be expressed in any units of length. Radio and television signals have relatively long wavelengths and are usually expressed in meters. They also have extremely small photon energies because of the inverse energy-wavelength relationship. For higher energy photons, such as light and x-ray, two smaller length units are used. These are:

$$1 \text{ Angstrom unit (Å)} = 10^{-10} \text{ m}$$

$$1 \text{ nanometer (nm)} = 10^{-9} \text{ m}$$

The angstrom unit is generally preferred for x-ray length and the nanometer is used for light. A nanometer is equivalent to a millimicron, which is used in some literature.

Since velocity (c) is essentially constant, the wavelength is related to the frequency of the radiation in the following manner:

$$\lambda = \frac{c}{f}$$

Since there is a specific relationship between wavelength and frequency, and between frequency and photon energy, it follows that wavelength and photon energy should also be related. By combining the two relationships in the following manner, the relationship between photon energy and wave length is obtained:

$$E = hf = \frac{hc}{\lambda}$$

By introducing the appropriate values for h and c, this can be written as:

$$E(\text{keV}) = \frac{12.4}{\lambda(\text{Å})}$$

This is a relationship that allows one to convert radiation photon energy into wavelength and vice versa. In some literature, x-ray photon energy spectra are given in terms of wavelength rather than photon energy. This causes the spectrum curve to have an entirely different appearance, as shown in Figure 5. By using the relationship given above, it is possible to convert a spectrum of one kind into the other. Since energy and wavelength are inversely related, the highest energy on the spectrum corresponds to the shortest wavelength.

In most instances, light photons are classified according to their

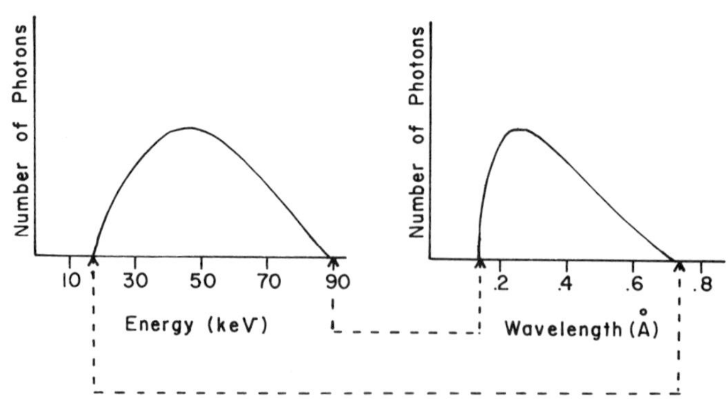

Figure 5. Two methods for drawing the same x-ray spectrum. One uses a photon energy scale and the other uses wavelength.

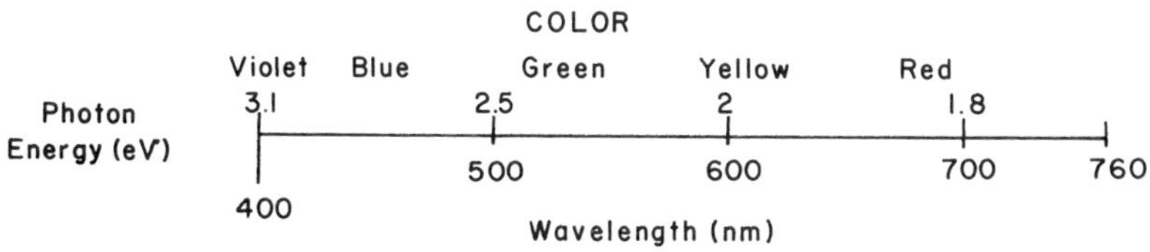

Figure 6. The visible light spectrum showing the relationship of color, wavelength, and photon energy.

wavelength. Another characteristic of light that is directly associated with the wavelength is color, as illustrated in Figure 6. The difference between red and blue light is just a difference in wavelength (and photon energy).

In summary, the four basic physical characteristics of electromagnetic photons are energy, wavelength, frequency, and velocity. The velocity of all radiation is essentially the same. The other three characteristics are interrelated so that if the value of one is known the others can be easily determined. Although a given photon can be completely described by specifying the value for any one of the three characteristics, certain characteristics are generally preferred for certain types of radiation. For example, radio signals are usually classified by frequency, light by wavelength, and x-ray photons according to their energies. The interrelationships among the photon characteristics are summarized in Figure 7.

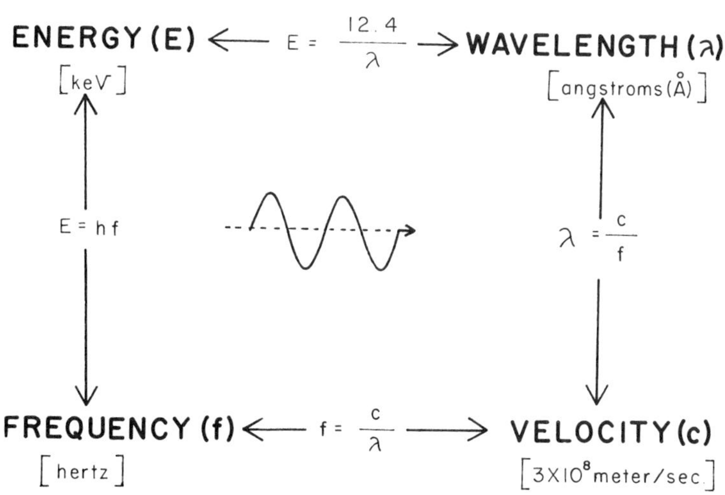

Figure 7. The relationship of the four basic physical characteristics of a photon.

Chapter III
Electrons and the Structure of Matter

X-ray photons begin and end their "lives" within various materials or matter. Both the birth and death of x-ray photons involve the interchange of energy with very small particles found within the atoms. These small particles are the electrons. In addition to being intimately involved in the formation and the absorption of photons, the electrons are the major transporters of energy between several of the components in the x-ray system. In fact, the electron might be considered the "lifeblood" of our modern civilization. It is the transporter of much of the energy we use, and is also an important part of most of our communications systems.

Electrons are the smallest particles found in the structure of matter. An electron has a mass of 9.1×10^{-28} grams (g) which means it would take 10.9×10^{26} electrons to have the same weight as one cubic centimeter (cc) of water. The question might be raised as to how such a small particle can be the foundation of our modern technology. The answer is simple—numbers. As will be seen later, tremendous numbers of electrons are involved in most applications. For example, when a 100-watt light bulb is turned on, electrons race through the wires carrying energy to it at the rate of 5.2×10^{18} electrons per second.

In addition to their mass, which is relatively small, all electrons carry a 1-unit negative electrical charge. It is the charge of an electron that gives it the ability to interact with other electrons and particles within the atoms.

ELECTRON ENERGY

Because an electron has both mass and electrical charge, it can possess energy. There are several different types of energy that an electron can

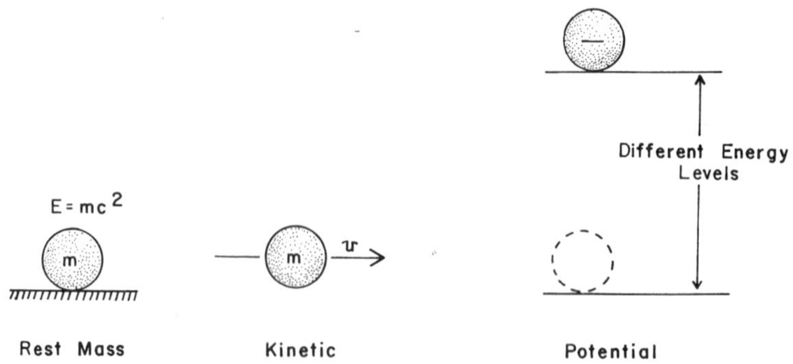

Figure 1. The three types of energy associated with electrons.

have, as shown in Figure 1. It is the ability of an electron to take up, transport, and give up energy that makes it useful in the x-ray system.

Rest-Mass Energy

Even when an electron is at rest and has no apparent motion, it still has energy. In fact, according to the laws of physics, any object has some energy just because of its mass. Under certain conditions, mass can be converted into energy and vice versa. Einstein's famous equation:

$$E = mc^2$$

predicts the amount of energy that could be obtained, if an object with a mass, m, is completely converted. In this relationship, c is the speed of light. Although it is not possible with our present technology to convert most objects into energy, it can happen to electrons. There are certain radioactive materials which emit particles, positrons, which can completely annihilate electrons. When this happens, the electron's mass is completely converted into energy, and according to Einstein's relationship each electron will yield 510 keV. This energy appears as a photon. Although this type of electron interaction does not occur in x-ray systems, it does take place in some diagnostic procedures which use radioactive positron emitters.

Kinetic Energy

Kinetic energy is energy associated with motion. It is a type of energy that a moving automobile or baseball has. When electrons are moving, they also have kinetic energy.

Generally, the quantity of kinetic energy that an object has is related to its mass and its velocity. For large objects, like baseballs and cars, the energy is proportional to the mass of the object and the square of the velocity. Doubling the velocity of such an object increases the kinetic energy by a factor of 4. In many situations, electrons travel with extremely high velocities which approach the velocity of light. At these high velocities, the simple relationship between energy and velocity given above cannot be used. One of the theories of relativity states that the mass of an object, such as electrons, changes at high velocities. The relationship between energy and velocity is somewhat complex, but is shown graphically in Figure 2. Electrons within the typical x-ray tube can have energies in excess of 100 keV. This means that they are traveling with velocities of more than half the speed of light.

Potential Energy

Potential energy is the type of energy possessed by an object because of its location or configuration. Potential energy is essentially a relative quantity. That is, an object in one location or configuration will have more or less energy than when it's located elsewhere. Although there is generally not a position of absolute zero potential energy, certain locations are often designated as the zero energy level for reference purposes.

Water captured behind the dam in a mountain lake has potential energy with respect to the water in the spillway below the dam. As the water moves from a position of high potential energy (the lake) to the one of lower potential energy (the spillway), the energy that it loses is transferred to turbines, which, in turn, convert it to a more useful form.

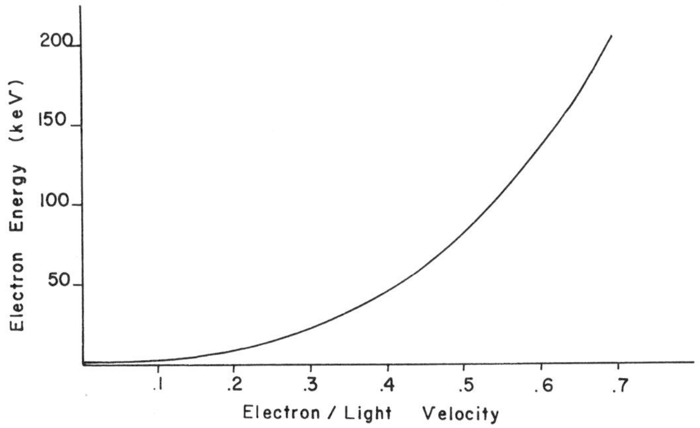

Figure 2. The relationship between electron kinetic energy and electron velocity. The electron velocity is expressed as a fraction of the velocity of light.

Electrons can have two forms of potential energy. One form is related to an electron's location within an electrical circuit, and the other is related to the electron's location within an atom. Both types of potential energy will be discussed in detail later. One important aspect of electron potential energy is that energy from some source is required to raise an electron to a higher energy level, and when an electron moves to a lower potential energy position it gives up energy.

ENERGY TRANSFER

Because electrons are too small to see, it is sometimes difficult to visualize what is meant by the various types of electron energy. Perhaps it is easier to grasp the concepts of energy types by considering the stone shown in Figure 3. Here the stone is used to demonstrate the various types of energy that also apply to electrons.

Potential energy will be considered first. It should be recalled that potential energy is generally a relative quantity. In this picture, the ground level has been arbitrarily designated as the zero potential energy position. When the stone is raised above the ground, it will be at a higher energy level. If the stone is placed in a hole below the surface, its potential energy would be negative with respect to the ground level. However, its energy would still be positive with respect to a position in the bottom of a deeper hole.

The stone at position A in Figure 3 has zero potential energy (rela-

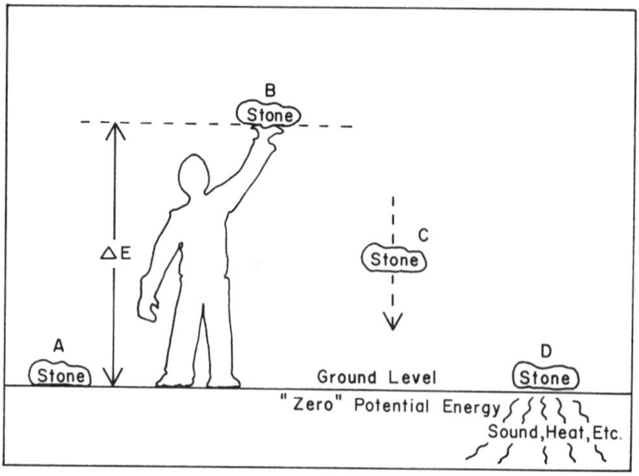

Figure 3. The transfer of energy from one type and form to another.

tively speaking), zero kinetic energy because it is not moving, and a rest-mass energy proportional to its mass. The rest-mass energy of a stone is of no practical use and will not be discussed further. When the man picks up the stone and raises it to position B, he increases its potential energy with respect to position A. The energy gained by the stone comes from the man. It will be shown later that electrons can be raised to higher potential energy levels by devices called power supplies. The additional potential energy possessed by the stone at B can be used to do work or can be converted into other forms of energy. If the stone were connected to a simple pulley arrangement and allowed to fall back to the ground, it could perform work by raising an object fastened to the other end of the rope. If the man releases the stone at B and allows it to fall back to the ground, what happens to its energy? It is converted into kinetic energy. As the stone moves downward, decreasing its potential energy, which is proportional to its distance above the ground, it is constantly increasing its speed and kinetic energy. Just before it hits the ground, its newly gained kinetic energy will be just equal to the potential energy supplied by the man. Electrons undergo a similar process within x-ray tubes where they swap potential for kinetic energy. Just as the stone reaches the surface of the ground, it will have more energy than when it was resting at position A. However, when it comes to rest on the ground at D, its energy level is the same as at A. The extra energy that was originally supplied by the man must be accounted for. In this situation, this energy is converted into other forms, such as sound, a small amount of heat, and mechanical energy used to alter the shape of the ground. When high speed electrons collide with certain materials, they also lose their kinetic energy. Their energy is converted into heat and x-radiation.

In this illustration, a visible stone has been used to illustrate the types of energy and energy transformations which apply to invisible electrons. The actual electron energy transformations will be discussed in detail later.

STRUCTURE OF MATTER

As illustrated in Figure 4, matter is where x-ray photons begin and end. Only within matter can a high speed electron give up its energy to form an x-ray photon, or a photon transfer its energy to an electron. The rate at which these interactions occur depends heavily on certain characteristics of the material. Later discussions will explore in depth both of these two very important interactions, the formation of x-ray photons by electron bombardment, and the absorption of x-ray energy. The present discussion deals only with the characteristics of the source and absorber materials which affect the interactions.

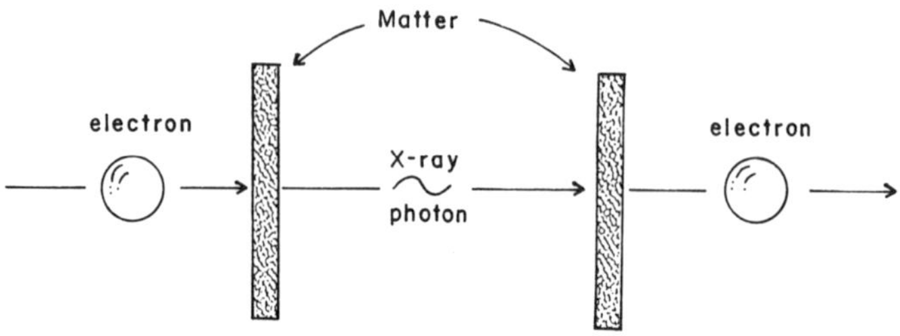

Figure 4. The role of matter with respect to the creation and absorption of x-ray photons.

It is not surprising that an important characteristic of matter, with respect to x-ray interactions, is the electron content. In addition to the concentration of electrons in a given material, the strength with which they are bound within the matter has much to do with x-ray interactions. These two general factors, electron concentration and binding, are generally related to two more common physical parameters, density and atomic number. As indicated in Figure 5, the density is the "concentration" of matter in a given volume expressed in the units of grams per cubic centimeter, whereas the atomic number is a specification of the number of electrons in each atom. It will also be shown that the electron binding is strongly related to atomic number.

Atomic Structure

The diagram of the atom, shown in Figure 5, represents the accepted model for the structure of an atom. The center portion, made up of neutrons and protons, is the nucleus. Essentially all of the weight of an atom, and matter, is contained within the nucleus. Since protons and neutrons have

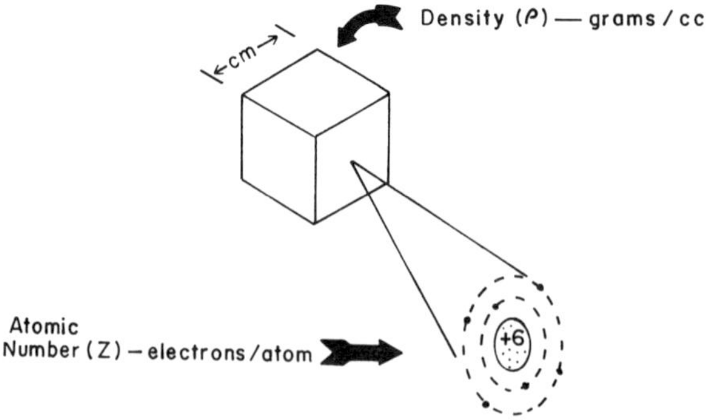

Figure 5. The important physical characteristics of matter that relate to x-ray interactions.

about the same mass, approximately one atomic mass unit (amu) each, the atomic weight is approximately proportional to the total number of neutrons and protons within the nucleus. The atom depicted in Figure 5 is carbon, which contains 6 protons and 6 neutrons and has an atomic weight of 12 amu. For most elements the actual atomic weight differs slightly from the sum of neutrons and protons, due to a mass-energy conversion which takes place in the formation of a nucleus. One significant aspect of the atomic weight is that it provides a means of comparing the mass of various materials on an atom-for-atom basis. It is also the key to determining the number of atoms of a substance contained in a given mass or volume. The number of atoms in a gram of material is inversely related to the atomic weight. Specifically, the relationship is

$$\text{atoms per gram} = \frac{\text{Avogadro's number (N)}}{\text{atomic weight (A)}}$$

where Avogadro's number has a value of 6.02×10^{23}.

Since the mass of an object, assuming uniform density, is the product of its volume and density, ρ, an expression for the number of atoms per cubic centimeter is

$$\text{atoms per cc} = \frac{\rho \text{N}}{\text{A}}$$

This relationship shows that the concentration of atoms in a substance is directly proportional to the density and inversely related to the atomic weight.

Neutrons have no electrical charge, but protons carry a positive charge of 1 unit each. The carbon nucleus in Figure 5, which contains 6 protons, has a total charge of +6 units. The number of protons contained in a nucleus is the atomic number. Z is the symbol for atomic number.

The electrons are located in orbits (sometimes referred to as shells) surrounding the nucleus. The various electron shells are designated by letters of the alphabet, beginning with K for the innermost shell. Progressing away from the nucleus, the other shells would be L, M, etc. A given atom will have only enough shells to accommodate its allotted number of electrons. The number of electrons in an atom is the same as the number of protons, i.e., the atomic number. Since each electron carries a negative 1-unit charge, the total charge of all electrons exactly cancels the positive charge of the nucleus. This gives the normal non-ionized atom a neutral or zero electrical charge. It is the atomic number which establishes the chemical identity of a substance. Each chemical element has its unique atomic number. For example, all atoms with 6 protons and an atomic number of 6 are carbon. Atomic numbers range from 1 for hydrogen to slightly over 100 for some of the rare elements like mendelevium and nobelium.

There is a rather rigid order in which the electrons are assigned to the various shells. Normally, the shells are filled in order, beginning with the innermost or K shell. The carbon atom in Figure 5 has only a K and L shell. Each shell, regardless of the atomic number, has a maximum number of electrons which it can hold. The K shell can contain, at the most, 2 electrons, the L 8, the M 18.

Electron Energy Levels

Electrons are bound to the positive nucleus of an atom by their negative electrical charge. The strength of this binding can be expressed in terms of energy. This so-called binding energy of an electron is equal to the amount of energy that would be required to remove the electron from the atom. Binding energy is a form of electron potential energy. As with any form of potential energy, some point must be designated as the zero energy level. In the case of electrons, a location outside of the atom where the electron is no longer under the influence of the nucleus is designated as the zero point. This can be compared to a golf ball resting on the ground. For the golf ball, the ground level would be designated as zero energy level. When an electron enters an atom, it drops to a lower energy level, just as the golf ball does when it rolls into a hole. Electrons within atoms are generally considered to have negative energy, since energy from some source must be added to raise them to the zero level. Likewise, the golf ball in the hole has negative energy with respect to the surface of the ground. It takes energy from some source to lift it back to zero level.

The concept of electron energy levels can be illustrated by using an energy level diagram of the type shown in Figure 6. It should be noticed that this diagram represents the electrons as being down in a hole. The electrons near the bottom are at the lowest energy level and would have the greatest binding energy.

As discussed previously, the electrons are arranged within the atoms in definite layers, or shells. Each shell is a different energy level. The K shell, which is closest to the nucleus, is at the lowest energy level. The diagram in Figure 6 is for tungsten, which has an atomic number of 74. Only the K, L, and M electron levels are shown. Additional electrons are located in the N and O shells. These shells would be located above the M shell and slightly below the zero energy level. It should be noticed that there is a significant energy difference between the various shells. All of

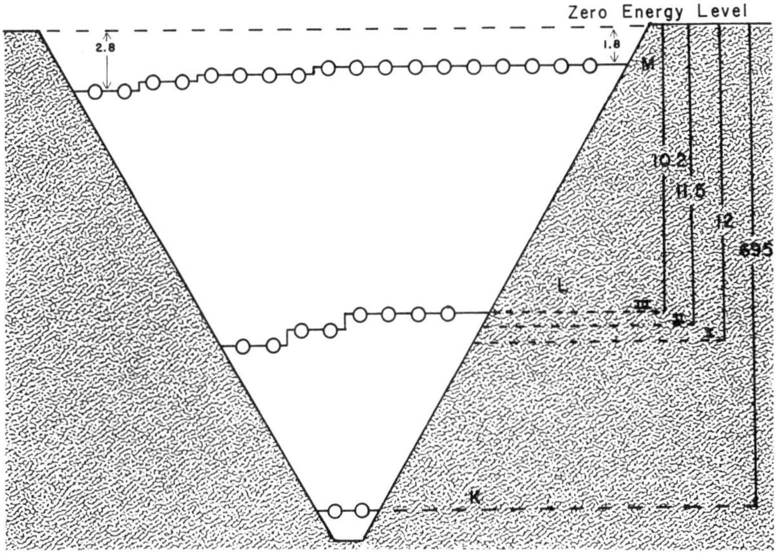

Figure 6. An energy level diagram of electrons within the tungsten atom.

the shells, except K, are subdivided into additional energy levels. For example, the L shell is divided into three levels, which are designated LI, LII, and LIII.

The binding energy for electrons in a specific shell, such as K, is related to atomic number. K shell electrons in the larger atoms are deeper within the atomic structure and have greater binding energies, as indicated in Figure 7. It should be noticed that only the K shell electrons for the higher atomic number elements have binding energies which are in the same range as the energies of diagnostic x-ray photons. This is significant in several types of interactions which will be discussed later. The binding energy of the L shell electrons is always much less than for the K, but it also increases with atomic number. For most substances the binding energy of the outermost electrons is in the range of 5 to 20 eV. These obviously are the electrons that are the easiest to remove from an atom. The removal of an electron from an atom is ionization. Since x-ray photons have sufficient energy to remove electrons from atoms, they can be considered as a form of ionizing radiation. Visible light, which has photon energies below the minimum binding energy in most atoms, cannot produce ionization.

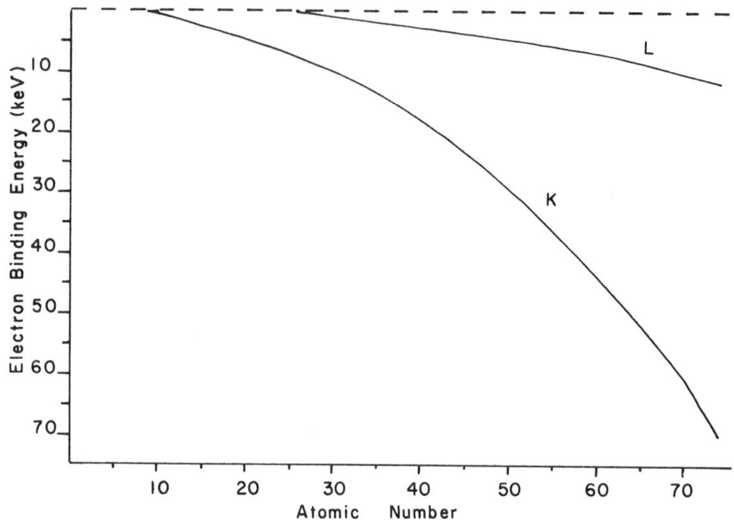

Figure 7. The relationship between K and L shell electron binding energy and atomic number.

Electron Concentration

X-ray photons are absorbed when they collide with electrons. As a photon passes through matter, its chance of being absorbed generally depends on the concentration of available electrons within the material. The concentration, or number of electrons per cubic centimeter, is given by

$$\text{Electrons per cc} = \rho N(Z/A)$$

This relationship is derived by multiplying the expression given previously for the number of atoms per cubic centimeter by the atomic number, which is the number of electrons per atom. Several comments concerning this relationship are in order. Avogadro's number, N, always has the same value and obviously does not change from element to element. Z and A have unique values for each chemical element. It should be noticed, however, that the number of electrons per cubic centimeter depends only on the ratio of Z to A. The elements with lower atomic numbers have approximately 1 neutron for each photon in the nucleus. The value of Z/A is approximately 0.5. As the atomic number and atomic weight are increased, the ratio of neutrons within the nucleus also increases. This produces a decrease in the Z/A ratio. This change is relatively small, however. Lead, which has an atomic number of 82 and an atomic weight of 207, has a Z/A ratio of 0.4. For most materials encountered in x-ray applications, the Z/A ratio varies by less than 20%. The single exception to this is hydrogen. Normal hydrogen contains no neutrons and has a nucleus that consists of a single proton. The Z/A ratio, therefore, has a value of 1.

Since Avogadro's number is constant, and the Z/A ratio is essentially constant, the only factor that can significantly alter the electron concentration is the density of the material. Most materials, especially pure elements, have more or less unique density values. In compounds and mixtures the density depends on the relative concentration of the various elements.

The fact that electron concentration does not significantly change with atomic number might suggest that atomic number has little to do with electron–x-ray interactions. This is, however, not the case. As x-ray photons pass through matter, the chance of interaction depends not only on electron concentration, but also on how firmly the electrons are bound within the atomic structure. There are certain types of interactions that occur only with firmly bound electrons. Since the binding energy of electrons increases with atomic number, the concentration of highly bound electrons increases significantly with increased atomic number.

Atomic number is essentially a characteristic of the atom and has a value that is unique to each chemical element. Many materials, such as human tissue, are not a single chemical element, but a conglomerate of compounds and mixtures. With respect to x-ray interactions, it is possible to define an effective atomic number, Z_{eff}, for compounds and mixtures. The effective atomic number is given by:

$$Z_{eff} = \sqrt[2.94]{f_1Z_1^{\ 2.94} + f_2Z_2^{\ 2.94} + f_3Z_3^{\ 2.94} + - -}$$

In this relationship, f is the fraction of the total number of electrons associated with each element. The exponent, 2.94, is derived from the relationship between x-ray interactions and atomic number, which will be discussed later.

Water, which is a major component of the human body, can be used to demonstrate the concept of effective atomic number. The water molecule contains 2 atoms of hydrogen, which have 1 electron each, and 1 oxygen atom with 8 electrons. The electron fractions, f, are therefore 0.2 for hydrogen and 0.8 for oxygen. Substitution of these values in the above relationship gives an effective atomic number for water of:

$$\begin{aligned} Z &= \sqrt[2.94]{0.2 \cdot 1^{2.94} + 0.8 \cdot 8^{2.94}} \\ &= 7.42 \end{aligned}$$

Table 1. Physical characteristics of materials involved in x-ray interactions

Material	Atomic number[a] (Z)	K electron binding energy (keV)	Density (g/cc)	Application
Beryllium	4.0		1.85	Low absorbing tube window
Fat	5.92		0.91	Body tissue
Water	7.42		1.0	Tissue "equivalent"
Muscle	7.46		1.0	Body tissue
Air	7.64		0.00129	
Aluminum	13.0		2.7	X-ray filter and penetration reference
Bone (femur)	14.0		1.87	Body tissue
Calcium	20.0		1.55	Body deposits
Copper	29.0	8.9	8.94	X-ray filter
Molybdenum	42.0	20.0	10.22	X-ray source
Silver	47.0	25.5	10.5	Absorber in film
Iodine	53.0	33.2	4.94	Contrast medium and receptor absorber
Xenon	54.0	34.5	0.0059	Receptor absorber
Barium	56.0	37.4	3.5	Contrast medium and receptor absorber
Lanthanun	56.0	38.9	6.15	Receptor absorber
Gadolinium	64.0	50.2	7.95	Receptor absorber
Tungsten	74.0	69.5	19.3	X-ray source
Lead	82.0	88.0	11.34	X-ray absorber for shielding

[a]Effective Z of tissues from Spiers (1946).

In x-ray systems a variety of materials are involved in x-ray interactions. Many of these materials are listed in Table 1, along with their principal physical characteristics and relationship to the x-ray system.

REFERENCE

Spiers, F. W. 1946. Effective atomic number and energy absorption in tissues. Br. J. Radiol. 19:218.

Chapter IV

Radiation Quantities and Units

Over the years a number of different quantities and associated units have been used for describing amounts of radiation. The variety of quantities tends to create some degree of confusion among radiation workers. It is the intent of this chapter to introduce those quantities and units that will be encountered by persons working in diagnostic radiology and to show the application of each and its relationship to the others. It is important to recognize that each quantity expresses a different aspect of x-radiation. For example, some quantities are associated with the concentration of radiation, some with the total amount of radiation in a beam, and others with the biological impact produced by the radiation. Since diagnostic x-ray systems utilize light to expose film and to view the final images, it is appropriate also to consider the basic quantities and units associated with this type of radiation.

RADIATION CONCENTRATION

The term concentration is used here to imply the amount of radiation delivered to some point within the x-ray beam. It can be described either with respect to the quantity of radiation passing through a small area or the quantity absorbed in a small specified volume or mass of material.

Photon Fluence

Photon fluence, ϕ, is the number of photons that pass through a 1-unit area as shown in Figure 1. An important parameter with respect to x-ray image quality is the photon fluence at the receptor surface. A low photon fluence will cause the image to have a noisy or mottled appearance. The details of this basic limitation to image quality will be discussed in a later chapter.

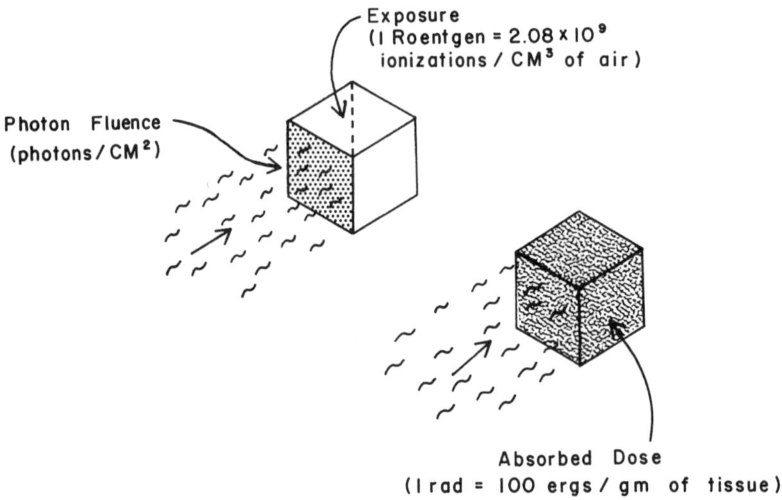

Figure 1. An illustration of the three important radiation quantities, photon fluence, exposure, and absorbed dose.

Another way of expressing the amount of x-radiation that passes through a given unit area is in terms of the energy fluence, ψ, which is the total energy that passes through the area and is usually specified in the units of ergs per square centimeter. It is the total of the individual photon energies. This is equivalent to multiplying the photon fluence by the average photon energy. Energy fluence, although not a commonly used quantity, is useful in specifying the actual energy content of an x-ray beam.

Exposure

The most common radiation quantity is exposure, X, which is expressed in the special units of roentgens, R. Exposure expresses the amount of radiation delivered to a point. Actually, it is an expression of the amount of ionization produced in air by the radiation at the point in question.

As x-radiation passes through air, some of the photons are absorbed. Some of the energy lost by the photons removes electrons from the atoms and produces ionization. The quantity of ionization produced can be expressed either as the number of atoms ionized or in terms of the total electric charge of the ions. The roentgen is defined as the amount of exposure that will produce a quantity of ions, of one sign, which has a total electrical charge of 2.58×10^{-4} coulombs per kg of air. An alternate expression for the roentgen that is somewhat easier to visualize is in terms of the number of ionizations produced in 1 cc of air. The electrical charge of 1 electron (one ionization) is 1.6×10^{-19} coulombs. One coulomb of charge is equivalent to 6.24×10^{18} electrons or ions. Multiplying this number by the total charge associated with 1 R gives 1.61×10^{15} ionizations per g of air. At standard temperature and pressure ((STP) 0° C, 760 mm Hg) air has a density of 0.001293 g per cc. Introducing this factor shows that 1 R will produce 2.082×10^{9} ionizations per cc at STP. Changes in temperature or atmospheric pressure will alter the number of ionizations per cubic centimeter of air, but not per gram.

Exposure is not equivalent to the actual energy of an x-ray beam, but the two quantities are related. The main advantage of exposure as a radiation quantity is that it is relatively easy to measure. The quantity of ionization produced in air by radiation can be determined by using an ionization chamber. The relationship between photon fluence and exposure is shown in Figure 2. The units used are photons per square millimeter per microroentgen. These units are chosen because of their applicability to the general radiation levels reaching x-ray image receptors. The relationship between photon fluence and exposure depends on the energy of the individual x-ray photons. This is largely because the rate of photon absorption in air changes with photon energy. At the lower photon energies, the absorption rate is relatively high and it takes fewer photons incident on a volume of air to produce a given quantity of ionization. At higher energies, fewer photons are absorbed within a given air volume, but each one loses more energy and produces more ionization and exposure.

Absorbed Dose

Both exposure and fluence indicate the quantity of radiation delivered to a point, but in no way indicate the amount of energy absorbed by tissue located there. The quantity for absorbed radiation energy is absorbed dose, D, and the basic unit is the rad, which comes from *r*adiation *a*bsorbed *d*ose. One rad is equivalent to the absorption of 100 ergs of energy per gram of material. This would be approximately the same quantity of energy absorbed in 1 cc of muscle tissue, since it has a density of approximately 1 g per cc. Absorbed dose expresses the quantity of energy that is taken out of an x-ray beam by an absorbing material. This is quite different from exposure and fluence, which are related to the quantity of radiation passing through an area.

Although exposure and absorbed dose are entirely different quantities, they are related. The dose absorbed by tissue is proportional to the expo-

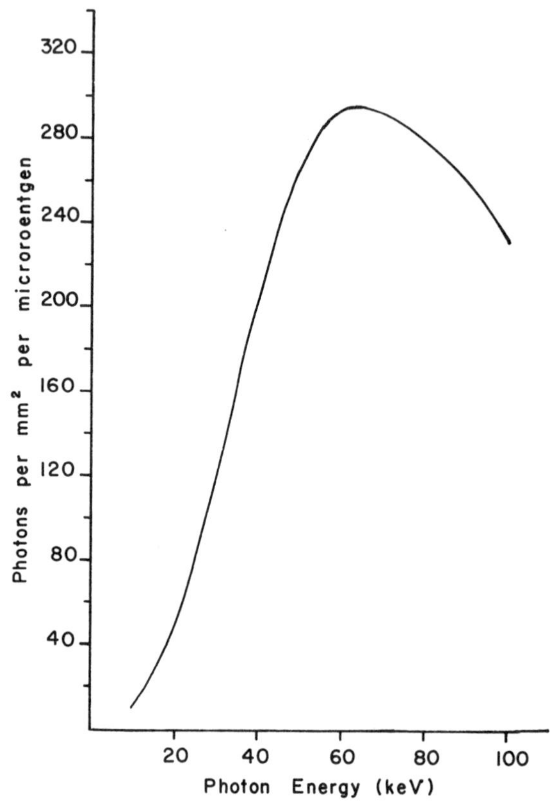

Figure 2. The relationship of photon fluence to exposure over the diagnostic energy range.

sure reaching it, as given by:

$$\text{Dose (rads)} = f \cdot \text{exposure (R)}$$

The f factor has the units of rads per roentgen. The value of f depends on the atomic number of the absorbing material, i.e., tissue, and the energy of the x-ray photons. Values of f are shown for several tissues in Figure 3. It should be noticed that the f factor values for muscle change by only a few percentage over the diagnostic energy range. For bone, however, the value is greater and exhibits a more pronounced dependence on photon energy. The significance is that, when a portion of the body receives a certain exposure, the absorbed dose is greater in bone than in the soft tissue.

The quantities that express the concentration of radiation can be summarized as follows. Exposure is the easiest to measure and is the quantity

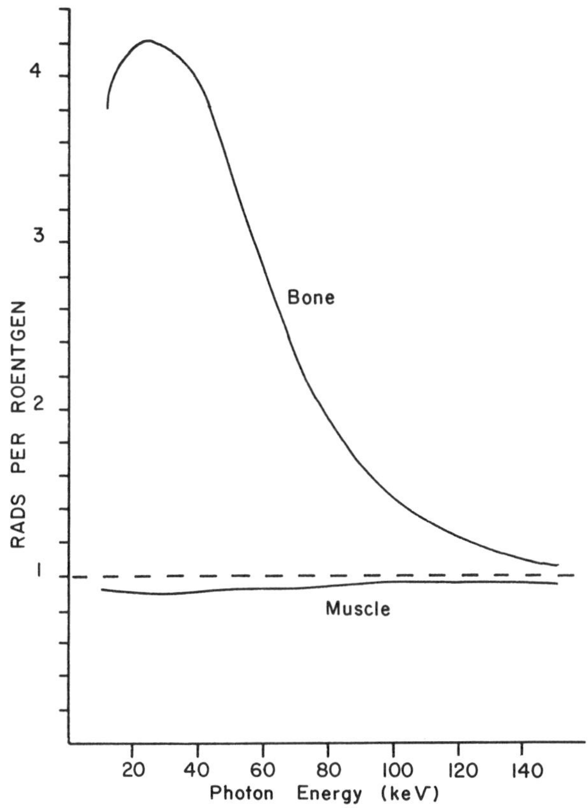

Figure 3. The relationship of absorbed dose to exposure in body tissues over the diagnostic energy range.

generally used to describe the amount of radiation delivered to some point within the x-ray beam. The concentration of photons, i.e., the fluence, at a point of known exposure can be determined by using the graph in Figure 2. The absorbed dose can be determined by multiplying the exposure by the appropriate f factor value from Figure 3.

Inverse-Square Relationship

As radiation leaves a source, it spreads out and passes through larger areas. Simple geometrical relationships can be used, as in Figure 4, to show that the cross-sectional area of an x-ray beam is proportional to the square of the distance between the source and the area. As the x-ray beam progresses away from the source, the radiation must cover a larger area. This means

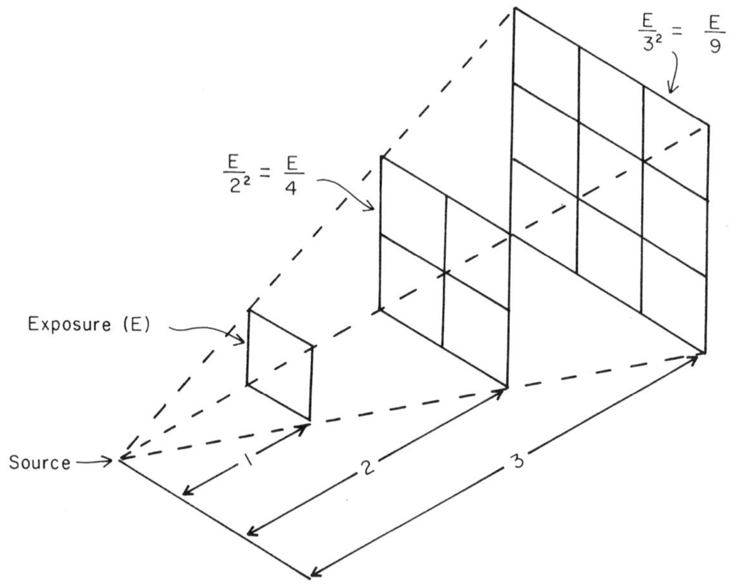

Figure 4. An illustration of the inverse-square law.

that the concentration of the radiation, either in terms of exposure or fluence, decreases with distance. Specifically, the exposure at points along the axis of an x-ray beam is inversely proportional to the square of the distance between the source and the respective point. This is illustrated in Figure 4. If an x-ray beam is delivering a certain exposure at a distance of 1 m, the radiation will cover the area shown. At a distance of 2 m from the source, the area of the beam will have increased by a factor of 4, and the exposure, i.e., the concentration, will have decreased by a factor of 4. At a distance of 3 m, the exposure will be one-ninth of the value at 1 m.

The radiation exposure produced by an x-ray machine operating with specified parameters is typically stated for a distance of 1 m (X_m). The exposure (X_d) to points at other distances is given by:

$$X_d = \frac{X_m}{d^2}$$

where d is the source-to-point distance in meters.

TOTAL RADIATION

In specifying the amount of radiation delivered to or absorbed by the human body, a very important distinction must be made. This is the difference between the radiation to a specific point, i.e., exposure, dose, or fluence, and the total amount of radiation imparted to the body. The total radiation delivered can be expressed in terms of both exposure and absorbed dose, as indicated in Figure 5.

Surface Integral Exposure

Consider two patients undergoing x-ray examinations. Each receives an entrance surface exposure of 1 R. However, the field size, i.e., x-ray beam area, is much larger for one patient than the other. Have they both received the same amount of radiation? In terms of exposure to a specific point, yes. In terms of total radiation, no. One roentgen delivered to a large area is much more radiation than 1 R delivered to a smaller area. The quantity that can be used to describe the total amount of radiation delivered is the surface integral exposure, SIE, which has the units of roentgens-square centimeters ($R \cdot cm^2$).

If the radiation exposure is uniform over the entire area, the SIE is just the product of the exposure in roentgens and the exposure area in square centimeters. In cases where the exposure is not the same at all points in the exposed area, the SIE can be found by adding the exposure values for each individual square centimeter of exposed surface. Mathematically, this is the process of integrating the exposure over the surface area.

The SIE can be measured during x-ray examinations by placing a special type of ionization chamber in the x-ray beam. The significance of SIE is that it describes total radiation imparted to a patient, whereas exposure only indicates the concentration of radiation at a specified point.

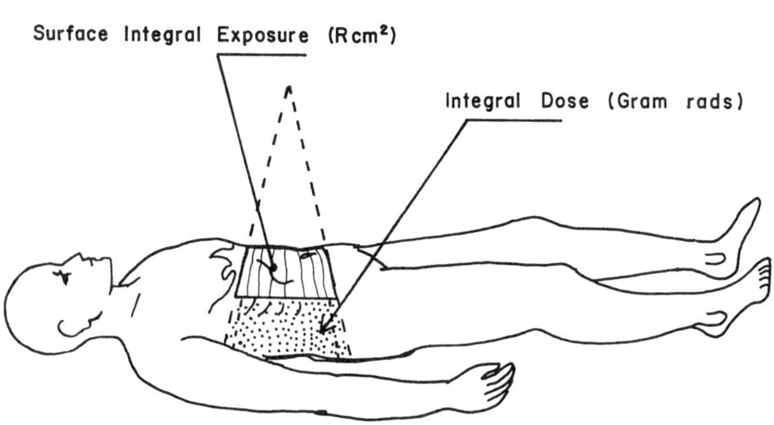

Figure 5. The total radiation imparted to the body.

Integral Dose

The integral dose, ID, is the total amount of energy absorbed by the body. The unit used is the gram-rad. One gram-rad is equivalent to 100 ergs. The relationship between integral dose and absorbed dose is quite similar to the relationship between surface integral exposure and exposure. Whereas absorbed dose (rads) specifies the concentration of energy absorbed at a specific point, the integral dose describes the total energy absorbed throughout the irradiated volume of the patient's body. Mathematically, the integral dose could be found by totaling the absorbed dose of each gram of irradiated tissue.

In most x-ray examinations, where the beam is confined to the body, a major portion (as much as 95%) of the total x-ray beam energy is absorbed by the patient. The integral dose is, therefore, approximately equal to the total x-ray beam energy.

The integral dose, or total energy absorbed by the body, is perhaps the most significant quantity with respect to biological radiation effects that are not limited to small critical organs.

BIOLOGICAL IMPACT

When x-ray energy is absorbed by living tissue, many different types of biological responses can occur. The extent of biological impact of the radiation depends on many factors, including the quantity of energy absorbed, i.e., the dose, the type of radiation involved, and the time period over which the radiation is delivered. For many biological effects, the change in biological impact with different exposure times is generally considered to be much less significant than changing the other two factors. The general relationship of biological impact to absorbed dose is shown in Figure 6.

Because different types of radiations vary in their effectiveness for producing biological changes, it becomes necessary to introduce additional quantities and units for specifying biological impact.

Dose Equivalent

In situations concerning the generally undesirable effects of radiation on the human body, the quantity for specifying the radiation biological impact is the dose equivalent, DE. The unit for dose equivalent is the rem. Dose equivalent is found by multiplying the absorbed dose, in rads, by the quality factor (QF) of the radiation. The QF is a characteristic of the radiation that expresses its effectiveness in producing biological damage per unit of absorbed dose. The quality factor, QF, depends directly on a

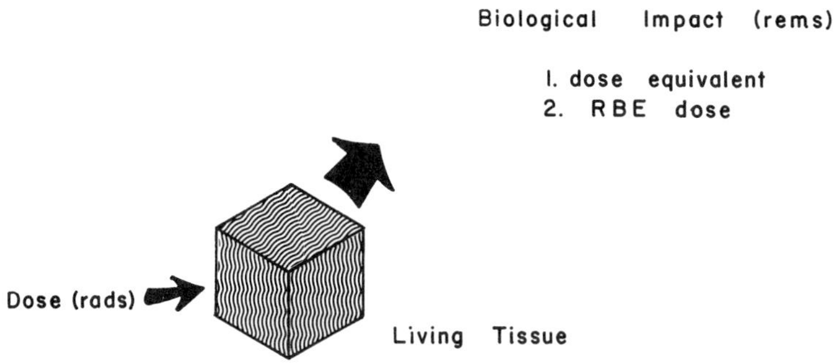

Figure 6. Conceptual relationship of biological impact to absorbed dose.

characteristic of the radiation that is designated the linear energy transfer (LET). The LET describes the rate at which various types of radiation deposit energy along the path of the radiation particles. In the case of x-radiation, the particles that actually transfer the radiation energy to the tissue are electrons. As the energetic electrons, created by the absorption of x-ray photons, pass through tissue, they deposit energy along their tracks. The rate at which energy is deposited, typically in the units of kiloelectronvolts per micron of path length, is the LET of the radiation. The LET associated with the absorption of x-rays is generally in the range of 1 to 10 keV per micron (μm) of electron path. The quality factor of this type of radiation has a value of 1. Other types of radiation, such as alpha particles, deposit energy at a higher rate along their path. This increased value for the LET causes more radiation damage per rad of absorbed dose. This increased biological impact would be reflected in a higher value for the radiation's QF.

With respect to personal exposure and radiation protection, the significant quantity is the dose equivalent in rems. However, the quantity that is the easiest to measure with most instrumentation is exposure in roentgens. The relationship between these two quantities is:

$$\text{Dose equivalent (rem)} = \text{exposure (R)} \cdot f \cdot QF$$

X-radiation of the type used for diagnostic purposes has an f factor value and a QF value that are very close to 1. In soft tissue, an exposure of 1 R would produce an absorbed dose of approximately 1 rad, which in turn would be a dose equivalent of approximately 1 rem.

Relative Biological Effectiveness (RBE) Dose

When specific biological effects, rather than general biological damage, are being considered, the quantity used to express the impact of the radiation is the RBE dose. The unit for RBE dose is the rem, the same as for dose equivalent. The RBE dose is found by multiplying the absorbed dose, in rads, by a factor that describes the relative effectiveness of the radiation for producing a given effect. This factor has been designated as the RBE of the radiation. Like the quality factor, the RBE value generally depends on the LET of the radiation. Unlike the quality factor, however, there can be different RBE values for the same radiation if different biological effects are being considered.

RBE values express the relative effectiveness of different types of radiation with respect to 200-keV x-rays. In other words, the RBE of 200-keV x-rays for all biological effects has a value of 1. The RBE for diagnostic quality x-rays and most biological effects usually has a value that is not greatly different from 1.

LIGHT

The vast majority of x-ray systems convert the x-ray image into light, which is recorded by the film. The purpose of this section is to define some of the basic light quantities and units that might be encountered in radiology. These can be conveniently divided into two categories—those that express the amount of light emitted by a source and those that describe the amount of light falling on a surface, such as a piece of film. The relationships of several light quantities and units are shown in Figure 7.

Luminance

Luminance is the light quantity that is generally referred to as brightness. It describes the amount of light that is being emitted from the surface of the light source. The basic unit of luminance (brightness) is the nit, which is equivalent to 1 candela per m^2 of source area.

The concept of luminance is somewhat easier to understand if it is related to the number of light photons involved. The quantity for specifying an amount of light is the lumen. One lumen of light with wavelengths encountered in x-ray imaging systems (540 nm) is equivalent to 3.8×10^{15} photons per sec. Another factor that determines luminance is the concentration of light in a given direction. This can be described in terms of a cone or solid angle that is measured in units of steradians.

If a light source produces an intensity of 1 candela per m^2 of surface area, it has a luminance of 1 nit. Perhaps it is more realistic to consider the quantity of light that would be emitted from a 1 mm^2 area of a source, such as the output screen of an image intensifier. One millimeter square is 10^{-6} m^2. If the intensifier has a luminance (brightness) of 1 nit, the intensity from

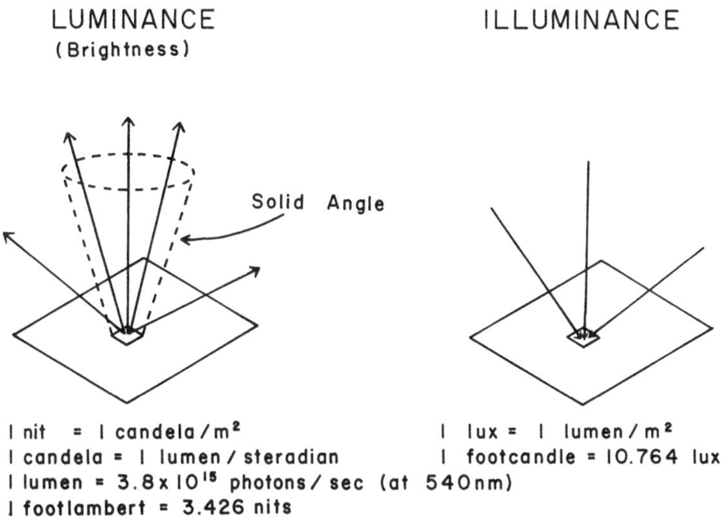

Figure 7. Light quantities and units encountered in radiology.

an area of 1 mm^2 would be 10^{-6} lumen in a 1-unit solid angle. This would be equivalent to 3.8×10^9 photons per sec, leaving the 1-mm^2 area through a cone (solid angle) of 1 steradian.

Another unit that is often used for specifying luminance is the footlambert, which is equivalent to 3.426 nits.

Illuminance

Illuminance is a specification of the quantity of light falling on or illuminating a surface. The basic unit is the lux. A surface has an illuminance of 1 lux when it receives 1 lumen per m^2 of surface area. Consider a small area on a piece of film that is 1 mm^2. For light with a wavelength of 540 nm, there are 3.8×10^{15} photons per sec per lumen. An illuminance of 1 lux to the film would be equivalent to 3.8×10^9 photons per sec to a 1-mm^2 area. The total light exposure to a film is found by multiplying the illuminance, in lux, by the exposure time, in seconds, and is expressed in units of lux-seconds.

One very important characteristic of an x-ray imaging system is the efficiency with which it transfers light from the output of the image intensifier tube to the surface of the film. This is the subject of a later chapter.

Another unit used in some literature for specifying illuminance is the footcandle, which is equivalent to 10.764 lux.

REFERENCES

International Commission on Radiation Units and Measurements. 1970. Linear energy transfer, ICRU Report 16. International Commission on Radiation Units and Measurements, Washington, D.C.

International Commission on Radiation Units and Measurements. 1970. Radiation dosimetry: x-rays generated at potentials of 5 to 150 kV, ICRU Report 17. International Commission on Radiation Units and Measurements, Washington, D.C.

International Commission on Radiation Units and Measurements. 1971. Radiation quantities and units, ICRU Report 19. International Commission on Radiation Units and Measurements, Washington, D.C.

United States Department of Health, Education and Welfare. 1970. Radiological Health Handbook. United States Government Printing Office, Washington, D.C.

Chapter V
Electronic Concepts

One of the major roles of electrons is the movement of energy. In the x-ray machine, electrons are used to move energy from the power supply to the x-ray tube. This chapter is concerned with basic electrical concepts and simple circuits as they apply to x-ray apparatus.

In the previous chapter it was shown that electrons are contained within the atoms. Electrons that are bound to an atom cannot be readily moved and used to transport energy. There are certain materials, however, that contain a significant number of "free" or very loosely bound electrons. These materials are known as conductors. Most metals are good conductors. Copper is used for most electrical conductors (wires) because it is a good conductor, relatively inexpensive, and has desirable mechanical properties, such as flexibility and strength. In an electrical circuit the wires, or conductors, are actually the source of electrons. A piece of wire, even if it is not connected to an electrical circuit, is essentially "filled" with electrons. If an additional electron is pushed into one end of the wire, it will push electrons ahead of it and an electron will be pushed out of the other end of the wire, if there is a place for it to go. The situation is very much like a water pipe; if water is forced in one end, it pushes an equal quantity out at the other. A conductor then provides both the electrons and a pathway over which they can move.

ELECTRON QUANTITIES

Current

When an electrical circuit is in operation, electrons are continuously moving or flowing through the conductor. The number of electrons that move past a given point per second is referred to as the current. Since, in the typical circuit, the number of electrons per second is quite large, a more useful unit than the number of electrons is desirable. The basic unit of

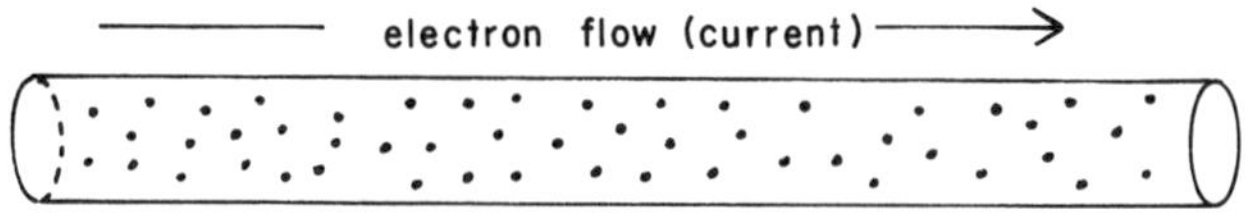

Figure 1. Electrons in a section of conductor or wire.

current is the ampere (A). One ampere is defined as the flow of 6.25×10^{18} electrons per sec. In x-ray tubes, the current is typically a fraction of 1 ampere and the milliampere (mA) is a more appropriate unit. As indicated in Figure 1, a current of 1 mA is equal to the flow of 6.25×10^{15} electrons per sec past a given point.

Electron Quantity and Charge

In addition to knowing the rate at which electrons are flowing through a circuit, i.e., the current, it is often necessary to know the total quantity in a given period of time. In x-ray work the most appropriate unit for specifying electron quantity is the milliampere-second (mAs). The total quantity of electrons passing a point (MAS) is the product of the current (MA) and the time in seconds (S). Since a current of 1 mA is a flow of electrons per sec, it follows that 1 mA·s is a "cluster" of 6.25×10^{15} electrons, as shown in Figure 1.[1]

It should be recalled that all electrons carry a negative electrical charge of the same size. In some situations the quantity of electrons might be specified in terms of the total electrical charge. If extra electrons are added to an object, it is said to have acquired a negative charge. However, if some of the free electrons are removed from an object, a positive charge is created. In either case, the total charge on the object is directly proportional to the number of electrons moved. Generally speaking, charge is just a way of describing a quantity of electrons. The basic unit of charge is the coulomb, which is equivalent to the total charge of 6.25×10^{18} electrons. By comparing numbers, it is seen that 1 coulomb is equivalent to 1,000 mAs.

[1]Note that "mAs" will be used throughout as the unit of measure for milliamperes—seconds and that the abbreviation "MAS" will be used when "tube current" is meant in a more general sense.

Voltage

In earlier discussions it was pointed out that electrons could exist at different potential energy levels, either because of their different positions within the atom, or because of their different locations within an electrical circuit. Consider the two wires or conductors shown in Figure 2. The electrons contained in one of the conductors are at a higher potential energy level than the electrons in the other. Generally, the electrons in the negative conductor are considered as being at the higher energy level. An electrical quantity that indicates the difference in electron potential energy between two points within a circuit is the voltage. Another name that might be used in place of voltage is potential difference, suggesting a difference in potential energy. The unit used for voltage, or potential difference, is the volt. The difference in electron potential energy between two conductors is directly proportional to the voltage. Each electron will have an energy difference of 1 eV for each volt. In fact, this is the origin of the energy unit, the electron volt. It is the quantity of energy that an electron gains or loses, depending on direction, when it moves between two points in a circuit that are 1 V "apart."

The arrows indicating electron flow in Figure 2 show directions electrons will move if the conductors are part of a complete circuit.

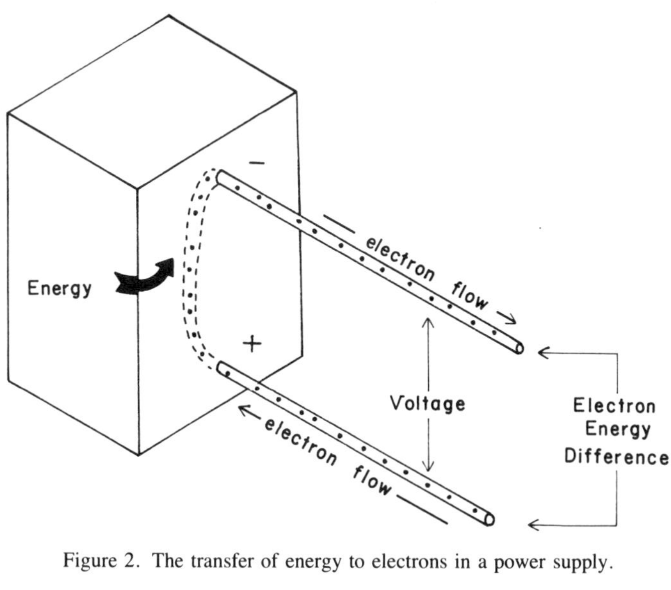

Figure 2. The transfer of energy to electrons in a power supply.

ELECTRICAL COMPONENTS

Power Supplies

In order to move an electron from one point within a circuit to another that is at a higher energy level, energy must be transferred to the electron. The device, shown in Figure 2, in which this energy transfer occurs is generally referred to as a power supply. Typical examples of power supplies are batteries and generators. A battery contains potential chemical energy, which is converted and transferred to the electrons. A generator takes mechanical energy, as from a turbine or automobile engine, and transfers it to electrons.

In effect, the power supply is an electron pump. The positive terminal is the inlet, and after the electrons are "pumped up" to a higher energy level they are expelled at the negative terminal. It should be recognized that the power supply is not the source of the electrons, just as the human heart is not the source of the circulating blood. The function of a power supply is quite analogous to that of the heart. It pumps the electrons (blood) to a higher voltage (pressure) and causes the electrons (blood) to circulate.

The important characteristic of a power supply is the amount of voltage that it can develop. Power supplies are generally designed to provide a voltage that is appropriate for their intended application. A flashlight battery produces 1.5 volts, whereas the power supply in an x-ray machine might produce 100,000 volts (100 kV) or more. Each electron that passes through a flashlight battery gains only 1.5 eV of energy, compared to the 100 keV of energy gained in the x-ray apparatus.

Loads

Whereas power supplies are devices that transfer energy to electrons, there are also devices that remove or take away the electron's energy. These devices are generally designated electrical loads. Figure 3 illustrates the basic idea of a load. As electrons flow through a load device, they lose their potential energy. In all cases, the energy lost by the electrons is converted into some other energy form. Common examples of electrical loads are light bulbs, which convert electron energy into light and heat; motors, which convert to mechanical energy; and x-ray tubes, where the energy from the electrons appears as x-radiation and heat. The energy lost by each electron that flows through a load depends on the voltage between the two conductors. The voltage, in turn, is generally determined by the power supply that is pumping electrons through the load.

Loads remove energy from the electrons by creating a certain amount of resistance or impedance to their flow. The basic characteristic of a load

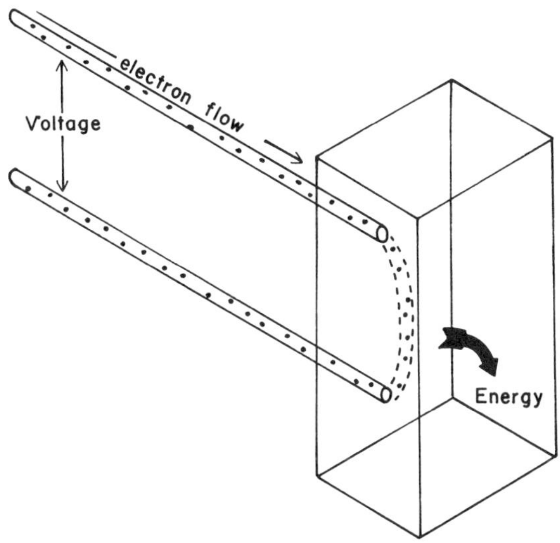

Figure 3. The loss of energy by electrons flowing through a load device.

device is the amount of impedance that it presents to electron flow. Electrical impedance is expressed in the units of ohms. A given load device is designed to have a certain impedance value.

One important aspect of a load's impedance is that it determines the amount of current that flows through the load for a given applied voltage. This relationship, known as Ohm's law, can be stated as follows:

$$\text{Current (A)} = \frac{\text{voltage (V)}}{\text{impedance (ohms)}}$$

It should be noticed that the electron flow, or current, is inversely related to the load impedance. If the same voltage is applied to two loads with different impedances, more current will flow through the load with the lower impedance. The current is also proportional to the applied voltage. If the voltage applied to a load is changed, the current flow will change proportionally. This is assuming, of course, that the impedance of the load remains unchanged.

There are several different types of impedance. Some types can impede current flow without removing energy from the electrons. The most common type, however, converts electron energy into heat. This form of impedance is called resistance.

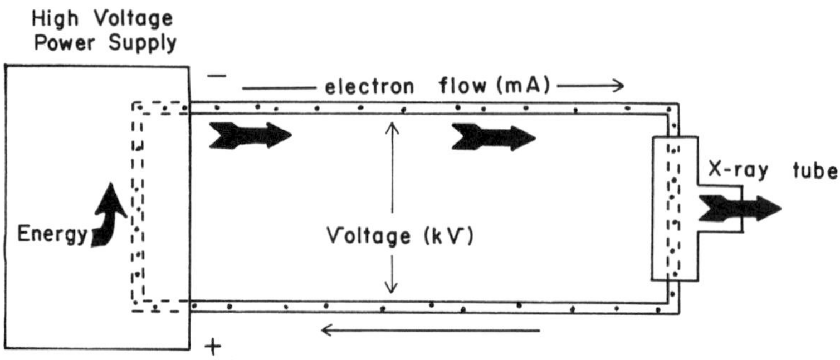

Figure 4. The basic x-ray machine circuit showing electron flow and the transfer of energy.

Circuits

An electrical circuit consists of various devices connected by conductors in a way that will permit electrons to flow between the components. The simplest circuit must contain at least two components, a power supply and a load. The basic circuit shown in Figure 4 is found in all x-ray machines. The power supply that gives energy to the electrons and pumps them through the circuit is discussed in detail in Chapter VII. The voltage between the two conductors in the x-ray circuit is typically in the range of 30,000 to 120,000 V (30 to 120 kV) and in radiology this kilovoltage is referred to as the KV.[2] The kilovoltage is generally adjustable and an appropriate value can be selected by the operator of the x-ray equipment.

In this circuit, the x-ray tube is the load. It is the place where the electrons lose their energy. The energy lost by electrons in passing through an x-ray tube is converted into heat and x-ray energy.

In the language of the x-ray worker, the electron flow or current through the circuit is referred to as the MA. This is because the value is typically expressed in the units of milliamperes (mA).

The electron flow, or MA, through the circuit is controlled by the x-ray tube. An x-ray tube is a glass container from which all air has been removed. As shown in Figure 5, the tube contains two elements through which the electrons flow. The element through which the electrons enter the x-ray tube from the negative conductor is designated as the cathode. From the cathode, the electrons flow through the vacuum space to the anode. From the anode the electrons leave the tube and return to the positive conductor of the circuit. Since a vacuum contains no electrons of

[2]Note that "kV" will be used throughout as the unit of measure for kilovolts and that the abbreviation "KV" will be used when "Kilovoltage" is meant in a more general sense.

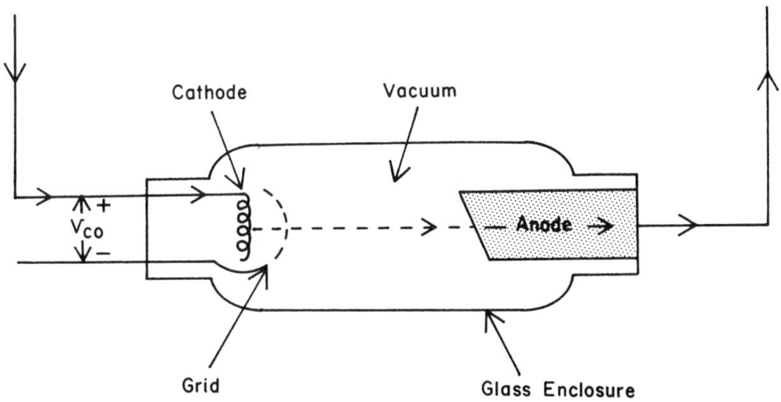

Figure 5. The basic components of an x-ray tube. Arrows indicate direction of the electron flow.

its own, it can become conductive only by the emission of electrons from the cathode. In all electronic tubes, the cathode is considered the source of electrons. Actually, it is the source only in the sense that the electrons enter the tube at the cathode and are emitted from it into the vacuum space. The cathode is generally metallic and is a good electrical conductor, but some means must be provided to remove the electrons. Normally, electrons will not flow from a conductor into the surrounding space. There are several ways to cause a cathode to emit electrons. In most x-ray tubes, electron emission from the cathode is produced by heating. Actually, the cathode is a small electrical heater. In this type of tube, the electron current (or MA) is controlled by changing the temperature of the heated cathode. The MA control of the x-ray machine is just a temperature control for the cathode. It is very similar to the control of an electric stove. Increasing the temperature increases the rate at which electrons are emitted and a higher tube current, or MA, results.

Actually, two factors control the flow of electrons from the cathode to the anode. One is the rate of emission from a cathode and the other is the voltage applied between cathode and anode. If no voltage is present, any electrons that are emitted will cluster around the cathode and retard further emission. In normal x-ray tube operation, the cathode is turned on, i.e., heated, before the KV is applied to the tube. Generally speaking, applying the KV turns the x-ray tube on and off, whereas the cathode temperature controls the actual current that flows.

Under some operating conditions, the KV might not be sufficiently high to collect all of the electrons emitted by the cathode. This condition allows electrons to accumulate near the cathode and form a "space charge." This retards electron emission and current flow. Operation of a tube in this condition is referred to as being space-charge limited.

Some x-ray tubes do not use a heated cathode but rely on the positive voltage of the anode to "pull" the electrons out of the cathode. This is referred to as field emission because of the very strong electrical field that must be present near the cathode before emission will occur.

In some x-ray tubes, a third element is added for the purpose of turning the current on and off. This element is a grid. The grid is a conductor located quite close to the cathode. If a cutoff voltage, V_{co}, is applied to the grid, it will halt electron emission from the cathode. The advantage of using a grid-controlled x-ray tube is that the tube current can be turned on and off very rapidly. This is useful when it is necessary to produce a pulsed x-ray beam, such as in cineradiography.

Conductor Size and Insulation

The typical electrical conductor, or cable, consists of two types of materials, conductor and insulator, as shown in Figure 6. The size of the cable or wire, i.e., cross-sectional area, determines the maximum current that can pass through it without undesirable effects occurring. The size of electrical conductors is generally specified in gauge numbers. The

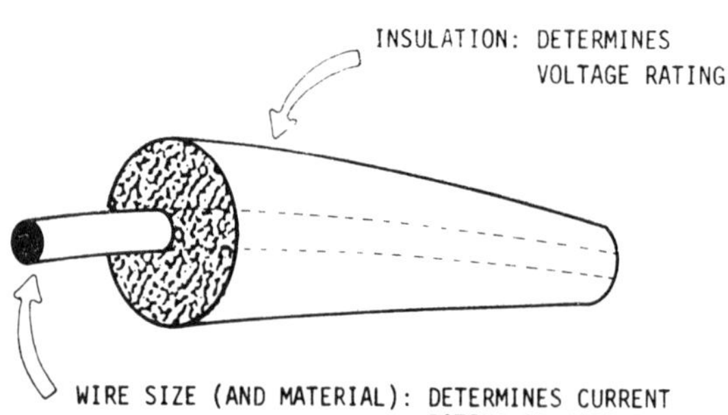

Number 14 (Gauge) Copper: 15 Amperes
Number 12 (Gauge) Copper: 20 Amperes
Number 2 or 3 Gauge Copper: 100 Amperes

Figure 6. The characteristics of a conductor that determine current and voltage capacity.

maximum recommended capacity of several copper conductor sizes is given in Figure 6. The passage of excessive current through a conductor will cause electrons to lose energy (voltage) and will also cause heat to be generated in the wire. Although copper is the most common conductor material, cables constructed of other materials are sometimes used.

The insulation surrounding the conductor prevents electrons from leaving the wire and flowing to objects that are in contact with the cable. The thickness of insulation required depends on the voltage between the conductor and other nearby objects. Voltage is like a pressure to electrons. If the voltage on a conductor exceeds the capacity of the insulation, electrons will break through and actually rupture the insulating material.

The electrical conductors that bring energy to the x-ray department are large copper conductors with relatively thin insulation. They are designed to carry high currents (several hundred amperes) at only 200 or 300 V. On the other hand, the cables that connect x-ray tubes to the power supply generally carry currents of less than 1 amp, but the voltages typically exceed 100,000 V. For that reason the relatively small conductor is surrounded by a very thick layer of insulation, giving the cable the appearance of being very large.

ELECTRICAL ENERGY TRANSFER

The major function of many electrical circuits is the transfer of energy. An excellent example is the circuit that connects the x-ray tube to the high voltage power supply, as shown in Figure 4. When the circuit is in operation, electrons circulate through the circuit, as indicated. This electron flow is the circuit's current. The electrons leave the high voltage power supply at the negative terminal, move through a conductor to the negative terminal (cathode) of the x-ray tube, through the tube, and then return to the positive terminal of the power supply. As each electron makes the trip, it moves a quantity of energy from the power supply to the x-ray tube. The quantity of energy for *each* electron is directly proportional to the voltage of the circuit. One electron will move 1 eV of energy for each volt difference between the two conductors. As an example, if the circuit voltage is 100 kV, electrons arriving at the x-ray tube will have 100 keV more energy than when they leave the anode terminal. This difference in energy is equal to the energy lost by the electrons in moving through the x-ray tube, where it is converted into heat and x-radiation.

Of special interest is the total amount of energy that is transferred from the power supply to the tube during a single x-ray exposure. This is simply the product of the energy carried by each electron and the number of electrons flowing through the circuit during the exposure time. Since the energy carried by a single electron is proportional to circuit voltage and the number of electrons is proportional to the MAS, an expression for the quantity of energy transferred is:

$$\text{Energy (J)} = \text{KV} \times \text{MAS}$$

In this relationship, it is assumed that the voltage remains constant throughout the exposure. Situations in which this is not true do occur in x-ray circuits and are discussed later.

Another important quantity is the power or rate at which energy is being transferred. The power is proportional to the number of electrons per second flowing through the circuit. This, of course, is the current. The relationship is:

$$\text{Power (watts)} = \text{voltage} \times \text{current (ampere)}$$

$$\text{Power (watts)} = \text{KV} \times \text{MA}$$

The first equation above is the relationship involving the basic units of volts and amperes. The second equation is more useful for the x-ray circuit, where the current is in milliamperes and the voltage in kilovolts. Since 1 mA is 0.001 ampere and 1 kV is 1,000 V, the product of MA and KV is still watts.

Alternating Current

In some electrical circuits, the voltage and current remain constant with respect to time. In these circuits the current is always flowing in the same direction. These are generally designated as direct current or DC circuits. A battery is an example of a power supply that produces a direct current.

There are power supplies, however, that produce voltages that are constantly changing with time. Since, in most circuits, the current is more or less proportional to the voltage, the current also changes value. In most circuits of this type, the voltage periodically changes polarity and the current changes or alternates direction of flow. This would be designated an alternating current or AC circuit. The electricity distributed by the power companies is AC. There are certain advantages to AC in that transformers can be used for stepping voltages up or down, and many motors are designed for AC operation.

If a graph of the instantaneous values of either the AC voltage or current is plotted with respect to time, it will generally be similar to the one shown in Figure 7. This representation of the voltage with respect to time is known as the waveform. Most AC power sources produce voltages with

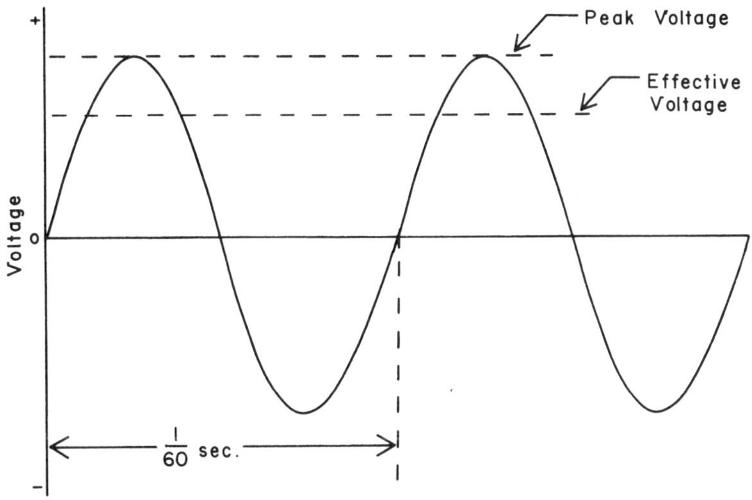

Figure 7. The typical waveform of an alternating voltage.

the so-called sine-wave waveform, shown in Figure 7. This name is derived from the mathematical description of its shape.

One characteristic of an alternating voltage is its frequency. The frequency is the rate at which it changes through one complete cycle. The time of one complete cycle is the period. The frequency is the reciprocal of the period. For example, the electricity distributed in the United States goes through one complete cycle in 0.0166 sec and has a frequency of 60 cycles per sec. The unit for frequency is the hertz, which is 1 cycle per sec.

During one voltage cycle, the actual voltage is changing continuously. At two times during the period it reaches a peak value, but remains there for a very short time. This means that for most of the period the circuit voltage is less than the peak value. For the purpose of energy and power calculations, an effective voltage value, rather than the peak value, should be used. For the sine-wave voltage, as shown in Figure 7, the effective value is 70.7% (0.707) of the peak voltage. This is the waveform factor, and its value depends on the actual shape of the voltage waveform. The relationship of effective to peak voltage is shown in Figure 7.

Chapter VI

Production of X-rays

It has been shown that x-ray energy is in the form of individual photons. The most distinguishing characteristic of a photon is its individual energy. X-ray photons with energies ranging from about 20 to 110 keV are used to form diagnostic images. In some examinations, such as computed tomography and radiography of the chest, higher energy photons are often used. This chapter will consider the mechanisms by which x-ray photons with energies suitable for diagnostic examinations can be produced.

Energy is required to produce x-ray photons, since photons are simply units of energy. The source of energy used for the production of x-rays is high speed electrons. In short, if a high speed electron with an energy of, say, 100 keV is suddenly stopped or significantly slowed down, the energy it loses can appear as an x-ray photon.

In order to produce x-ray photons under controlled conditions, three things are required: 1) a source of free electrons (a cathode); 2) a means of accelerating the electrons to high speeds (high voltage); 3) a material that can slow down the electrons and cause their energy to appear as photons (an anode). This all occurs within the x-ray tube, as shown in Figure 1. The element within the x-ray tube that emits electrons is the cathode. A very high electrical voltage is applied between the cathode and the other element within the tube, the anode or target. Since the anode is positive with respect to the cathode, the electrons are attracted to the anode. Their speed and kinetic energy when they reach the anode surface depend on the applied voltage. They will gain 1 keV of energy for each kilovolt of applied electrical potential. For example, if the applied voltage is 100 kV (100,000 V), each electron will have a kinetic energy of 100 keV when it reaches the anode.

When the electrons strike the anode, they lose their energy. Most of

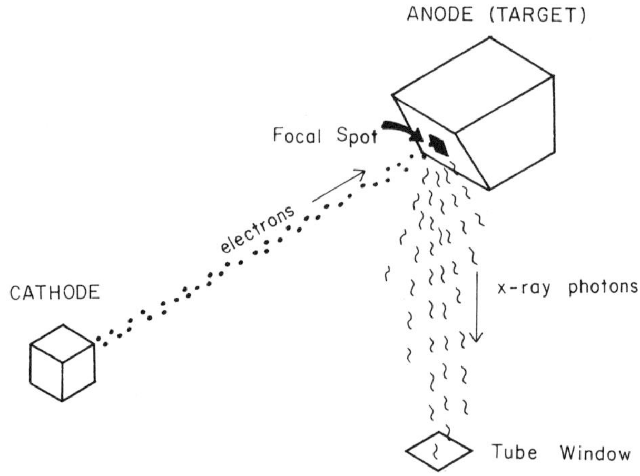

Figure 1. The basic components of an x-ray tube that are associated with x-ray production.

the electrons lose their energy in a series of small steps. This energy appears as heat within the anode. However, a few of the electrons will encounter conditions that will take away a large portion of their kinetic energy in one step. This is the energy that will appear as x-ray photons. In x-ray tubes used in diagnostic procedures, approximately 1% of the total electron energy is converted into x-ray. Most of it appears as heat. Also, the x-ray photons are emitted from the focal spot in all directions. Only a small fraction of the photons generated pass through the tube window and make up the useful x-ray beam.

There are two types of interactions between the high speed electrons and the anode material that can produce x-ray photons. Both of these are illustrated in Figure 2.

Bremsstrahlung

The most significant type of interaction, regarding the number of photons produced, is the so-called Bremsstrahlung process. Bremsstrahlung is German for "braking radiation" and is a good description of the process. Electrons that penetrate the anode material and pass close to a nucleus are deflected and slowed down by the attractive force from the nucleus. The energy lost by the electron during this encounter appears in the form of an x-ray photon. All electrons do not produce photons of the same energy. Only a few photons are produced that have energies close to that of the bombarding electrons. Most of the photons generated will have lower energies. Although the reason for this is somewhat complex, a simplified

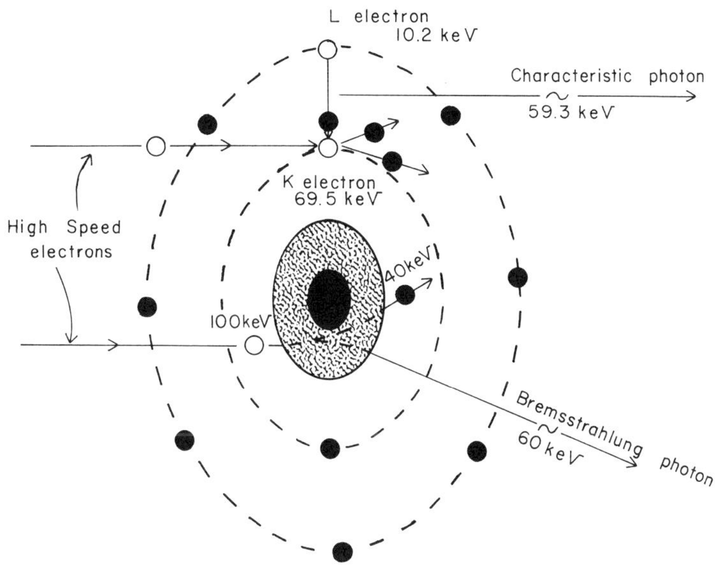

Figure 2. The two types of electron-atom interactions that produce x-ray photons.

model for the Bremsstrahlung interaction is shown in Figure 3. First, it is assumed that there is a space, or field, surrounding the nucleus in which electrons will experience the "braking" force. This field can be divided into zones as illustrated. This then gives the nuclear field area the "appearance" of a target with the actual nucleus located in the center. An electron striking anywhere within the target will experience some braking action and will produce an x-ray photon. Those electrons striking nearest the center will be subjected to the greatest force and will, therefore, lose the most energy and produce the highest energy photons. The electrons hitting in the outer zones experience weaker interactions and produce lower energy photons. Assuming that the zones have essentially the same width, they will have different areas. The area of a given zone depends on its distance from the nucleus. Since the number of electrons hitting a given zone depends on the total area within the zone, it is obvious that the outer zones will capture more electrons and create more photons. From this model an x-ray energy spectrum, such as the one shown in Figure 3, could be predicted.

The basic Bremsstrahlung spectrum has a maximum photon energy that corresponds to the energy of the incident electrons. This is 70 keV for the example shown. The number of photons produced increases for a

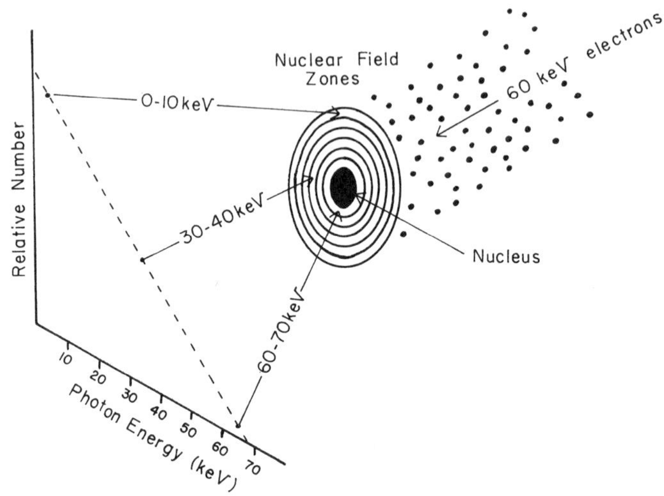

Figure 3. A model for Bremsstrahlung production and the associated photon energy spectrum.

decrease in photon energy below this point. It should be mentioned, however, that the x-ray spectrum emerging from the tube will generally look quite different from the one shown here, for reasons to be discussed later.

The ideal situation would be for most of the electrons to create x-ray photons rather than heat. The fraction of the total electron energy that is converted into x-ray energy generally depends on two factors. One is the atomic number (Z) of the anode material; the other is the energy of the electrons. Most x-ray tubes use tungsten, which has an atomic number of 74, as the anode material. In addition to having a high atomic number, tungsten has several other characteristics that make it suited for this purpose. Tungsten is almost unique in its ability to maintain its strength at high temperatures, and it has a high melting point and relatively low rate of evaporation. For many years pure tungsten was used as the anode material. In recent years an alloy of tungsten and rhenium has been used as the target material. This alloy is used only for the surface of some anodes. Most of the anode body under the tungsten-rhenium surface on many tubes is manufactured from a material that is relatively light weight and has good heat storage capability. Two such materials are molybdenum and graphite. The use of molybdenum as an anode base material should not be confused with anodes, which also have molybdenum surfaces. Such tubes are often used in mammography, for reasons to be discussed later.

The reason for using a rhenium-tungsten alloy is to improve the long-term radiation output of tubes. X-ray tubes with pure tungsten anodes suffer from reduced radiation output with usage. This is significantly improved in tubes using rhenium alloys.

Characteristic Radiation

A second type of interaction between the high speed electrons and the anode material also produces x-ray photons. This type of interaction, also illustrated in Figure 2, involves a collision between the high speed electron and one of the orbital electrons in the atom. The interaction can occur only if the incoming electron has a kinetic energy greater than the binding energy of the electron within the atom. When this condition exists and the collision occurs, the electron is dislodged from the atom. When the orbital electron is removed, it leaves a vacancy that will be filled by an electron from a higher energy level. As the filling electron moves down from a higher energy level to fill the vacancy, it will give up energy, which is emitted in the form of an x-ray photon. This is known as characteristic radiation, because the energy of the photon is a characteristic of the chemical element which serves as the anode material. In the example shown, the electron dislodges a K electron, which has a binding energy of 69.5 keV. The vacancy is filled by an electron from the L shell, which has a binding energy of 10.2 keV. The characteristic x-ray photon, therefore, will have an energy equal to the difference between these two levels, or 59.3 keV.

Actually, a given anode material will give rise to several different characteristic x-ray energies. This is because electrons at different energy levels, K, L, etc., can be dislodged by the bombarding electrons and the vacancies can be filled from different energy levels. The electronic energy levels in tungsten are shown in Figure 4, along with some of the energy changes that give rise to characteristic photons. Although filling L shell vacancies does generate photons, their energies are too low to be of any use in diagnostic imaging. Each characteristic energy is given a designation, which indicates the shell in which the vacancy occurred, with a subscript, which shows the origin of the filling electron. A subscript alpha (α) denotes filling from one of the L shell electrons and beta (β) indicates filling from either the M or N shells.

The spectrum of the significant characteristic radiation from tungsten is shown in Figure 4. Characteristic radiation produces a line spectrum with several discrete energies, whereas Bremsstrahlung produces a continuous spectrum of photon energies over some specific range. The number of photons created at each characteristic energy is different because the probability for filling a K-shelled vacancy is different from shell to shell.

Molybdenum anode tubes produce two rather intense characteristic

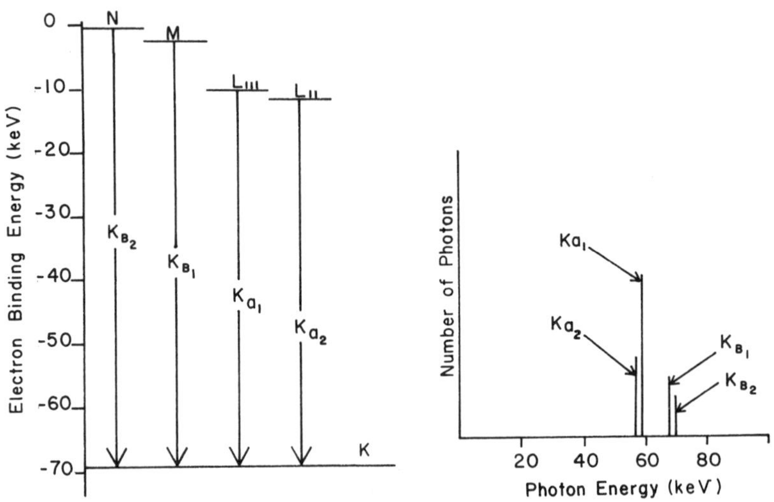

Figure 4. Electron energy levels in tungsten and the associated characteristic x-ray spectrum.

x-ray energies. These are K-alpha radiation, at 17.9 keV, and K-beta, which occurs at 19.5 keV.

X-RAY SPECTRUM

The x-ray beam that emerges from a tube will have a spectrum of photon energies that is determined by several factors. A typical spectrum is in Figure 5. The spectrum is made up of photons resulting from both Bremsstrahlung and characteristic interactions. A significant number of the lower energy photons are absorbed or filtered out as they attempt to pass through the anode surface, x-ray tube window, or added beam filter material. X-ray beam filtration will be discussed more extensively in Chapter X. The amount of filtration is generally dependent on the composition and thickness of material through which the x-ray beam passes and is what generally determines the shape of the low energy side of the spectrum curve.

The high energy side of the spectrum is controlled by the kilovoltage applied to the x-ray tube. This is because the kilovoltage establishes the energy of the electrons as they reach the anode, and no x-ray photon can be created with an energy greater than that of the electrons. The maximum photon energy, therefore, in kiloelectronvolts (or KeV), is numerically equal to the maximum applied potential in kilovolts. In some x-ray equipment the voltage applied to the tube might vary during the exposure. The maximum

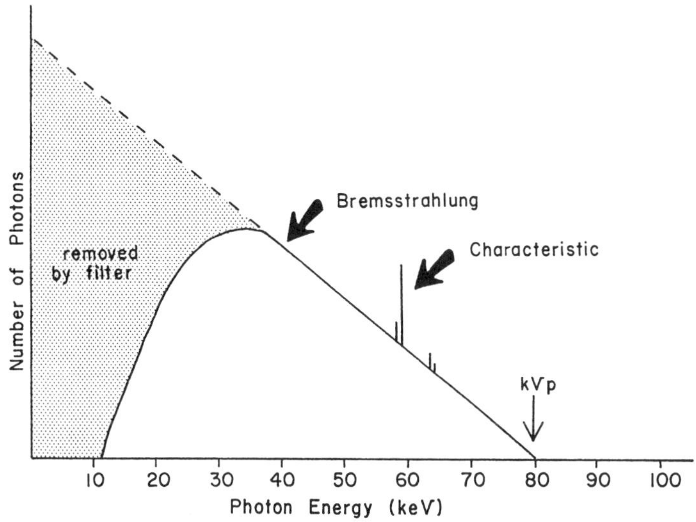

Figure 5. A typical photon energy spectrum from a machine operating at kVp = 80.

photon energy is determined by the maximum or peak voltage during the exposure time. This value is generally referred to as the kilovolt peak (KVP) and is one of the adjustable factors on the x-ray equipment.

In addition to establishing the maximum x-ray photon energy, the KVP plays a major role in determining the quantity of radiation that will be produced for a given number of electrons, such as 1 mAs, striking the anode. It was stated earlier that the general efficiency of x-ray production by the Bremsstrahlung process is increased by increasing the energy of the bombarding electrons. Since the electron energy is determined by the KVP, it follows that the KVP will affect x-ray production efficiency.

Changing the kVp will generally alter the Bremsstrahlung spectrum, as shown in Figure 6. The total area under the spectrum curve represents the number of photons produced. If no filtration is present where the spectrum is essentially a triangle, it can be shown that the amount of radiation produced is approximately proportional to the KVP squared. However, with the presence of filtration, increasing the KVP also increases the relative penetration of the photons and a smaller percentage will be filtered out. This results in an even greater increase in radiation output with KVP.

The KVP value also has a strong influence on the production of characteristic radiation. First of all, no characteristic radiation is produced if the

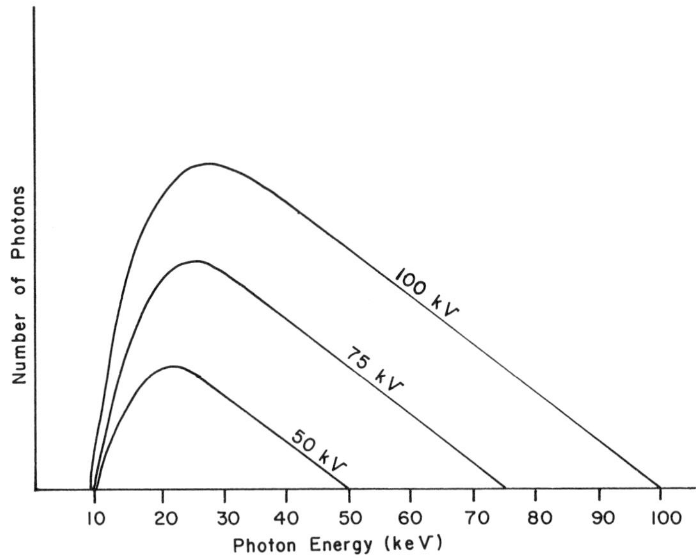

Figure 6. Comparison of photon energy spectra produced at different kVp values.

KVP is less (numerically) than the binding energy of the K shell electrons. When the kilovoltage is increased above this threshold level, the quantity of characteristic radiation is generally proportional to the difference between the operating kilovoltage and threshold kilovoltage.

The relative composition of an x-ray spectrum with respect to Bremsstrahlung and characteristic radiation depends on the anode material, kilovoltage, and filtration. In a tungsten anode tube no characteristic radiation is produced when the KVP is less than 69.5. At some of the higher kilovoltage values generally used in diagnostic examinations, the characteristic radiation might contribute as much as 25% of the total radiation. In molybdenum target tubes operated under certain conditions of KVP and filtration, the characteristic radiation can be a major part of the total output.

EFFICIENCY AND EFFICACY

Only a small fraction of the energy delivered to the anode by the electrons is converted into x-radiation. Most of the electron energy is absorbed and converted into heat. The efficiency of x-ray production is defined as the total x-ray energy expressed as a fraction of the total energy imparted to the anode. The two factors which determine production efficiency are the voltage applied to the tube, KV, and the atomic number of the anode, Z. An approximate relationship is:

$$\text{Efficiency} = \text{KV} \cdot \text{Z} \cdot 10^{-6}$$

It is interesting to observe that for a tungsten anode (atomic number of 74) and an applied voltage of 100 kV, the efficiency is less than 1%.

For a single x-ray exposure, the energy imparted to the anode is given by:

$$\text{Energy (J)} = \text{KV} \cdot \text{MAS}$$

where MAS is the quantity of electrons passed through the tube. Multiplying this expression for energy by the efficiency gives an expression for the amount of x-ray energy produced as follows:

$$\text{X-ray energy (J)} = \text{KV}^2 \cdot \text{MAS} \cdot \text{Z} \cdot 10^{-6}$$

This equation indicates that the quantity of x-rays produced, in terms of energy, increases in proportion to the square of the KV. This was illustrated previously in Figure 6. In practice, one is more concerned with the quantity of radiation which actually comes out of the tube. Since increasing the KV increases the average photon energy, the beam becomes more penetrating and a larger fraction will pass through the filter or other absorbing material. The effect of this is that the x-ray output will generally increase with KV more than that indicated by the above relationship.

The above relationship is helpful in identifying the factors that control x-ray production. It is somewhat limited, however, in that it expresses x-ray production in terms of energy rather than exposure. Also, it does not contain a factor relating to the fraction of x-ray energy produced which is emitted in the direction of the useful beam. In most applications the useful beam is only a small fraction of the total x-ray energy produced. The largest portion of the energy is absorbed within the tube or by the beam collimators. A more useful parameter is the x-ray efficacy, E_x, of the x-ray tube. This quantity is defined as the amount of exposure, in milliroentgens, delivered to a point in the center of the useful x-ray beam at a distance of 1 m from the focal spot for 1 mAs of electrons passing through the tube. The efficacy value expresses the ability of a tube to convert electronic energy into x-ray exposure. A knowledge of the efficacy value for a given tube permits the determination of both patient and film exposures by methods to be discussed in later chapters. Like x-ray energy output, efficacy of a tube depends on a number of factors including 1) KVP; 2) volt-

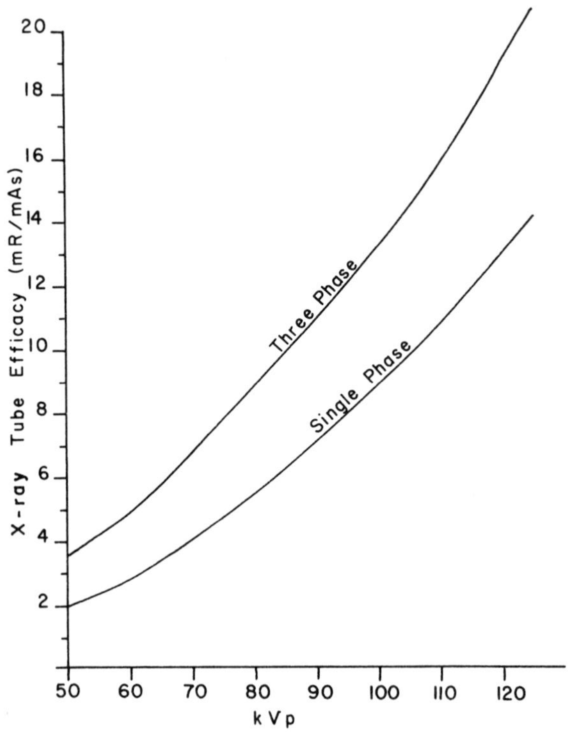

Figure 7. Typical x-ray tube efficacy values.

age waveform; 3) anode material; 4) filtration; 5) tube age and anode surface damage.

The efficacy value for a particular tube can be readily determined by methods to be discussed in a later chapter. Figure 7 gives typical efficacy values for tungsten anode tubes with normal filtration.

Chapter VII

Energizing and Controlling the X-ray Tube

The production of x-rays requires high energy (speed) electrons. In the x-ray tube, the electrons are accelerated to high energies by the high voltage (kilovoltage) which is applied between the cathode and anode. Diagnostic x-ray equipment generally requires an adjustable high voltage ranging from approximately 40 to 120 kV. Other voltages can be found in special applications. For example, mammography is typically performed with tube potentials in the 28- to 40-kV range and some chest examinations are conducted using 350 kV.

The maximum voltage available from the power line coming into the building is only a few hundred volts. It is necessary to increase the voltage, alter its waveform, and apply it to the x-ray tube in a controlled manner in order to produce useful x-radiation. This is the function of that part of the x-ray system that is generally designated as the power supply. The typical power supply circuit provides the following functions:

1. Produces the required high voltage (KV).
2. Changes the waveform of the voltage (alternating current (AC) to DC).
3. Provides for the adjustment of the high voltage (KV).
4. Provides for adjustment of x-ray tube current (MA).
5. Provides for selection of focal spot size.
6. Controls the exposure time.

These functions will now be considered in detail.

KILOVOLTAGE PRODUCTION AND CONTROL

Much of the power supply circuitry is used to produce and control the high voltage that is applied to the tube. The power supply contains several components that provide this specific function.

The Transformer

The transformer is a device that can step an electrical voltage either up or down. In the x-ray machine the kilovoltage is produced by stepping up the incoming power line voltage with a transformer. This discussion of transformer principles will make use of the x-ray high voltage transformer as an example.

Physically, a transformer consists of two coils of wire, as shown in Figure 1. One coil, designated as the primary, is the input to the transformer. This coil is connected to an electrical power source, such as the power line. The other coil, the secondary, is the output from the transformer and is what produces the high voltage.

There is no direct flow of electrons between the primary and secondary coils. They are coupled together by the magnetic field produced by current passing through the primary coil. The transformer is based on two physical principles involving the interaction between electrons and magnetic fields. Simply stated, these are: 1) when electrons flow through a coil of wire, a magnetic field is created around the coil; 2) electrons within a coil of wire will receive energy if the coil is placed in a *changing* magnetic field.

The key to transformer operation is that the primary coil must produce a constantly changing magnetic field in order to boost the energy of the electrons in the secondary coil. This occurs when the primary of the transformer is connected to an AC source. When AC is applied to the input of a transformer, the primary coil produces a constantly pulsing magnetic field. It is this pulsing magnetic field that pumps the electrons through the secondary coil. An electron in the secondary coil will gain a certain amount of energy each time it goes around one loop or turn on the coil. Therefore, the total energy gained by an electron as it passes through the secondary coil is proportional to the number of turns (N_s) on the coil. Since the energy of an electron is directly related to the voltage, it follows that the output voltage from a transformer is proportional to the number of turns on the secondary coil.

The most important characteristic of a transformer is the relationship of the output to the input voltage. This relationship, the voltage step-up ratio, is determined by the ratio of the number of turns on the secondary

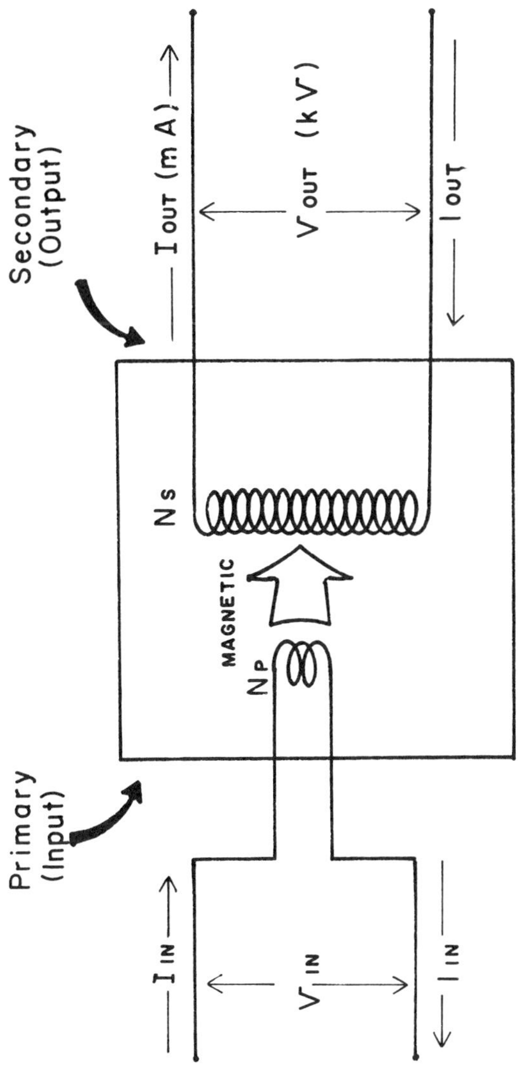

Figure 1. The basic diagram of a high voltage transformer.

coil with respect to the primary. A transformer is designed to give a certain voltage step-up ratio. The high voltage-producing transformers in x-ray equipment have step-up ratios of approximately 1,000:1, or they produce 1 kV for each volt applied to the primary. The voltage relationship can be written as:

$$\text{Voltage out} = \text{voltage in} \times \frac{\text{secondary turns}}{\text{primary turns}}$$

The transformer is a device in which electrons flowing through the primary coil lose energy which, in turn, is transferred to the electrons in the secondary coil. At first, it would appear that the transformer is performing the impossible task of creating energy, since an electron gains more in the secondary than is lost by an electron passing through the primary. This does not happen, of course, and the answer is that there are many more electrons flowing through the primary circuit, in comparison to the secondary. Many electrons pass through the primary coil, each one losing a certain amount of energy. This total energy is transferred to a smaller number of electrons in the secondary, so that an individual secondary electron gets much more energy than was lost by an individual primary electron. For a transformer, it can generally be said that the total energy out is equal to the total energy in. This neglects any energy loss that may occur within the transformer and is generally quite small. In terms of power, the relationship is:

$$\text{Power out} = \text{power in}$$

$$V_o I_o = V_{in} I_{in}$$

Since more electrons must flow through the primary than the secondary, the primary current will be much greater than the secondary current, which is typically the x-ray tube MA. Assuming the equality of input and output power, the following current relationship is obtained.

$$I_{in} = I_o \frac{V_o}{V_{in}}$$

For example, if a transformer has a voltage step-up of 1,000 to 1, the input (primary) to output (secondary) current will also be 1,000 to one. For each milliampere of x-ray tube current, 1 ampere of power line current will be required. When the equipment is operating at 500 mA, a power line current of approximately 500 A will be required. This is why most x-ray equipment must be connected to special electrical circuits that have the capacity to deliver high currents.

The transformer could be described as a device that converts a high input current to a high output voltage, where the product of voltage and current, i.e., the power on each side, is essentially the same.

There are applications in which transformers are used to step a voltage down and increase the current. This is achieved by building the transformer with fewer number of turns on the secondary with respect to the primary.

In most x-ray apparatus, it is desirable to change the voltage (KV) applied to the tube. This is generally done by using the type of transformer illustrated in Figure 2. This, the so-called autotransformer, has a movable contact on the secondary coil which permits the effective number of turns to be changed. Since the output voltage is proportional to the number of turns on the secondary, the output voltage can be adjusted by moving the contact. The typical system will have an autotransformer which applies an adjustable voltage to the input of the high voltage (step-up) transformer. The autotransformer does not produce any significant increase in voltage. In fact, most autotransformers give a slight voltage reduction. Autotransformers often use a combined primary-secondary coil, but the principle is the same as if the two coils were completely separated, as shown.

The question is often raised as to the possibility of putting an adjustable contact on the secondary of the high voltage transformer for the purpose of KV selection. There would be many problems with this. High voltage, such as generated in the transformer, requires extensive insulation. This is normally achieved by placing the high voltage transformer in a completely enclosed tank of oil. There is no practical way to connect the KV selector switch, located on the control console, to the high voltage circuit without interfering with the insulation.

Rectification

The output voltage from the high voltage transformer is AC and changes polarity 60 times per sec. If this voltage were applied to an x-ray tube, the anode would be positive with respect to the cathode only half of the time. During the other half of the voltage cycle, the cathode would be positive and would tend to attract electrons from the anode. Although the anode

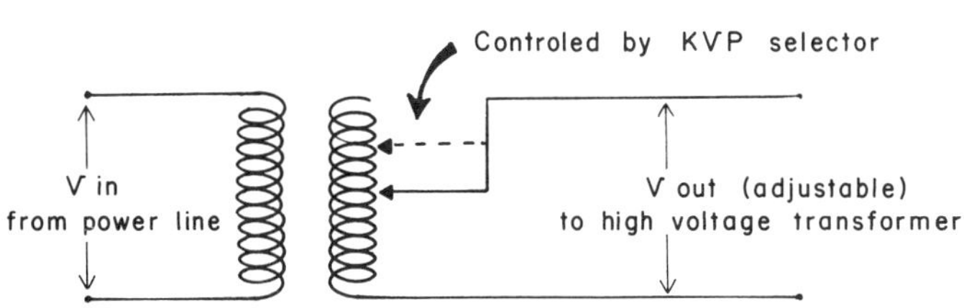

Figure 2. Diagram of an autotransformer.

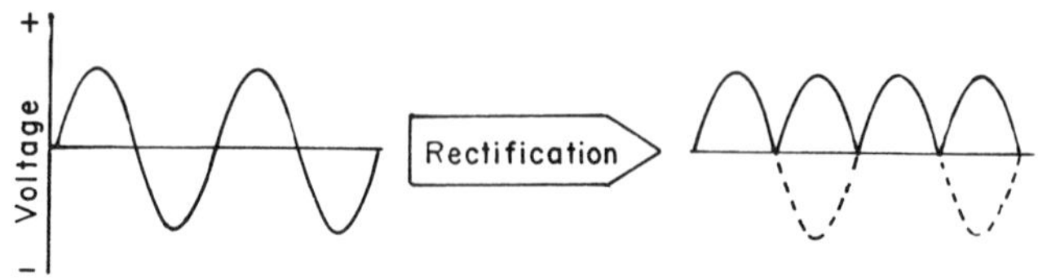

Figure 3. The change in voltage waveform produced by rectification.

does not emit electrons, unless it is very hot, this reversed voltage is generally undesirable. A circuit is needed which will take the voltage during one-half of the cycle and reverse its polarity, as illustrated in Figure 3. This procedure is called rectification.

The typical rectification circuit is made up of several individual components known as rectifiers. A rectifier is a relatively simple two-terminal device which will permit electrons to flow through it in one direction, but not the other. It can be compared to the valves of the heart, which permit blood to flow in one direction, but not the other. In fact, in some countries, rectifiers are referred to as valves. Earlier, x-ray equipment used vacuum tube rectifiers, but now most rectifiers are of the solid state type.

A typical rectifier circuit is shown in Figure 4. It should be noticed that the circuit has two input points to which the incoming voltage from the

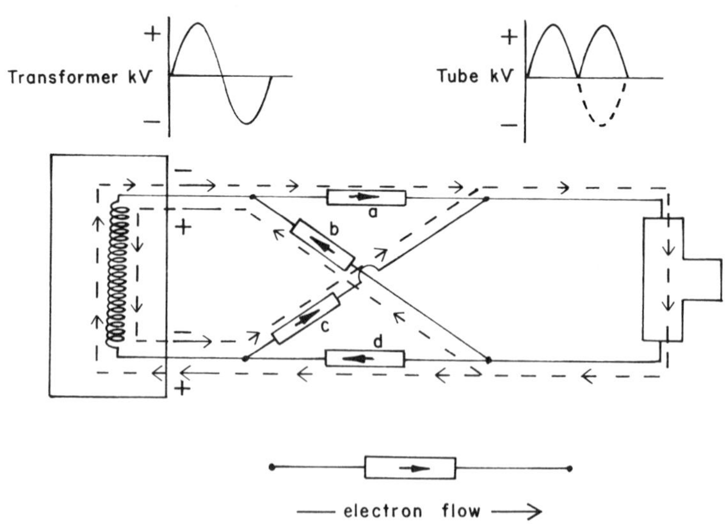

Figure 4. A typical x-ray machine rectifier circuit.

transformer is applied, and two output points, across which the rectified output voltage will appear and be applied to the tube. The circuit contains four rectifiers, labeled a, b, c, and d in Figure 4. Electrons (current) can flow through a rectifier only in the direction indicated by the arrow. The waveform shown indicates the polarity of the lower terminals with respect to the upper. The operation of this circuit can be understood easily by considering the following sequence of events.

During the first half of the voltage cycle, the upper transformer terminal is negative and the electrons are flowing into the rectifier circuit at that point. From there, they can only flow through rectifier a and on to the x-ray tube. They enter the tube at the cathode terminal, leave by means of the anode, and return by the lower conductor to the rectifier circuit. At that point it would appear that they have two possible pathways to follow. They will, however, flow only through rectifier d because the lower transformer terminal is positive and is more attractive to them than the upper negative terminal. During this part of the voltage cycle, rectifiers b and c do not conduct. During the second half of the cycle, the polarity of the voltage from the transformer is reversed and the lower terminal is negative. The electrons now leave the transformer at this point, pass through rectifier c and on to the cathode end of the x-ray tube. The electrons leaving the x-ray tube by means of the lower conductor will choose to pass to rectifier b because of the attraction of the upper transformer terminal which is now positive.

In effect, the rectifier circuit takes an alternating polarity voltage and reverses one-half of it so that the outcoming voltage always has the same polarity. In this particular circuit, the cathode of the x-ray tube is always receiving a negative voltage with respect to the anode. This particular circuit consisting of four rectifier elements connected as shown is known as a bridge rectifier. Since it makes use of all of the voltage waveform, it is classified as a full wave rectifier.

It is possible to construct a rectifier circuit consisting only of one rectifier element. The disadvantage is that it will conduct only during one-half of the cycle. That type is classified as a half wave rectifier. This type of rectification is found only in some smaller x-ray machines, such as used in dentistry. In most such apparatus the x-ray tube itself serves as the rectifier.

Both the full wave and half wave circuits discussed up to this point use single high voltage transformers and are classified as single phase apparatus. The basic disadvantage of single phase operation is that the kilovoltage (KV) applied to the x-ray tube is constantly changing, or pulsing, throughout the exposure.

VOLTAGE WAVEFORM AND X-RAY PRODUCTION

In Chapter VI it was shown that the rate of x-ray production was strongly dependent on the voltage applied to the tube. The spectrum shown in Figure 5 is for x-rays produced with a constant high voltage (potential) applied to the tube. When an x-ray tube receives its voltage from either a half wave or full wave single phase power supply, the kilovoltage is changing at all times, as shown in Figure 4. This means that both the quantity and energy spectrum of x-rays produced changes constantly with time throughout the cycle. It is helpful to step through the following sequence of events, as illustrated in Figure 5. At the beginning of the voltage cycle (time equal to 0) the KV is 0 and no x-rays would be produced. A short time later, when the KV has increased to 25, the simplified x-ray spectrum would be approximately that shown as line a. Most of the x-ray photons that are produced are of such low energy that they are absorbed before leaving the tube. When the KV reaches 50, the spectrum, represented by line b, has undergone two significant changes. First, the total number of photons produced, which is proportional to the total area under line b, has increased by a factor of 4; and second, there are more high energy photons which can penetrate out of the tube. When the kilovoltage reaches 75, the KVP, x-ray

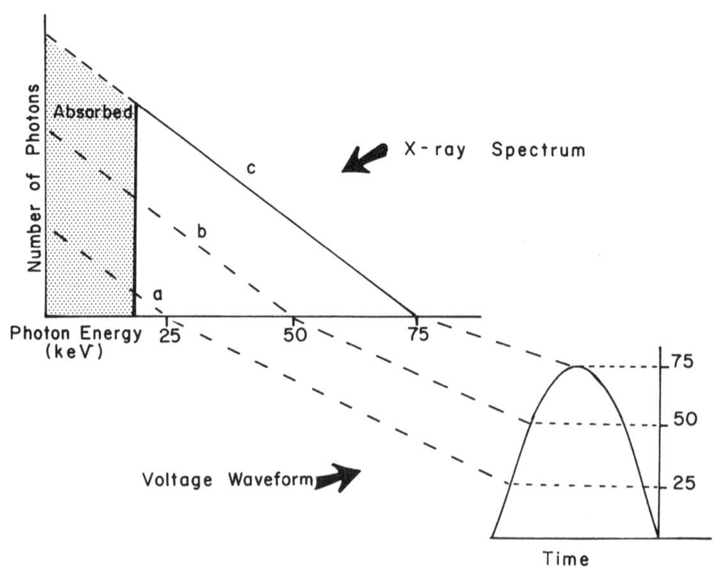

Figure 5. The relationship of the x-ray spectrum to voltage waveform.

production is at its maximum rate. The spectrum under line c would be the approximate spectrum from the x-ray tube if the KV remained constant at 75. However, when the voltage is changing as shown, the output from the tube would be a spectrum of photon energies which is an average of all of the instantaneous spectra. In comparison to the constant potential spectrum, line c, the total number of photons will be less and their average or effective energy will also be decreased.

The rate at which exposure is delivered to the receptor varies significantly with time for single phase equipment, as shown in Figure 6. Most of the exposure is produced during a small portion of the voltage cycle, when the voltage is near the KVP value. Several factors contribute to this effect. One that has already been mentioned is that the efficiency of x-ray production increases with voltage and gives more exposure per milliampere-second at the higher voltage levels. The second factor, also mentioned previously, is that the photons produced at the higher tube voltages have higher average energies and are more penetrating. A third factor is that the tube current (MA) is also changing with time during the voltage cycle. When an x-ray machine is set at a certain MA value, the stated value is usually the average throughout the exposure time. In single phase equipment, the MA value changes significantly during the voltage cycle. The overall effect is that the x-ray exposure is delivered to the receptor in a series of pulses. Between the pulses there is a period of time in which no significant exposure is delivered. This means that, generally, the total exposure time must be longer for single phase equipment than for systems that develop a constant high voltage or potential. Constant potential x-ray

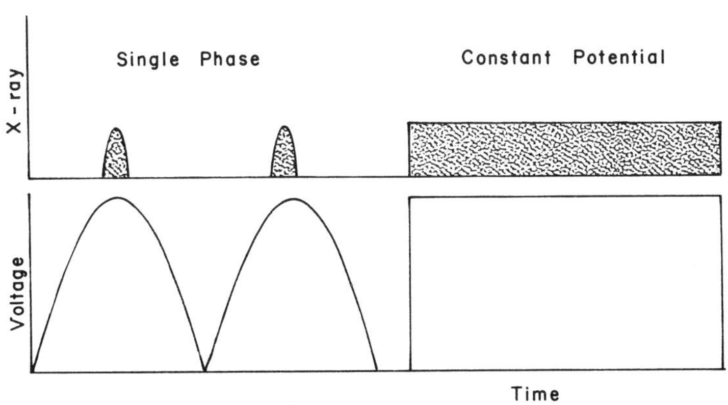

Figure 6. Comparison of x-ray output from single phase and constant potential x-ray equipment.

equipment can deliver a given film exposure in a much shorter total exposure time.

Three-Phase Power

One of the most practical means of obtaining essentially constant voltage and high average current is to use three-phase electrical power. The concept of three-phase electricity can best be understood by considering it as three separate incoming power circuits, as shown in Figure 7. Although this illustration shows six conductors coming in, this is not necessary in reality, because the power lines can be shared by two circuits. Each circuit, or "phase," delivers a voltage that can be transformed and rectified in the conventional manner. The important characteristic of a three-phase power system is that the waveforms or cycles in one circuit are out of step, or phase, with respect to the other two. This means that the voltage in the three circuits will peak at different times. In an actual circuit the three voltage waveforms are combined, as shown in Figure 7. They are not actually added, but are combined in a manner so that the output voltage at any instant is equal to whichever phase is highest at that time. Since the voltage will drop only a few percent before it is picked up by another

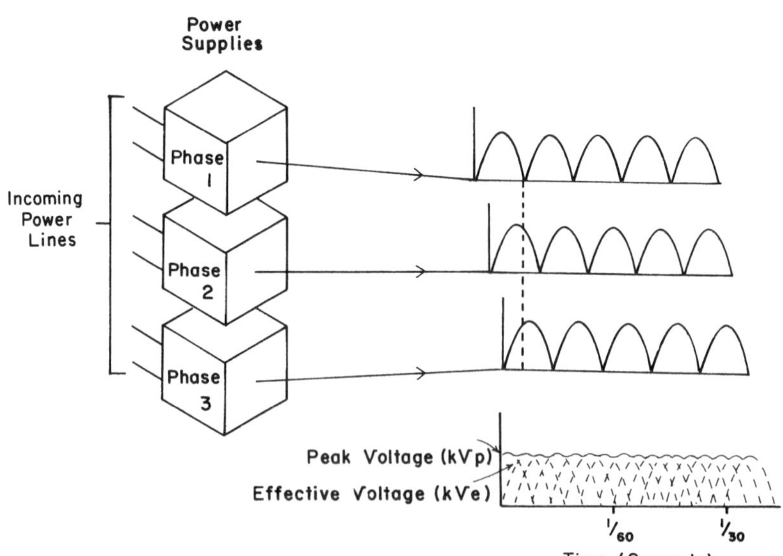

Figure 7. The time relationship of voltage waveforms in a three-phase power system.

phase, the overall effective voltage is quite close to the peak voltage. This is not the case for single-phase power, as illustrated in Figure 8.

The voltage variation over the period of a cycle is designated as the ripple and is expressed as a percentage. The typical ripple levels for several different power supply circuits are shown in Figure 8.

One way of classifying power supply circuits is according to the number of pulses that they produce in the period of one cycle, i.e., 1/60th

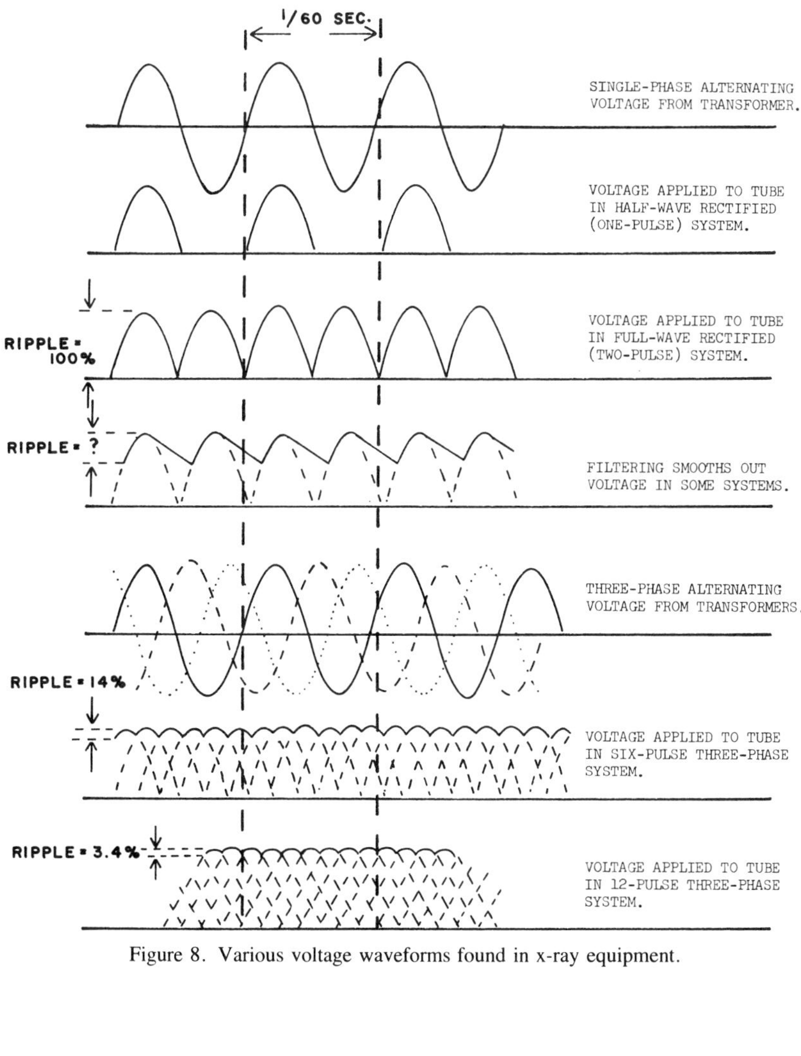

Figure 8. Various voltage waveforms found in x-ray equipment.

of a second. By using a somewhat complex circuit of transformers and rectifiers, it is possible to produce a 12-pulse machine that has a ripple level of less than 4%.

Capacitors

Although three-power power supplies produce output voltages with relatively small variations or ripple, even greater voltage constancy is desired in some applications. This is achieved by adding a capacitor to the circuit. The function of a capacitor is illustrated in Figure 9.

For all practical purposes, a capacitor can be described as a storage tank for electrons. When it is connected to a voltage source, electrons flow into the capacitor and it becomes ''charged.'' As the electrons flow in, the voltage of the capacitor increases until it reaches the voltage of the supply. Energy is actually stored in the capacitor when it is charged. The amount of energy is proportional to the voltage and the quantity of stored electrons. If a charged capacitor is then connected to another circuit, the capacitor becomes the source, and the electrons flow out and into the circuit.

When a capacitor is used to produce a constant voltage or potential, it is connected between the rectifier circuit and the x-ray tube, as shown in Figure 9. As the voltage rises toward its peak, electrons from the rectifier circuit flow both to the x-ray tube and into the capacitor. When the voltage from the rectifier circuit begins to fall, electrons flow out of the capacitor and into the x-ray tube. Within certain operational limits, this can maintain a constant potential across the tube. Capacitors can be used on either single-phase or three-phase equipment. On single-phase equipment, however, there is more of a limitation on the tube current that can be used without introducing ripples.

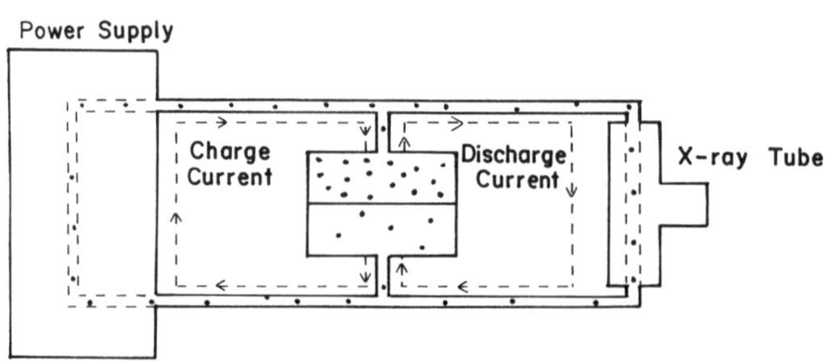

Figure 9. The basic function of a capacitor in an x-ray circuit.

CAPACITOR STORAGE POWER SUPPLIES

In the discussion of the high voltage transformer, it was pointed out that the current flowing into the power supply circuit must be greater than the tube current by a factor equal to the voltage step-up ratio. This is typically as high as 1,000:1. This would require 1 ampere of power line current for every 1 mA of tube current. The special circuits feeding permanently installed x-ray equipment are capable of these high currents. However, in other areas of the hospital where portable x-ray equipment is used, the normal electrical circuits are limited to currents of about 15 to 20 A. Many portable x-ray machines are now designed to overcome this basic limitation by using a capacitor as an electron energy storage device.

A simplified capacitor storage-discharge type power supply is shown in Figure 10. Most equipment of this type uses step-up transformers and rectifiers to produce the high voltage and to charge the capacitor. The electrons are pumped into the capacitor at a relatively low rate (current), so as not to overload the electrical circuit. Charging times can be as long as 10 to 20 sec. The current flow into the capacitor is typically just a few milliamperes. However, when it is discharged to the tube over a short

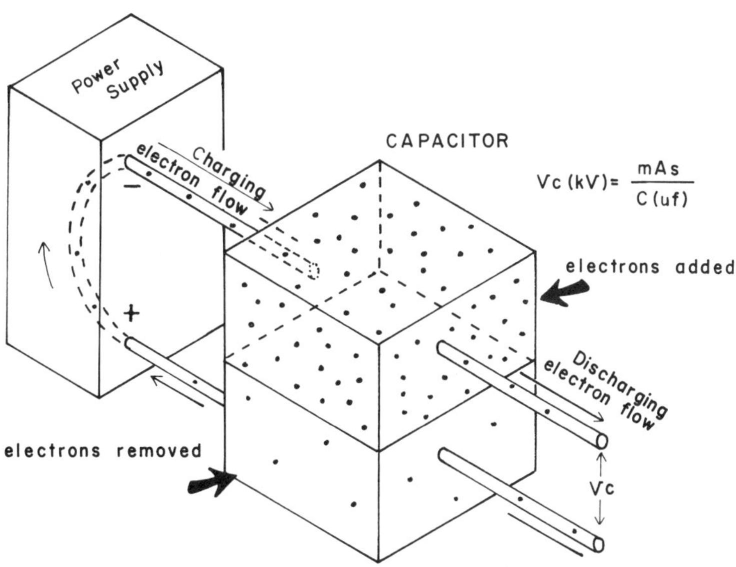

Figure 10. A capacitor storage power supply.

period of time, i.e., the exposure time, the current can be several hundred milliamperes.

The voltage across a capacitor is proportional to the quantity of electrons stored (MAS). The actual relationship depends on the size or capacity of the capacitor. Many machines use 1-microfarad (μF) capacitors which produce a voltage of 1 kV for each milliampere stored. The real significance of this is associated with the discharge part of the operation. As the electrons flow from the capacitor to the tube, the voltage drops at the rate of 1 kV per mAs. For example, as shown in Figure 11, if a machine is charged to 70 kV, and an exposure of 18 mAs made, the voltage will have dropped to 52 kV at the end of the exposure.

It should be noticed that the capacitor storage type x-ray equipment has a high voltage waveform unlike other power supplies. One important factor that should be remembered by equipment operators is that an attempt to get large mAs exposures will drop the kV to very low values by the time the exposure terminates. Since low tube voltages produce very little film exposure, but increase patient exposure, this type of operation should be avoided. Generally, the total MAS should be limited to approximately one-third of the initial KV value.

A means for turning the tube current on and off is included in the x-ray tube circuit. Most machines use a grid-control x-ray tube for this purpose.

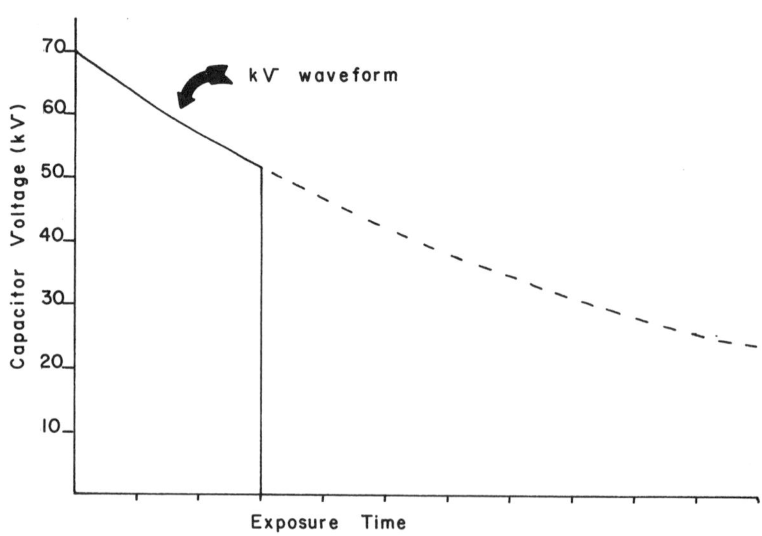

Figure 11. The waveform produced by a capacitor storage x-ray machine.

CONTROLLING THE TUBE CURRENT

It has been shown that the basic circuit within an x-ray machine is relatively simple in that it contains only two major components, the high voltage power supply and the x-ray tube. In circuits of this type the voltage value is determined by the characteristics of the power supply, and the current value is determined primarily by characteristics of the x-ray tube. This basic circuit is shown in Figure 12. In any electrical circuit the current is generally inversely proportional to the amount of impedance to electron flow contained in the circuit. If there were no impedance present, a so-called short circuit would exist and the current would increase to dangerously high levels. In the basic x-ray circuit essentially all of the impedance occurs at the surface of the cathode. When the cathode is cold, the electron flow from cathode to the vacuum space is completely impeded at the surface. This impedance is reduced by heating the cathode so that some electrons are emitted and produce a current flow. The amount of current is generally determined by the rate of electron emission, which in turn depends on the cathode temperature.

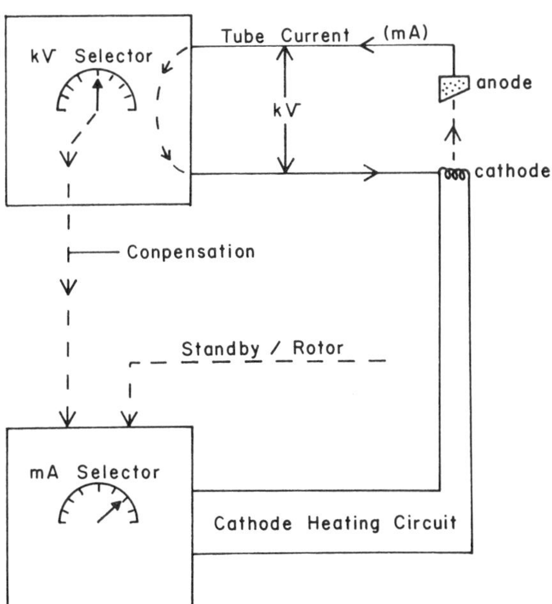

Figure 12. The circuit used to control tube current in an x-ray machine.

The cathode is heated electrically by a current from a separate low voltage power supply. The output of this supply is controlled by the MA selector. Increasing the MA selector setting passes more heating current through the cathode; this, in turn, increases the temperature, and the increased emission produces an increase in the x-ray tube current. It should be observed that there are actually two currents flowing through portions of the x-ray tube. One current, the MA, flows from the cathode to the anode and through the high voltage power supply. The other current flows only through the coils of the cathode. It is this current that controls the cathode-to-anode current.

The cathode temperature required to produce adequate thermionic emission, especially at high MA values, is relatively high. The temperature is sufficiently high, in many cases, to produce some evaporation of the tungsten cathode. Because of this, it is undesirable to keep the cathode at the high operating temperature except for the duration of the x-ray exposure. Most x-ray equipment operates with two levels of cathode heating. When the equipment is turned on, the cathode is heated to a standby level that hopefully will not produce significant evaporation. Just before the actual exposure is initiated, the cathode temperature is raised to a value that will give the appropriate tube current. In most radiographic equipment, this function is controlled by the same switch that activates the anode rotor. Maintaining the cathode temperature at full operating temperature unnecessarily can significantly shorten the x-ray tube lifetime.

Although it is true that the x-ray tube current is primarily controlled by cathode temperature, there are conditions under which it is influenced by the applied KV. An approximate relationship between tube current and KV is shown in Figure 13. At low KV values, some of the electrons which are emitted from the cathode are not attracted to the anode and form a so-called space charge. This build-up of electrons in the vicinity of a cathode in effect repels electrons at the cathode surface and reduces emission. Under this condition, the x-ray tube current is said to be space-charge limited. This can be especially significant at low kilovoltages, such as are used in mammography. This effect can be reduced by locating the cathode and anode closer together.

As the KV is increased, the space charge decreases and the x-ray tube current rises to a value limited by the cathode emission. At that point the tube is said to be saturated. Many x-ray tubes are operated below the point of complete saturation. This dependence of tube current on the KV is generally undesirable. Many x-ray machines contain a compensation circuit in order to minimize the effect. As indicated in Figure 12, the compensation is activated by the KV selector. As the KV is adjusted to higher

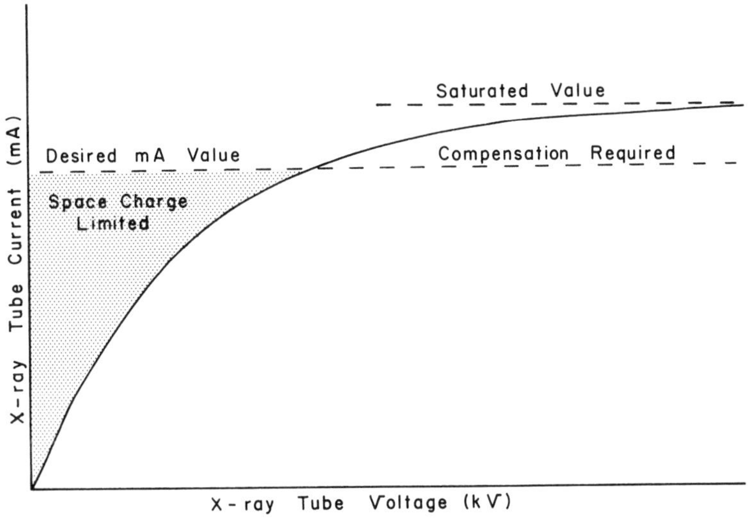

Figure 13. The general relationship between x-ray tube current and voltage for a fixed cathode temperature.

values, the compensation circuit causes the cathode temperature to be decreased. The lower emission compensates for the decreased space charge.

The x-ray tube current can be read or monitored by a meter located in the high voltage circuit. The major consideration is that it must be placed in the part of the circuit that is near ground voltage, or potential. This permits the meter to be located physically on the control console, without requiring extensive high voltage insulation.

Chapter VIII

Heat Production and Distribution

In order to produce x-radiation, it is necessary to transfer relatively large amounts of electrical energy to the x-ray tube. Only a small fraction (typically less than 1%) of the energy deposited in the x-ray tube is converted into x-rays. Most of the energy appears in the form of heat. This places a definite limitation on the use of x-ray apparatus. If excessive heat is transferred to the x-ray tube, the temperature will rise above critical values and the tube can be damaged. This damage can be in the form of a melted anode or a ruptured tube housing. In order to prevent this type of damage, the x-ray equipment operator must be aware of the quantity of heat being produced and its relationship to the heat capacity of the x-ray tube.

HEAT PRODUCTION

Heat is produced in the focal spot area by the bombarding electrons from the cathode. Since only a small fraction of the electron's energy is converted into x-radiation, it can be ignored in heat calculations. In a single exposure, the quantity of heat produced in the focal spot area is given by:

$$\text{Heat (J)} = \text{KVP} \cdot \text{MAS} \cdot w$$

In this relationship, w is the waveform factor. The value of this factor is determined by the waveform of the voltage applied to the x-ray tube. Values for most of the waveforms encountered in diagnostic x-ray machines are: constant potential, 1.0; 3-phase, 12-pulse, 0.99; 3-phase, 6-pulse, 0.96; single phase, 0.71.

The relationship between a quantity of heat expressed in heat units

(HU) and joules is given by:

$$\text{Heat (HU)} = 1.4 \cdot \text{heat (J)}$$

Since the product of the joules-to-heat unit conversion factor (1.4) and the waveform factor for single phase (0.71) is equal to 1, the following relationship is obtained:

$$\text{Heat (HU)} = \text{KVP} \cdot \text{MAS}$$

Here it is seen that for single-phase operation the heat produced in heat units is the product of the KVP and MAS. In fact, this is why the heat unit is used. In the earlier days of radiology, when most of the equipment was of the single-phase type, it was desirable to calculate heat quantities without having to use a waveform factor. This was achieved by introducing a new unit, the heat unit. For three-phase, six-pulse equipment, the heat in heat units is given by:

$$\text{Heat (HU)} = 1.35\ \text{KVP} \cdot \text{MAS}$$

The factor of 1.35 is the ratio of the waveform factors, 0.96/0.71.

The rate at which heat is produced in a tube is equivalent to the electrical power and is given by:

$$\text{Power (watts)} = \text{KVP} \cdot \text{MA} \cdot \text{w}$$

The total heat delivered during an exposure, in joules or watt-seconds, is the product of the power and the exposure time.

HEAT CAPACITY

In order to evaluate properly the problem of x-ray tube heating, it is necessary to understand clearly the relationship of three physical quantities: heat, temperature, and heat capacity. Heat is a form of energy and can be expressed in any energy units. However, in x-ray equipment, heat is usually expressed in the units of joules (watt-seconds) or in heat units.

Temperature is a physical quantity associated with an object which indicates its *relative* heat content. Temperature is specified in the units of degrees. Physical changes, such as melting, boiling, and evaporation are directly related to an object's temperature rather than its actual heat content.

For a given object, the relationship between temperature and heat content involves a third quantity, which is a characteristic of the object, and this is the object's heat capacity. The general relationship can be expressed as follows.

$$\text{Temperature} = \frac{\text{heat}}{\text{heat capacity}}$$

The heat capacity of an object is more or less proportional to its size, or mass, and a characteristic of the material known as the specific heat. As heat is added to an object, the temperature will increase. When a given amount of heat is added, the actual temperature increase is inversely proportional to the object's heat capacity. An object with a large heat capacity will experience a smaller temperature rise than an object with a small heat capacity. In other words, the temperature of an object is determined by the relationship of its heat content to its heat capacity. This is illustrated in Figure 1.

In x-ray tube operation the goal is never to exceed certain critical temperatures which will produce damage. This is achieved by keeping the heat content below specified critical values.

In most x-ray tubes there are three distinct areas with critical heat capacities, as shown in Figure 2. The area with the smallest capacity is the focal spot area, or focal spot track. This is the point at which the heat is produced within the tube. From this area the heat moves by conduction throughout the anode body and by radiation to the tube housing. Heat is also transferred from the anode body to the tube housing by radiation. Heat is removed from the tube housing by transfer to the surrounding atmosphere. When the tube is in operation, heat generally flows into and out of the three specific areas shown. Damage can occur if the heat content of any area exceeds its maximum heat capacity.

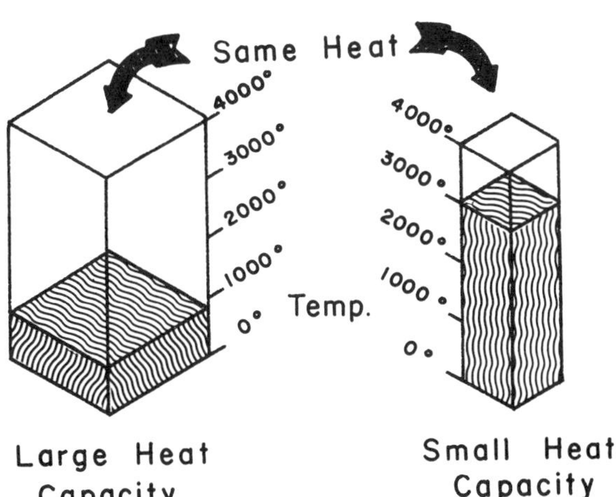

Figure 1. The relationship of heat, temperature, and heat capacity.

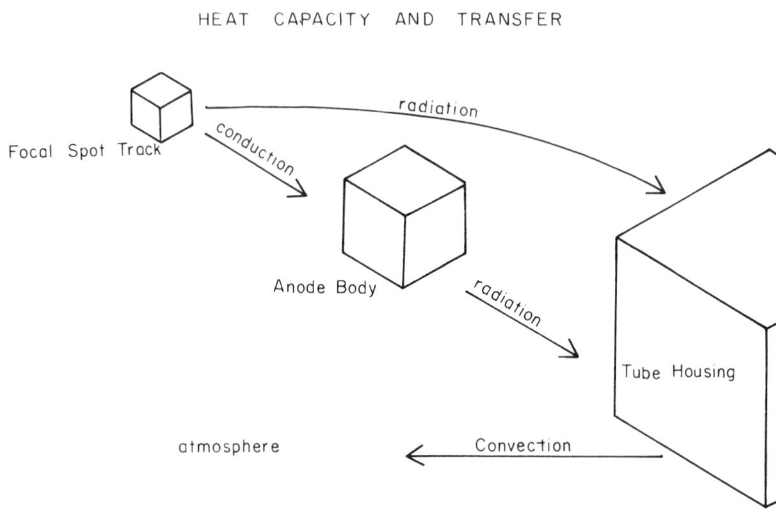

Figure 2. The three critical heat capacities in an x-ray tube.

FOCAL SPOT AREA

The maximum heat capacity of the focal spot area, or track, is the major limiting factor on single exposures. If the quantity of heat delivered during an individual exposure exceeds the track capacity, melting of the anode surface can occur, as shown in Figure 3. The capacity of a given focal spot track is generally specified by the manufacturer by means of a power versus exposure time curve, as shown in Figure 4. This type of curve shows the maximum power that can be delivered to the tube for a given exposure time, without producing overload. Graphs of this type are generally designated as tube rating charts. From this graph, it is seen that the safe power limit of a tube is inversely related to the exposure time. This is not surprising, since the total heat developed during an exposure is the product of power and exposure time. If a tube had one specific heat capacity, say 5,000 J, there would be many power-exposure time combinations which would equal this value, as shown by the dotted line in Figure 4. Since this line differs from the rating curve, it is obvious that the focal spot track does not have a unique heat capacity, but has one that depends on exposure time. In this example, for an exposure time of 0.1 sec, the power rating is 50,000 watts and the total heat capacity is 5,000 J. For shorter exposure times the power rating increases, but not enough to equal the same total

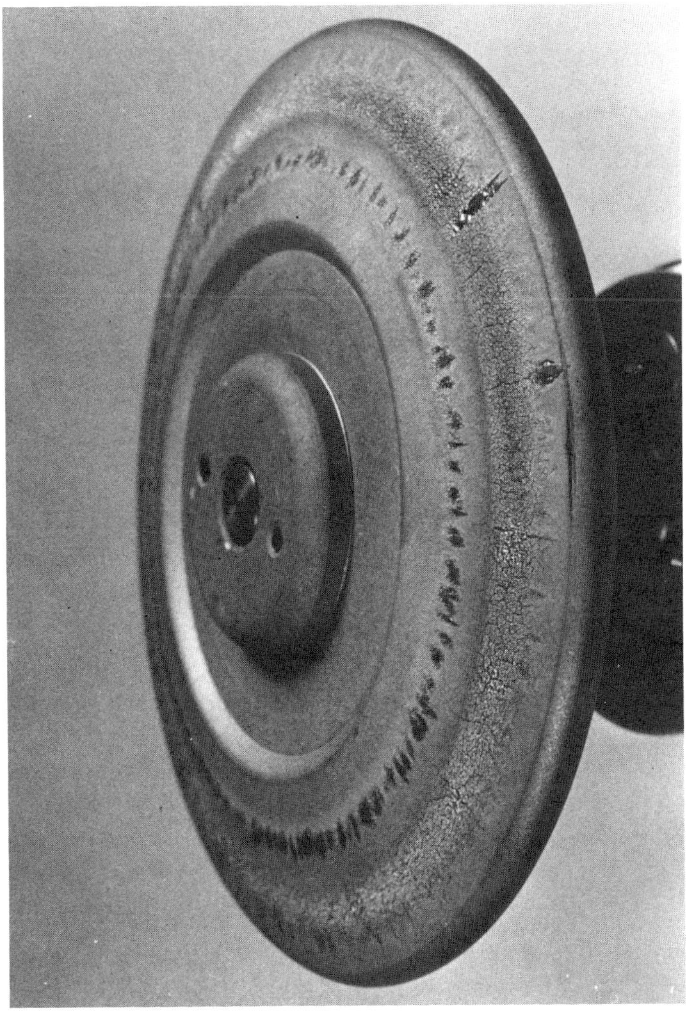

Figure 3. A rotating anode which has been damaged by overheating.

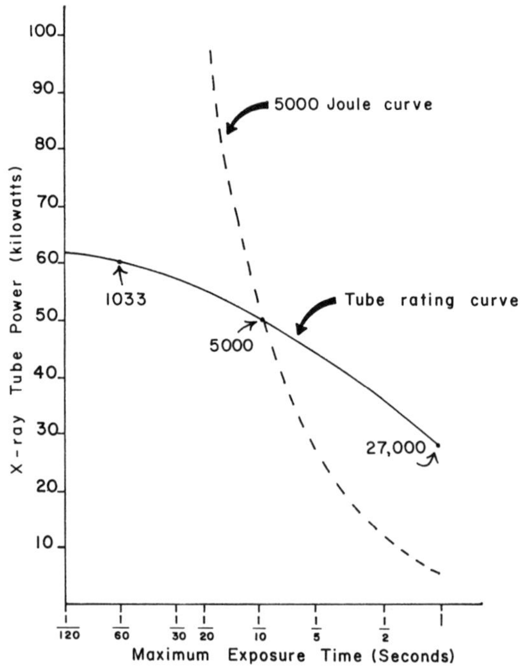

Figure 4. The rating curve of an x-ray machine. Total heat capacity at three different exposure times is indicated.

heat of 5,000 J. It is not just the total amount of heat delivered to the tube that is crucial, but also the time in which it is delivered.

X-ray tubes are often given single power ratings. It has just been shown that the actual power rating is dependent on exposure time. By general agreement, an exposure time of 0.1 sec is used for specifying a tube's power rating. Although this does not describe a tube's limitations at other exposure times, it does provide a means of comparing various tubes and operating conditions.

There are a number of different factors which determine the heat capacity of the focal track area. The focal spot track is that surface area of the anode that is bombarded by the electron beam. In stationary anode tubes, it is a small area with dimensions of a few millimeters. In the rotating anode tube, however, the focal spot track is much larger because of the movement of the anode with respect to the electron beam. Figure 5 shows a small section of a rotating anode.

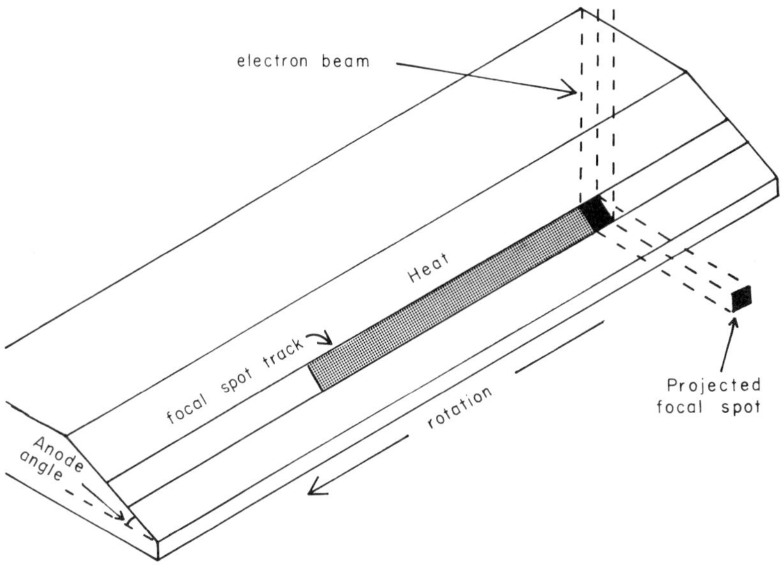

Figure 5. A section of a rotating anode showing relationship of focal spot track to electron beam and anode angle.

Focal Spot Size

From the standpoint of producing x-ray images with minimum blur, a small focal spot is desired. However, a small focal spot tends to concentrate the heat and give the focal spot track a lower heat capacity. The only advantage of a larger focal spot is increased capacity. Many x-ray tubes have two different focal spot sizes that can be selected by the operator. The small focal spot is generally used at relatively low power settings. The large focal spot is used when the machine must be operated at power levels which would exceed the rated capacity of the small focal spot. The specified size of an x-ray tube focal spot is the dimensions of the projected focal spot shown in Figure 5. It should be noticed that the actual focal spot, the area bombarded by the electron beam, is always larger than the projected or effective focal spot. For a given anode angle, the width of the focal spot track is directly proportional to the size of the projected spot. However, the relationship between heat capacity and specified focal spot size is somewhat different. In many tubes, doubling the focal spot size will increase the power rating by a factor of about 3.

Anode Angle

The actual relationship between focal spot width (and heat capacity) and the size of the projected focal spot is determined by the anode angle. Anode angles generally range from about 7 to 20 degrees. For a given focal spot size, the track width and heat capacity are inversely related to anode angle. Although anodes with small angles give maximum heat capacity, they have definite limitations with respect to the area which can be covered by the x-ray beam. There is generally a significant drop-off of x-ray intensity toward the anode end because of the so-called heel effect. In tubes with small angles this is more pronounced and limits the size of the useful beam. Figure 6 shows the nominal field coverage for different anode angles. The selection of an x-ray tube anode angle should be made by considering the trade-off between heat capacity and field of coverage.

Anode Rotation Speed

In rotating type tubes the anode assembly is mounted on bearings and actually forms the rotor of an electric motor. The x-ray tube is surrounded by a set of coils that form the stator of the motor. When the coils are energized from the power line, the rotor spins. The speed of rotation is determined by the frequency of the applied current. When the stator coils are operated from the 60-Hz power line, the speed of rotation will be approximately 3,000 rpm. By using a special power supply which produces

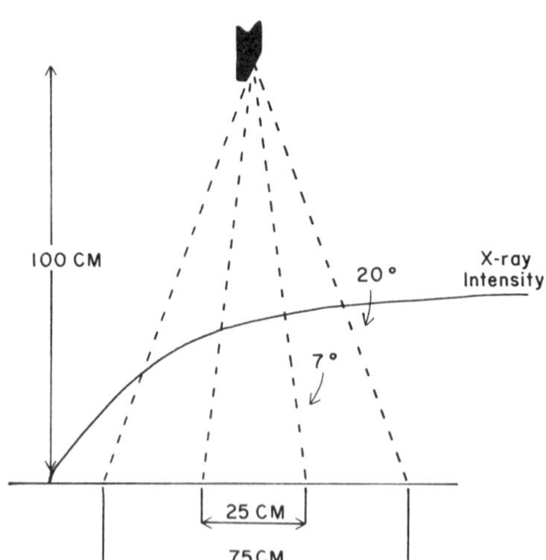

Figure 6. The variation of x-ray intensity due to the anode heel effect.

180 Hz current, rotation speeds of approximately 10,000 rpm can be obtained. This is commonly referred to as high speed rotation.

The effective length of the focal spot track is proportional to the speed of rotation for a given exposure time. High speed rotation simply spreads the heat over a longer track, especially for short exposure times. High speed rotation generally increases the power capacity of a tube by approximately 60%.

Kilovoltage Waveform

Another factor which affects the heat capacity of the focal spot track is the waveform of the kilovoltage. Single-phase power supplies deliver energy to the anode in pulses, as shown in Figure 7. On the other hand, three-phase power supplies deliver the heat at an essentially constant rate, as indicated. Figure 7 compares the temperatures produced by a single-phase and a three-phase machine delivering the same total heat. Because of the pulsating nature of the single-phase power, some points on the anode surface will be raised to a higher temperature than others. These hot spots will exceed the temperature produced by an equal amount of three-phase energy. When an x-ray tube is operated from a single-phase power supply, the maximum power must be less than for three-phase operation to keep the hot spots from exceeding the critical temperature. Or, in other words, three-phase operation increases the effective focal spot track heat capacity and rating of an x-ray tube.

The effect of kilovoltage waveform on tube rating should not be confused with the effect of waveform on heat production, which was discussed earlier. However, both factors should be considered together to determine whether there is any advantage to using three-phase power from the standpoint of tube heating. In comparing three-phase and single-phase operation, three factors should be considered:

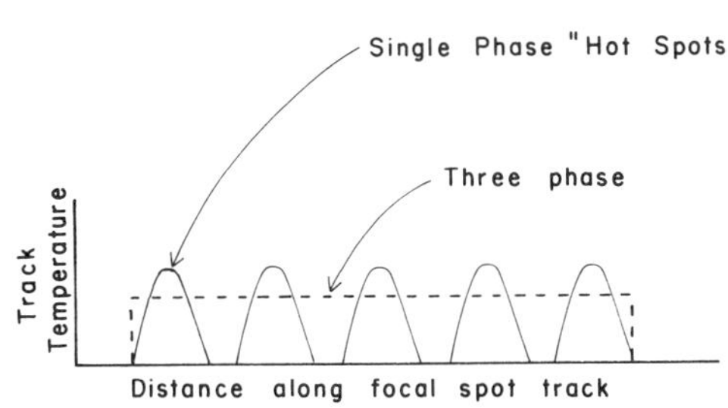

Figure 7. The approximate distribution of temperature along the focal spot track for single-phase and three-phase operation.

1. Three-phase operation permits a tube to be operated at a higher power level because of the uniform distribution of heat.
2. Three-phase operation produces more x-radiation and increased penetration at a given KVP and MAS setting.
3. Three-phase operation produces more heat for a given KVP and MAS setting.

The real advantage of three-phase operation is related to the first two factors listed above. Because of the increased efficiency of x-ray production and the increased penetrating ability of the radiation, lower values of either KVP or MAS are required to produce a given film exposure. This more than compensates for the increased heat production associated with three-phase operation. Additionally, the increased rating, or maximum permissible power, associated with the three-phase waveform adds to the advantage. Generally speaking, an x-ray tube can be operated at a higher power level when it is supplied from a three-phase power supply, and it will also be more efficient in producing radiation.

A rating chart for an x-ray tube operated with different waveforms and rotation speeds is shown in Figure 8. The highest power capacity is ob-

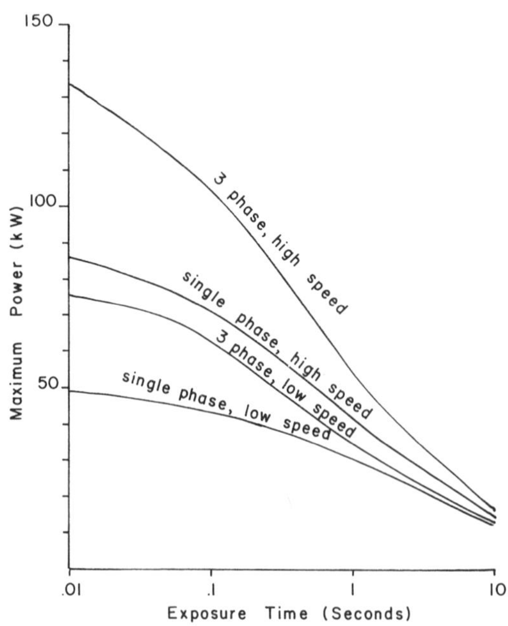

Figure 8. The rating curves for an x-ray tube operated under different conditions.

tained by using three-phase power and high speed rotation. It should be noticed that the real advantage of both three-phase and high speed operation occurs at relatively short exposure times. As the exposure time is increased, overlapping of the focal spot track and the diffusion of heat make the difference in power capacity much less significant.

The rating charts supplied by x-ray tube manufacturers are usually different in format from the one shown in Figure 8. It is a common practice to have a different chart for each of the four operating conditions (waveform and speed) shown. Also, the chart contains a number of different curves, each one representing a different KVP value. The vertical scale on such a rating chart, as shown in Figure 9, is tube current. Even though the format is different, a chart of this type is still a power rating chart. Each combination of KVP and tube current at a specific exposure time represents a constant power value. A chart of this type is easier to use, since it is not actually necessary to calculate the power. The rating chart is used to determine if the technical factors, KVP, MA, and exposure time for a given exposure will exceed the tube's rated capacity.

Most rotating anode tubes contain two focal spots. As mentioned

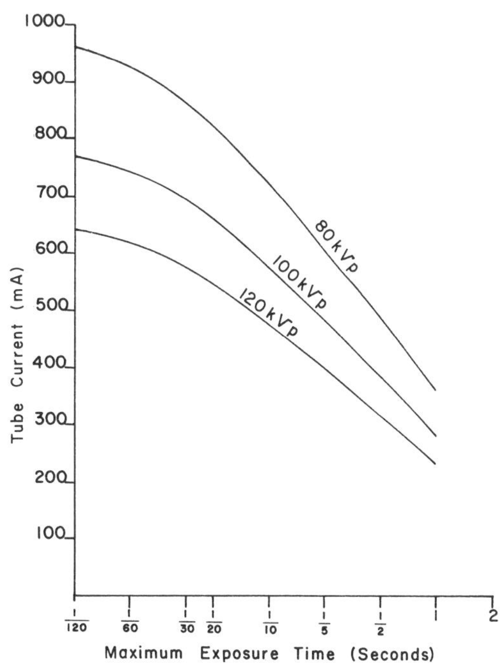

Figure 9. The conventional x-ray tube rating chart.

Table 1. Heat rating (in joules) for typical x-ray tube for exposure time of 0.1 sec and focal spot sizes of 0.7 mm and 1.5 mm

	Single-phase	Three-phase
3,600 rpm	700 (0.7 mm) 2,300 (1.5 mm)	1,050 (0.7 mm) 3,400 (1.5 mm)
10,800 rpm	1,100 (0.7 mm) 3,900 (1.5 mm)	1,700 (0.7 mm) 5,800 (1.5 mm)

previously, the size of the focal spot significantly affects the heat capacity. It should be remembered that a given x-ray tube actually has a number of different rating values, depending on focal spot size, rotation speed, and waveforms. Some typical values are shown in Table 1.

ANODE BODY

The focal spot track heat capacity is generally the limiting factor for single exposures. In a series of exposures the build-up of heat in the total anode can become significant. Excessive anode temperature can cause cracking or warping of the anode disc. The heat capacity of an anode is generally described graphically, as shown in Figure 10. This set of curves, often

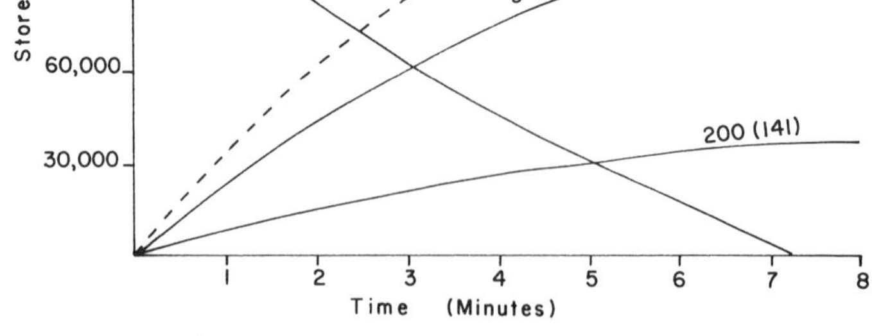

Figure 10. Anode heating and cooling curves.

referred to as the thermal characteristics of an anode, conveys several important pieces of information. The maximum heat capacity is indicated on the heat scale. The heating curves indicate the build-up of heat within the anode for various energy input rates. These curves apply primarily to the continuous operation of a tube, such as in fluoroscopy. For a given x-ray tube, there is a critical input rate that can cause the rated heat capacity to be exceeded after some period of time. This is generally indicated on the graph. If the heat input rate is less than this critical value, normal cooling prevents the total heat content from reaching the rated capacity.

The cooling curve can be used to estimate the amount of cooling time necessary between sets of exposures. It is used in the following manner. Suppose a fast sequence of exposures has produced a heat input of 90,000 HU. This is well over half of the anode storage capacity. Before a similar sequence of exposures can be made, the anode must cool down to a level where the added heat will not exceed the maximum capacity. For example, after an initial heat input of 90,000 HU, a cooling time of approximately 3.5 min will decrease the heat content to 30,000 HU. At this point, another set of exposures producing 90,000 HU could be produced.

Anode damage can occur if a high powered exposure is produced on a cold anode. It is generally recommended that tubes be warmed up by a series of low energy exposures to prevent this type of damage.

TUBE HOUSING

The third heat capacity that must be considered is that of the tube housing. Excessive heat in the housing can result in the rupture of the oil seals, or plugs. Like the anode, the housing capacity places a limitation on the extended use of the x-ray tube rather than on individual exposures. Since the housing is generally cooled by the movement of air or convection, its effective capacity can be increased by using forced air circulation.

The housing heat capacity is much larger than that of the anode and is typically over 1,000,000 HU. The time required for a housing to dissipate a given quantity of heat can be determined by cooling charts supplied by the manufacturer.

The heat characteristics of x-ray tubes should be considered when selecting tubes for specific applications. The characteristics should also be used as a guide to proper tube operation.

Chapter IX

Interaction of X-rays with Matter

It has been shown that x-ray photons are created by energetic electrons interacting with matter at the atomic level. Photons end their lives by a reverse type of interaction in which they transfer their energy to electrons contained in matter. X-ray interactions are important in diagnostic examinations for several reasons. It is the selected interaction of x-ray photons with the structure of the human body that produces the x-ray image. It is also the interaction of x-ray photons with the receptor that converts an x-ray image into one that can be viewed or recorded. One type of interaction, in particular, is generally undesirable because it alters the direction of photons. This, in turn, reduces the quality of most x-ray images and subjects the human body to another source of radiation exposure. This chapter will deal with the basic interactions which occur between x-ray photons and matter.

The discussion of photon interactions should begin by recalling that x-ray photons are individual units of energy. As an x-ray beam passes through matter, three possible fates await each individual photon, as shown in Figure 1:

1. It can interact with the matter and be completely absorbed.
2. It can interact and be scattered or deflected from its original direction.
3. It can penetrate the section of matter without interacting.

There is no way to predict what will happen to any individual photon. It is possible, however, to obtain information regarding the probability that a photon will be engaged in a certain type of interaction under various conditions. If a photon undergoes an interaction by being either absorbed or scattered, the beam is reduced in intensity and is said to be attenuated. The relative rate at which this occurs is expressed in terms of the linear attenuation coefficient (μ). The value of μ represents the fractional chance

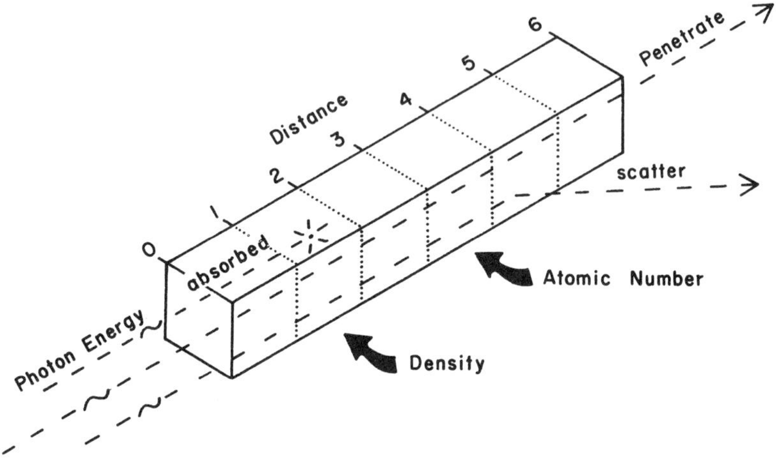

Figure 1. The three possible fates of x-ray photons passing through matter and the factors that influence them.

that a photon will be engaged in an interaction as it travels a stated distance. The attenuation coefficient is normally expressed in units of mm^{-1} (per millimeter) or cm^{-1} (per centimeter). For example, if the attenuation coefficient value for photons under a certain condition is 0.15 cm^{-1}, this means that the chance or probability of a photon interaction is 0.15 or 15 times out of 100 for each centimeter it travels.

The actual value of the attenuation coefficient depends on the characteristics of both the photons and the material through which they pass. The only characteristic of the radiation which is related to probability of interaction and the value of the attenuation coefficient is the energy of the individual photon. It will be shown in detail later that the chance of a photon interacting, and therefore the value of the attenuation coefficient, is more or less inversely related to photon energy. Generally speaking, low energy photons have a higher probability of interacting than high energy photons.

The two physical characteristics of matter which affect the value of the attenuation coefficient are density (ρ) and atomic number. Linear attenuation coefficient values are directly proportional to a material's density. The reason for this relationship is quite straightforward. It is recalled that the concentration of electrons (electrons per cubic centimeter) is primarily a function of a material's physical density (grams per cubic centimeter) and is essentially independent of other factors. The only exception is hydrogen. Because of this direct relationship between linear attenuation coefficient and material density, and because the density of some materials might vary, it is a common practice to report attenuation coefficient values that have been normalized by dividing by the material density. These are known as mass attenuation coefficients (μ/ρ).

As shown below, the value of the linear attenuation coefficient is the product of the material density and the mass attenuation coefficient. The value of the mass attenuation coefficient, in turn, is determined by the energy of the photons and the atomic number of the material.

$$\mu = \rho(\mu/\rho)$$

In diagnostic x-ray applications there are only two types of interactions between photons and matter which are of any significance. These are the so called photoelectric and Compton interactions. The total rate of attenuation is the sum of the rates for each type of interaction, or:

$$(\mu/\rho)_{\text{total}} = (\mu/\rho)_{\text{photoelectric}} + (\mu/\rho)_{\text{Compton}}$$

PHOTOELECTRIC INTERACTIONS

In the photoelectric interaction, as shown in Figure 2, a photon transfers all of its energy to an electron contained in one of the atomic shells. The electron is ejected from the atom by this energy and begins to pass through the surrounding matter. The electron rapidly transfers its energy and moves only a relatively short distance from its original location. The photon's energy is therefore deposited in the matter close to the site of the photoelectric interaction. The energy transfer is a definite two-step process. The photoelectric interaction in which the photon transfers its energy to the electron is the first step. The depositing of the energy in the surrounding matter by the electron is the second step. The details of energy transfer by electrons will be discussed later.

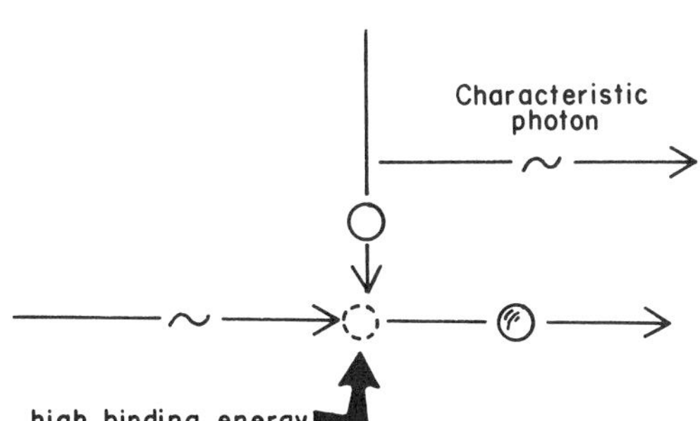

Figure 2. The photoelectric interaction.

It is generally said that photoelectric interactions occur with electrons which are bound firmly to the atom, that is, those which have a relatively high binding energy. It will be shown below that photoelectric interactions are most probable when the electron binding energy is just a little less than the energy of the photon. If an electron has a binding energy that is more than the energy of the photon, a photoelectric interaction cannot occur. This type of interaction is possible only when the photon has sufficient energy to overcome the binding energy and remove the electron from the atom.

The photon's energy is actually divided into two parts by the interaction. A portion of the energy is used to overcome the electron's binding energy and to remove it from the atom. The remaining energy is transferred to the electron as kinetic energy and is what is deposited near the site of interaction. Since the interaction creates a vacancy in one of the electron shells, typically the K or L, an electron will move down to fill in. The drop in binding energy of this second electron will give rise to a characteristic photon. The energy of the characteristic radiation depends on the binding energy of the electrons involved. Characteristic radiation which is initiated by an incoming photon is referred to as fluorescent radiation. Fluorescence, in general, is a process in which some of the energy of a photon is used to create a second photon of less energy. This is a process that converts x-ray into light photons. Whether the fluorescent radiation is light or x-ray depends on the binding energy levels in the absorbing material.

Dependence on Photon Energy

In a given material, the probability of photoelectric interaction occurring is strongly dependent on the energy of the photon and its relationship to the binding energy of the electrons. Figure 3 shows the relationship between the attenuation coefficient for iodine (Z 53) and photon energy. The coefficient has been normalized with respect to density. This graph shows two very significant features of the relationship. One is that the coefficient value, or the probability of photoelectric interactions, decreases rapidly with increased photon energy. It is generally said that the probability of photoelectric interactions is inversely proportional to the cube of the photon energy. This general relationship can be used to compare the photoelectric attenuation coefficients at two different photon energies. If the two energies are designated as low (l) and high (h), the relationship can be written as follows:

$$\frac{\mu_h}{\mu_l} = \left(\frac{E_l}{E_h}\right)^3$$

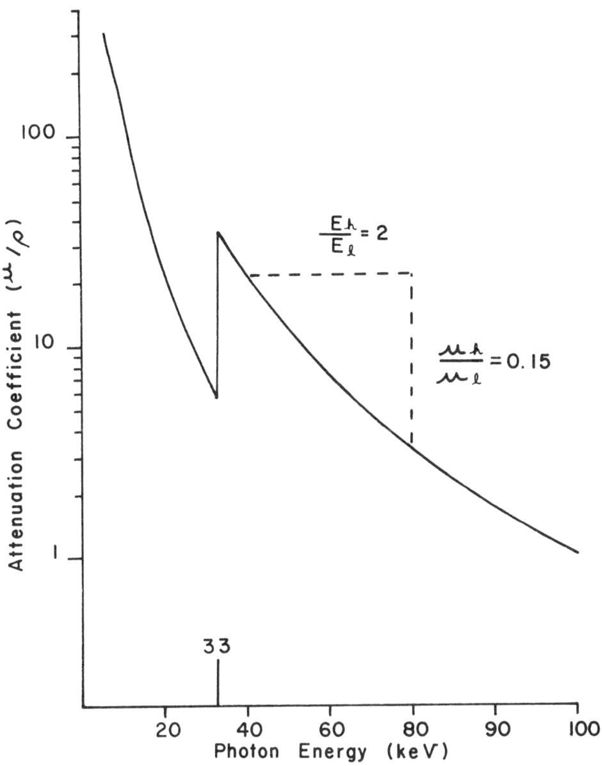

Figure 3. The relationship between the photoelectric attenuation coefficient for iodine and photon energy.

An example of this is shown in Figure 3. Here, the ratio of the attenuation coefficients at energies of 40 and 80 keV is being compared. According to the general relationship, this ratio would be:

$$\frac{\mu_h}{\mu_l} = \left(\frac{40}{80}\right)^3 = 0.125$$

In this case, the ratio of the measured attenuation coefficients is 0.15, which is quite close to the value of 0.125 found by using the above relationship.

The significant point is that the probability of photoelectric interactions occurring in a given material drops drastically as the photon energy is increased.

The other important feature of the attenuation coefficient-photon energy relationship shown in Figure 3 is that it has an abrupt change at one particular energy. This occurs at the binding energy of the shell electrons. The K electron binding energy is 33 keV for iodine. This particular feature of the attenuation coefficient curve is generally designated as the K, L, or M edge. The reason for a sudden change in the attenuation coefficient is apparent if it is recalled that photons must have energies which are equal to or slightly greater than the binding energy of the electrons with which they interact. When photons with energies less than 33 keV are passing through iodine, the interactions are primarily with the L shell electrons. They do not have sufficient energy to eject electrons from the K shell and the probability of interacting with the M and N shells is quite low because of the relatively large difference between the electron binding and photon energies. However, photons with energies slightly greater than 33 keV can also interact with the K shell electrons. This means that there are more electrons in the material which are now available for interactions. This produces the sudden increase in the attenuation coefficient. In the case of iodine, the attenuation coefficient abruptly jumps from a value of 5.6 to a value of 36, or increases by a factor of more than 6.

A similar change in the attenuation coefficient occurs at the L shell electron binding energy. For most elements, however, these are below 10 keV and are not within the useful portion of the x-ray spectrum.

Photoelectric interactions occur at the highest rate when the energy of the x-ray photons is just above the binding energy of the electrons.

Relationship to Atomic Number

The probability of photoelectric interactions occurring is very dependent on the atomic number of the material. Figure 4 shows the relationship between the attenuation coefficient and atomic number for photons with energies of 60 keV. The electron binding energies are less than 60 keV for atomic numbers less than 60. Therefore, the 60 keV photons are capable of interacting with all electrons. A basic explanation for the increase in photoelectric interactions with atomic number is that at the higher atomic numbers there are more electrons in the atoms with binding energies closer to the 60 keV photon energy.

COMPTON SCATTERING

A Compton interaction is one that absorbs only a portion of the energy and leaves a photon with reduced energy. This resulting photon leaves the site of the interaction in a direction different from that of the original photon, as

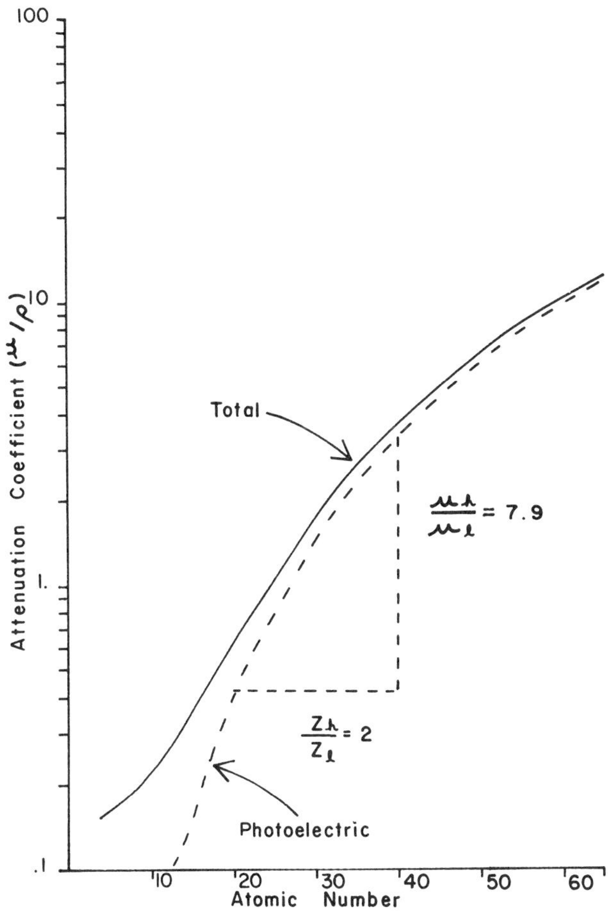

Figure 4. The relationship between attenuation coefficient and material atomic number for photons with an energy of 60 keV.

shown in Figure 5. Because of this change in photon direction, this type of interaction is classified as a scattering process. In effect, a portion of the incident radiation "bounces off" or is scattered by the material. This is extremely significant in some situations because the material within the primary x-ray beam becomes a radiation source. The scattered radiation is generally referred to as secondary radiation. The most significant source of scattered radiation in x-ray procedures is the patient's body. The portion of the patient's body which is within the primary x-ray beam becomes the

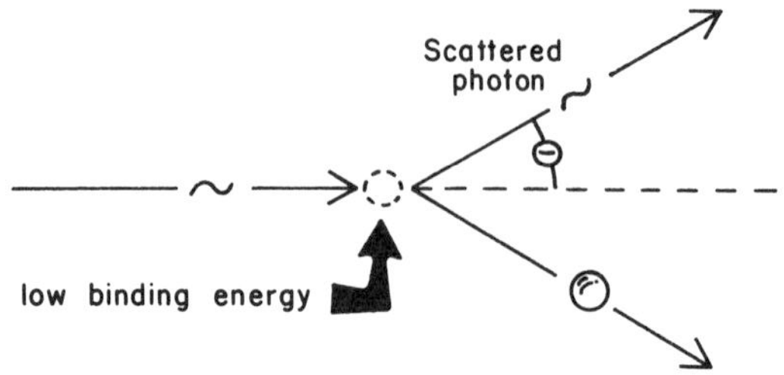

Figure 5. The Compton interaction.

source of scattered radiation. This has two undesirable consequences. The scattered radiation that continues in an essentially forward direction and reaches the image receptor decreases the quality of the image. The radiation that is scattered from the patient is the basic source of radiation exposure to the personnel conducting the examination.

There are actually two types of interactions that produce scattered radiation. One type, referred to by a variety of names, including coherent, Thompson, Rayleigh, classical, and elastic, is a pure scattering interaction and deposits no energy in the material. Although this type of interaction is possible at low photon energies, it is generally not significant in diagnostic procedures. The other type of interaction that produces scattered radiation and deposits some energy in the material is known as Compton scattering. It is the predominant type of interaction between the x-ray beam and the soft tissue of the body in most x-ray examinations. It is the only type of scattering interaction that will be considered in the following discussion.

Probability of Compton Interaction

Compton interactions can occur with the very loosely bound or essentially free electrons within the material. All of the electrons in low atomic number materials and the majority of electrons in high atomic number materials fall in this category. The characteristic of the material that affects the probability of Compton interactions is the number of available electrons. It was shown earlier that all materials, with the exception of hydrogen, have approximately the same number of electrons per gram of material. Since the concentration of electrons in a given volume is proportional to the density of the materials, the probability of Compton interactions follows the same pattern. The rate at which Compton interactions would occur within a cubic centimeter of material is proportional only to the physical density, and not the atomic number as in the case of photoelectric interactions. The major exception is in materials that contain a significant proportion of hydrogen. In these materials with more electrons per gram the probability of Compton interactions will be enhanced.

Compton interactions are more probable for lower energy photons. Figure 6 shows the general relationship between the Compton mass attenuation coefficient and photon energy. Although the chances of Compton interactions decrease with photon energy, the change is not as rapid as for photoelectric interactions, which are inversely related to the cube of the photon energy.

Direction of Scatter

The direction a scattered photon goes with respect to the original beam direction is described in terms of the scatter angle, θ. It is possible for photons to scatter in any direction. The direction in which an individual photon will scatter is purely a matter of chance. There is no way in which the angle of scatter for a specific photon can be predicted. However, there are certain directions that are more probable and that will occur with a greater frequency than others. The factor that can alter the overall scatter

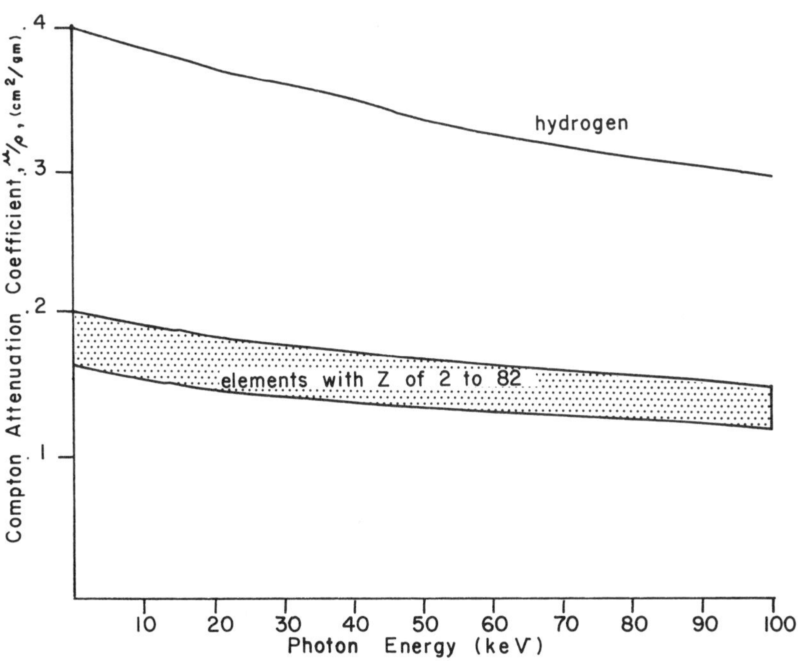

Figure 6. The relationship between Compton attenuation coefficient values and photon energy.

direction pattern is the energy of the original photon. In diagnostic examinations the most significant scatter will be in the forward direction. This would be an angle of scatter of only a few degrees. However, especially at the lower end of the energy spectrum, there is a significant amount of scatter in the reverse direction, i.e., backscatter. For the diagnostic photon energy range, the number of photons that scatter at right angles to the primary beam is in the range of one-third to one-half of the number which scatter in the forward direction. Increasing primary photon energy causes a general shift of scatter to the forward direction. However, in diagnostic procedures, there is always a significant amount of back- and sidescatter radiation.

Energy of Scattered Radiation

When a photon undergoes a Compton interaction, its energy is divided between the scattered secondary photon and the electron with which it interacts. The electron's kinetic energy is quickly absorbed by the material along its path. In other words, in a Compton interaction, part of the original photon's energy is absorbed and part is converted into scattered radiation.

The manner in which the energy is divided between scattered and absorbed radiation depends on two factors—the angle of scatter and the energy of the original photon. The relationship between the energy of the scattered radiation and the angle of scatter is a little complex and should be considered in two steps. The photon characteristic that is specifically related to a given scatter angle is its change in wavelength. It should be recalled that a photon's wavelength (λ) and energy (E) are inversely related as given by:

$$E = \frac{12.4}{\lambda}$$

Since photons lose energy in a Compton interaction, the wavelength always increases. The relationship between the change in a photon's wavelength, $\Delta\lambda$, and the angle of scatter is given by:

$$\Delta\lambda = 0.024(1 - \cos\theta)$$

For example, all photons scattered at an angle of 90 degrees, where the cosine has a value of 0, will undergo a wavelength change of 0.024 Å. Photons which scatter back at an angle of 180 degrees where the cosine has a value of -1 will undergo a wavelength change of 0.048 Å. This is the maximum wavelength change that can occur in a scattering interaction.

It is important to recognize the difference between a change in wavelength and a change in energy. Since higher energy photons have shorter wavelengths, a change of say 0.024 Å represents a larger energy change than it would for a lower energy photon. Figure 7 shows the relationship between wavelength change and energy change at different photon energies. This illustration shows the change in both energy and wavelength for photons undergoing right-angle (90-degree) scatter. All photons scattered at an angle of 90 degrees will undergo a wavelength change of 0.0243 Å. The change in energy associated with 90-degree scatter is not the same for all photons and depends on their original energy. The change in energy can be found as follows. For a 110-keV photon, the wavelength is given by:

$$\lambda = \frac{12.4}{100} = 0.1127 \text{ Å}$$

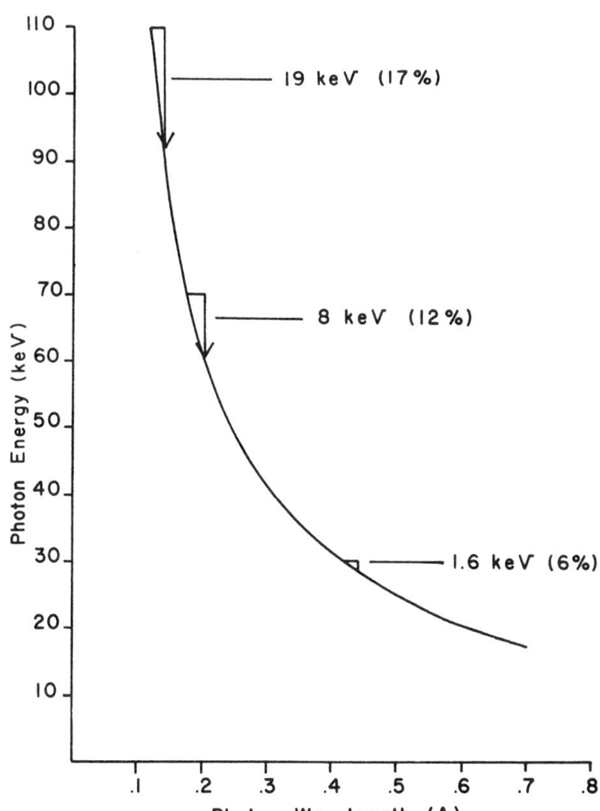

Figure 7. The change in photon energy and wavelength for right-angle (90-degree) scatter.

A scatter angle of 90 degrees will always increase the wavelength by 0.0243. Therefore, the wavelength of the scattered photon will be 0.1127 plus 0.0243 or 0.1370. The energy of a photon with this wavelength is given by:

$$E = \frac{12.4}{0.137} = 91 \text{ keV}$$

The 110-keV photons will lose 19 keV or 17% of their energy in the scattering process. Lower energy photons lose a smaller percentage of their energy as shown.

Figure 8 shows the energy of photons scattered at different angles. As mentioned previously, photons that scatter in the forward direction, that is, at small scatter angles, have energies that are only slightly less than those of the primary photons.

The significant factors relating to Compton interactions can be summarized as follows. The probability of Compton interactions is essentially independent of material atomic number and decreases slightly with increased photon energy. It is possible for a photon to scatter in any direction, but certain directions are generally more probable than others. The chance of being scattered in the forward direction increases with photon energy. A photon which is scattered in a given direction will experience an increase in wavelength by an amount uniquely related to the angle of scatter. A specific change in wavelength represents different energy changes, depending on the original photon energy.

The real significance of Compton interactions in radiology is that they create a source of secondary radiation, primarily within the patient's body.

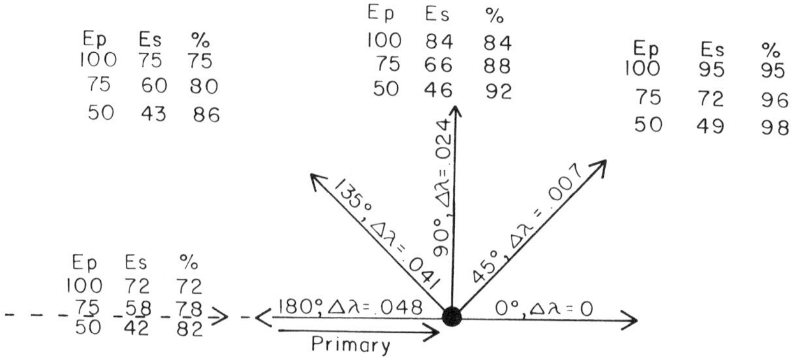

Figure 8. The energy of scattered radiation, E_s, for different primary photon energies, E_p, and scatter angles.

COMBINED INTERACTIONS

As x-ray photons pass through matter, there is a possibility of being involved in two types of interactions with the material electrons. The photoelectric interaction captures all of the photon energy and deposits it within the material, whereas the Compton interaction removes only a portion of the energy, and the remainder continues as scattered radiation. The combination of the two types of interactions produces the overall attenuation of the x-ray beam. It is now possible to consider the factors that determine which of the two interactions is most likely to occur in a given situation. The relative number of photoelectric interactions with respect to the Compton is determined by the energy of the photons and the atomic number of the material.

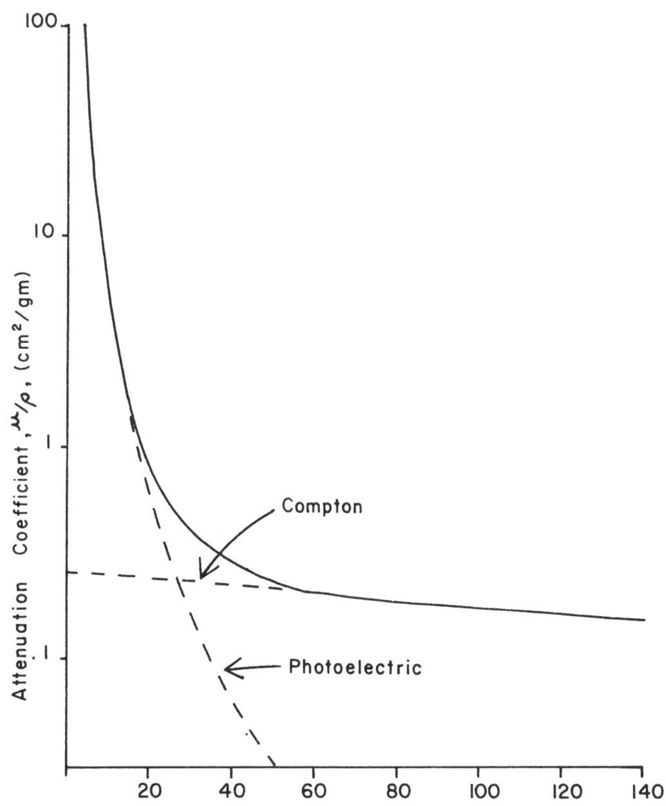

Figure 9. Photoelectric, Compton, and total attenuation coefficient values in soft tissue for different photon energies.

An excellent example of the combined effect of the two interactions in soft tissue is shown in Figure 9. This graph not only contains a plot of the total attenuation coefficient with respect to photon energy, but also the contribution of the two types of interactions. At the lower photon energies, photoelectric interactions are much more predominant than Compton. Over most of the energy range, the probability of both decreases with increased energy. However, the important thing to notice is that the decrease in photoelectric interactions is much greater. This is because the photoelectric rate changes in proportion to $1/E^3$, whereas Compton interactions are much less energy dependent. In soft tissue, the two lines cross at an energy of about 30 keV. At this energy, both photoelectric and Compton interactions occur in equal numbers. Below this energy, photoelectric interactions predominate. Above 30 keV Compton interactions become the significant process of x-ray attenuation. As photon energy is increased, two changes are occurring; the probability of both types of interactions decreases, but the fall-off in Compton is less and it becomes the predominant type of interaction.

The energy at which interactions change from predominantly photoelectric to Compton is a function of the atomic number of the material. Figure 10 shows this cross-over energy for several different materials. In higher atomic number materials, photoelectric interactions are more probable in general and they predominate up to higher photon energy. The conditions that cause photoelectric interactions to predominate over Compton are the same conditions that enhance photoelectric interactions, that is, low photon energies and materials with high atomic numbers.

The total attenuation coefficient value for materials involved in x-ray interactions can vary tremendously if photoelectric interactions are involved. A minimum value of approximately 0.15 cm^2 per g is established by Compton interactions. Photoelectric interactions can cause the total attenuation to increase to very high values. For example, at 30 KeV, lead (Z=82) has a mass attenuation coefficient of 30 cm^2 per g.

ELECTRON INTERACTION

Both photoelectric and Compton interactions dislodge electrons from the atoms within the material and give the electrons a considerable velocity. In the case of photoelectric interactions, the energy of the electron is equal to the energy of the incident photon less the binding energy of the electron within the atom. In Compton interactions, the relationship of the electron energy to that of the photon depends on the angle of scatter and the original photon energy, as discussed previously. The electrons set free by these

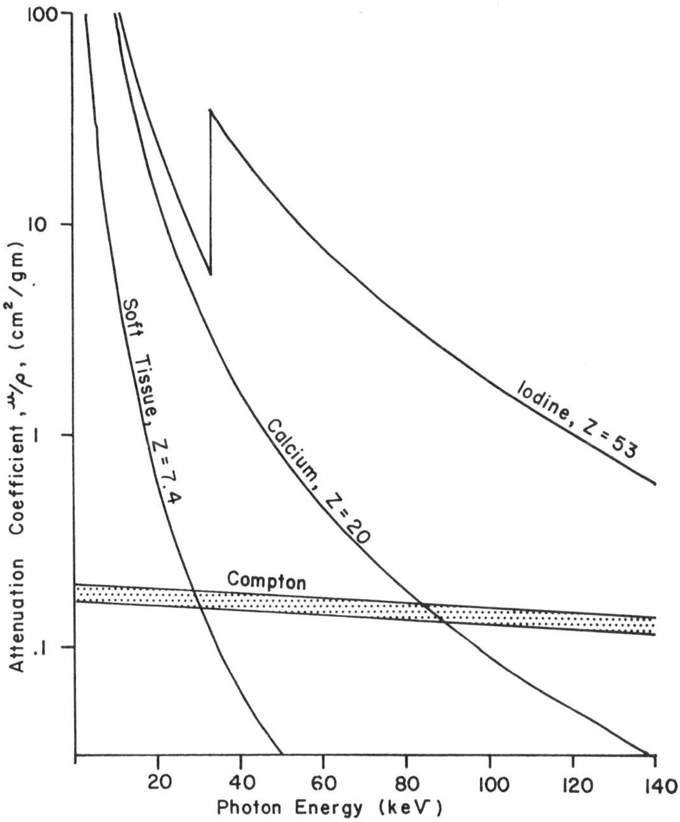

Figure 10. Photoelectric and Compton attenuation coefficient values for different materials and photon energies.

interactions will therefore have kinetic energies ranging from relatively low values up to a little below the energy of the incident photons.

As the electrons leave the site of the interaction, they immediately begin to transfer their energy to the surrounding material. Because the electron carries an electrical charge, it is able to interact with other electrons without actually touching them. As the electron passes through the material it in effect pushes the material electrons away from its path. If the force on an electron is sufficient to remove it from its atom, ionization results. In some cases the atomic or molecular structures might be raised to a higher energy level or excited state. Regardless of the type of interaction, the moving electron loses some of its energy. Most of the ionization produced by x-radiation is not a result of the direct x-ray photon interactions, but rather the interactions of the resulting energetic electrons with the material. For example, in air, radiation must expend an average energy of 33.4 eV per ionization. Consider a 50-keV x-ray photon undergoing a photoelectric interaction. The initial interaction of the photon ionizes 1 atom, but the resulting energetic electron ionizes approximately 1,500 additional atoms.

It is helpful to have some concept of the distance traveled by the electrons coming out of photoelectric and Compton interactions. The distance traveled or range of the electrons depends on their energy and the density and atomic number of the material. Since most x-ray photons interact with the soft tissue of the body, this is the only material that will be considered. Figure 11 shows the relationship between electron range and energy in water, which has approximately the same density and effective atomic number as soft tissue. Since the electrons lose their energy more or less continuously, and continue to move until all of their energy is dissipated, it is not surprising that the range is essentially proportional to their original energy. From this curve, it can be seen that the range of electrons formed in photoelectric and Compton interactions will, in most cases, be less than 0.1 mm. Or, in other words, most of the energy of an x-ray

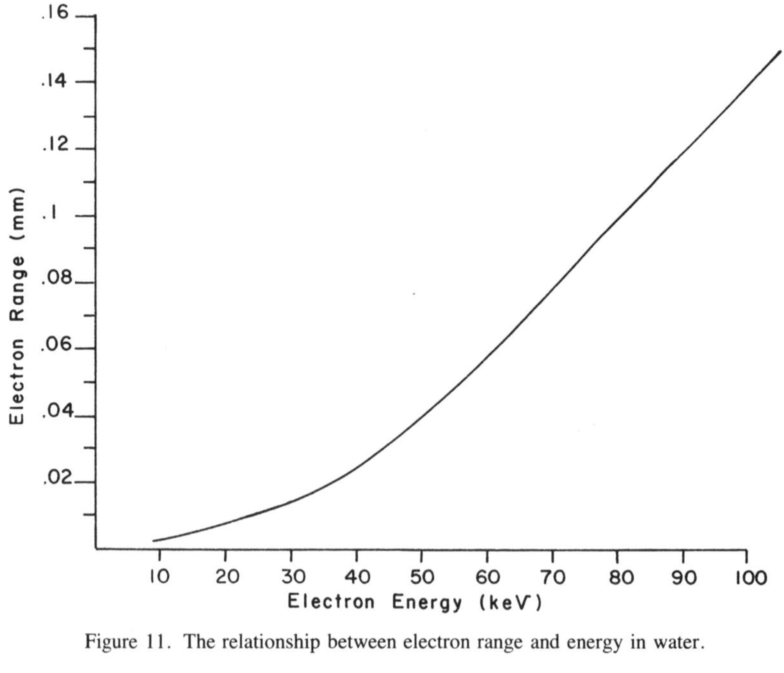

Figure 11. The relationship between electron range and energy in water.

photon is deposited very close to the site of interaction. An exception is the energy that is carried away from the site of interaction by characteristic and Compton photons.

In concluding this discussion of photon and electron interaction, a very important comparison should be made. An individual x-ray photon can travel a considerable distance through matter before it interacts. When it does interact it will typically have only one interaction in which it loses its energy. On the other hand, as an electron moves through matter, it is engaged in many interactions along its path and loses some energy in each one.

The probability of a photon penetrating a greater distance before interacting is generally increased with increased photon energy. However, it is not possible to predict the actual range of a photon. Even for photons of the same energy, some will travel a much greater distance than others before interacting. However, electrons of a specific energy have a rather definite range, as shown in Figure 11.

Chapter X

X-ray Penetration

The use of x-radiation in diagnostic medicine is based on the principle that some of the x-ray photons within an x-ray beam will not interact and will pass through or penetrate a given section of material. The last chapter introduced the two basic types of interactions between photons and matter that are of importance in diagnostic radiology and emphasized the factors that alter the probability of the various interactions occurring. In a given situation, the photons that are not involved in photoelectric and Compton interactions are the ones that penetrate the material. Any factor that increases the chance of photons interacting with matter decreases the fraction of photons that will penetrate.

The penetration, P, of an object is defined as the fraction of radiation that passes through the object. Another way of expressing it is that penetration is the fraction of the primary x-ray beam that is not involved in interactions within the object. This is illustrated in Figure 1. If an x-ray beam delivers an exposure, X_0, of 100 mR to a point without passing through an attenuating object and an exposure, X, of 5 mR when it passes through the object, the penetration, P, can be found as follows:

$$P = \frac{X}{X_0} = \frac{5 \text{ mR}}{100 \text{ mR}} = 0.05$$

Since penetration is a ratio of exposures, it does not have any units.

The above relationship can be rearranged to form an expression for the exposure through an object. For example, the question might be how much exposure would be delivered to a receptor when an x-ray machine is set to deliver 50 mR without the patient in the beam and it is known that the patient penetration is 0.02. In this case, the exposure to the receptor through the patient, X, can be found as follows:

$$X = X_0 \cdot P = 50 \text{ mR} \times 0.02 = 1.0 \text{ mR}$$

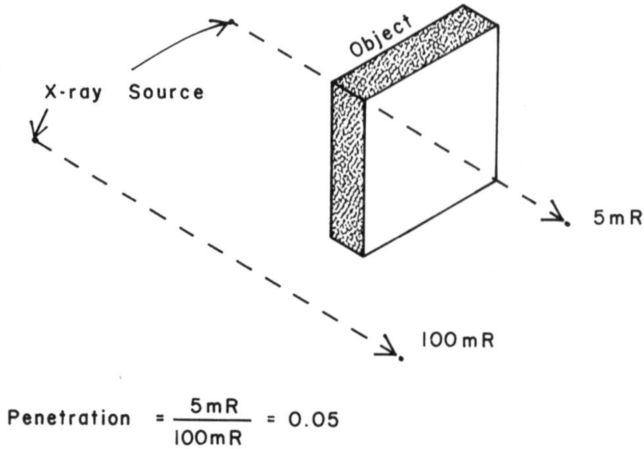

Figure 1. An illustration of the concept of penetration.

PENETRATION RATES

Penetration Factor

In the previous discussion of x-ray interactions (Chapter IX), the chance of an interaction occurring was described in terms of the attenuation coefficient, μ. It should be recalled that this specifies the probability or chance that an individual photon will be removed from the primary beam as it travels a distance of 1 unit (millimeter, centimeter, etc.).

Another very useful way of describing the penetrating ability of x-rays is by means of the penetration factor, p. The penetration factor is defined as the fraction of x-ray photons which pass through a 1 unit thick (millimeter or centimeter) section of an object without undergoing an interaction. The units for the penetration factor are per millimeter or per centimeter (mm^{-1} or cm^{-1}), depending on the material involved.

Although it is obvious that the value of the penetration factor is related to the attenuation coefficient, the exact form of the relationship needs some explanation. The fraction of photons that penetrates is equal to 1 minus the fraction that is involved in interactions. If this latter quantity is known, the penetration can be easily determined. At first it might appear that the attenuation coefficient value is equivalent to the fraction of photons that are attenuated. The logic of this is that if one photon has a probability of μ per centimeter of being attenuated, then the fraction of a large number of photons undergoing interactions would also be μ. This would lead to a relationship between penetration factor, p, and attenuation coefficient, μ, of the following form.

$$p = 1 - \mu$$

This relationship, although useful in illustrating the general concept of penetration, ignores one factor and is valid only for very small values of μ.

The factor that is not taken into account in the above relationship is that as photons interact and are removed from the x-ray beam, the overall rate of interactions decreases. At any point along the path of the x-ray beam, the rate, R, at which photons are interacting (photons per unit distance) is given by:

$$R = \mu N$$

where N is the number of photons passing that point. As the beam passes into the object, the number of photons at each point along the way is decreasing. Therefore, the rate at which photons are interacting decreases continuously and is not the same throughout the material.

A relationship that takes into account the decreasing rate of interactions along the path of the beam is given by:

$$p = e^{-\mu}$$

This is a so-called exponential relationship. In this equation, e is the symbol for Euler's number, which has a value of 2.718. For a given value of μ, the value of $e^{-\mu}$, the penetration factor, can be determined by referring to the tabulated values in Appendix I. For example, if a given material has an attenuation coefficient of 0.4 per centimeter, the penetration factor (per centimeter) is equal to $e^{-0.4}$. By referring to the table of exponential values, it is found that this is equivalent to 0.67. Or, in other words, the penetration factor is 0.67 (67%).

Two relationships between the attenuation coefficient and the penetration factor have been described. One is easier to visualize but does not take into account the effect of the decreasing number of photons on the overall attenuation rate. The other relationship is more precise but requires special tables, or a calculator with exponential functions to evaluate. The two expressions for the penetration factor are compared in Table 1 for a number of different values of μ. It is seen that when μ is relatively small, i.e., 0.1, the value of $1 - \mu$ is quite close to the value of $e^{-\mu}$. However, as the value of μ increases, the difference between the two expressions for penetration factor also increases. When the value of μ is relatively large, the use of $1 - \mu$ will underestimate the penetration.

It should be noticed that the penetration factor is inversely related to

Table 1. Comparison of attenuation coefficient and penetration factor values

Attenuation coefficient (μ)	Penetration factor		
	$e^{-\mu}$	$1 - \mu$	Error (%)
0.1	0.904	0.9	0.5
0.2	0.82	0.8	2.3
0.3	0.74	0.7	5.5
0.4	0.67	0.6	10.5
0.5	0.61	0.5	17.6
0.6	0.55	0.4	27.0

the attenuation coefficient. Factors that cause an increase in the value of the attenuation coefficient will produce a corresponding decrease in x-ray penetration.

Half-value Layer (HVL)

The two basic methods of describing the penetrating ability of an x-ray beam through a given material are compared in Figure 2. The penetration factor, p, specifies penetrating ability in terms of the fraction of photons that penetrate a specified thickness. A second method is to describe the penetrating ability in terms of the thickness of material associated with some specified amount of penetration. The most common penetration value

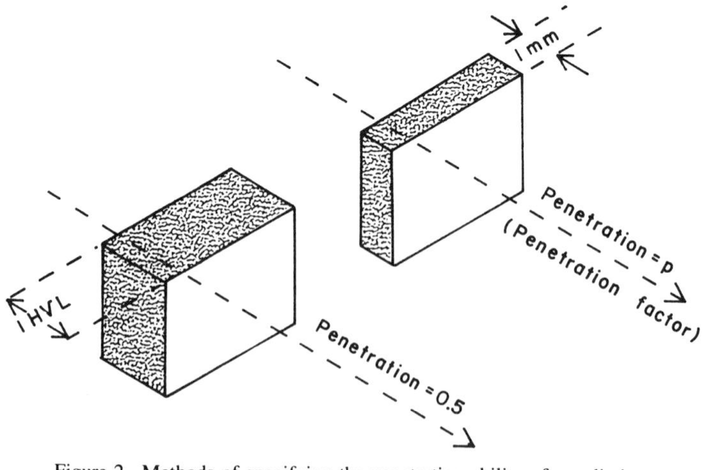

Figure 2. Methods of specifying the penetrating ability of x-radiation.

used is 0.5. Since this represents a penetration of one-half of the photons, the required thickness of material is designated as the half-value layer (HVL). In other words, 1 HVL is the thickness of a given material that will permit a penetration of exactly 0.5 or 50%. Radiation with a high penetrating ability will have a high HVL value because more thickness is required to reduce penetration to 0.5. The relationship between HVL and attenuation coefficient (μ) is given by:

$$\text{HVL} = \frac{0.693}{\mu}$$

This shows that the HVL is inversely proportional to the attenuation coefficient. The number, 0.693, is the exponent value that gives a penetration of 0.5 ($e^{-0.693} = 0.5$).

Any factor that changes the value of the attenuation coefficient will also cause a change in both the penetration factor and HVL. These three quantities are compared in Figure 3 for aluminum. Aluminum has two significant applications in an x-ray system. It is used as a material to filter x-ray beams and also as a reference material for measuring the penetrating ability of x-rays. The value of the attenuation coefficient decreases rather rapidly with increased photon energy and causes the penetrating ability expressed either in terms of the penetration factor, p, or the HVL to increase. This illustrates the increased penetrating ability of higher energy photons.

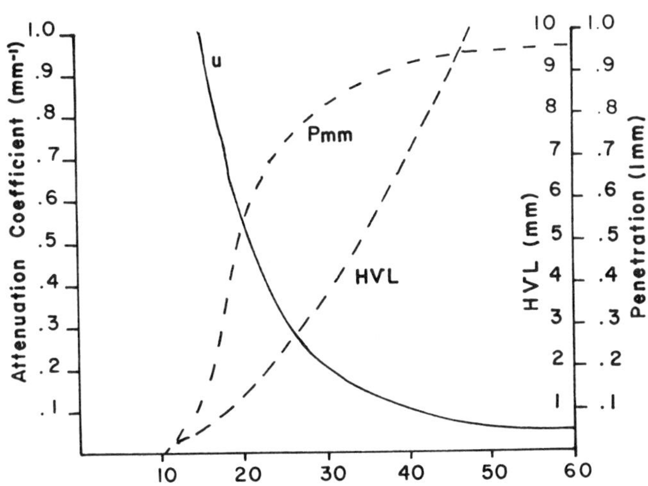

Figure 3. The relationship of attenuation coefficient, HVL, and penetration factor to photon energy. The values shown are for aluminum.

RELATIONSHIP OF PENETRATION TO THICKNESS

The penetration factor describes the fraction of x-ray photons that penetrate a thickness of 1 unit for a particular attenuation coefficient value. The penetration, P, through other thicknesses, x, is related to the penetration factor by:

$$P = p^x$$

The application of this relationship is illustrated in Figure 4. Consider a piece of material that is 7 cm thick. In Figure 4 the material has been sliced into 1-cm pieces, but this does not alter the relationship. Assume that for the photon energies and material being used, the attenuation coefficient has a value of 0.1 and the penetration factor is 0.904 per cm. This means that each centimeter thickness of material will pass 0.904 (90.4%) of the photons impinging upon it. If, in the example, the first centimeter slice is exposed to 100 photons, approximately 90 photons would penetrate. A fraction of these photons, 0.904, would be expected to penetrate the second layer. The penetration through the two layers combined would be 0.904 × 0.904 or 0.817 (rounded to 0.82). The fraction of photons that penetrates the third layer is also 0.904. Of the 100 photons that entered the first layer, only 82 will enter the third layer. The number of photons leaving the third layer would be 82 × 0.904, or approximately 74. The penetration through

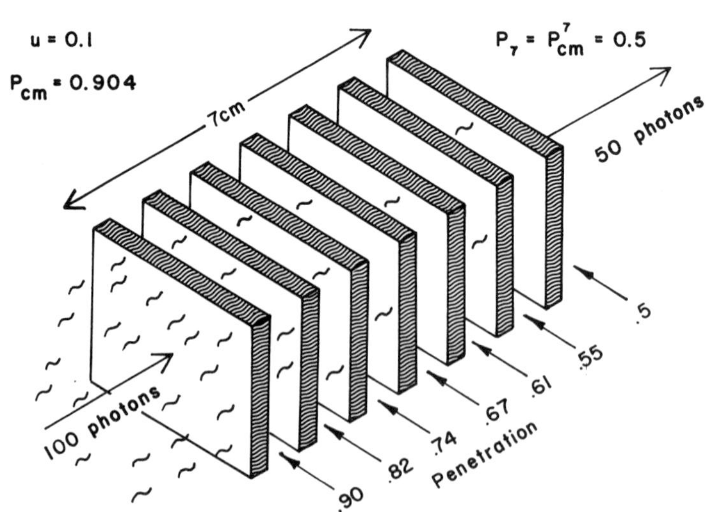

Figure 4. The penetration through various thicknesses.

3 cm of thickness is therefore 0.74. This procedure can be continued to arrive at a general expression for the penetration as follows:

$$1 \text{ cm}, P = p$$

$$2 \text{ cm}, P = p \cdot p = p^2$$

$$3 \text{ cm}, P = p \cdot p \cdot p = p^3$$

$$x \text{ cm}, P = p^x$$

The relationship between penetration and material thickness is shown graphically in Figure 5. The shape of this curve is characteristic of an exponential relationship. It should be noticed that the slope of a curve decreases with material thickness. At any point along the curve, the slope is proportional to the number of photons reaching that point, which is constantly decreasing with thickness. Relating this to the example shown in Figure 4 yields the following. In the first layer, 100 photons enter, 90 photons penetrate, and 10 photons interact with the material and are attenuated. However, in the seventh layer, 55 photons enter, 50 penetrate, and 5 are taken out of the beam by interactions. In the first layer, the approximate rate of attenuation is 10 photons per cm, whereas in the

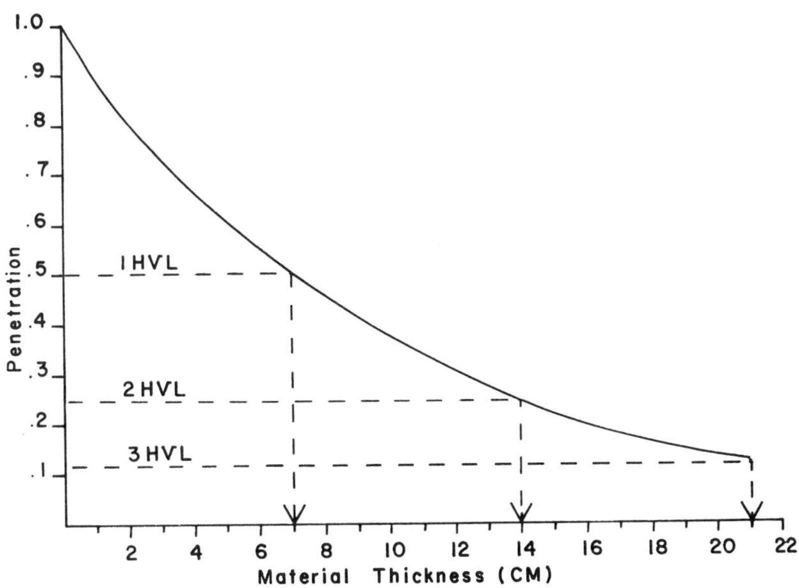

Figure 5. The relationship between penetration and material thickness.

seventh layer the rate is 5 photons per cm. The significant point is that each centimeter of thickness is attenuating the same fraction of photons but not the same number.

Figure 5 illustrates an important aspect of the HVL concept. If the penetration through a thickness of 1 HVL is 0.5 (50%), the penetration through a thickness of 2 HVLs is 0.5 × 0.5 or 25%. Each succeeding layer of material with a thickness of 1 HVL reduces the number of photons by a factor of 0.5. The relationship between penetration and thickness through material that is n half-value layers thick is:

$$P = (0.5)^n$$

An example using this relationship is in determining the penetration through lead shielding. Photons of 60 keV have an HVL in lead of 0.125 mm. The problem is to determine the penetration through a lead shield which is 0.5 mm thick. At this particular photon energy 0.5 mm is 4 HVLs and the penetration would be:

$$n = \frac{\text{thickness}}{\text{HVL}} = \frac{0.5}{0.125} = 4$$

$$P = (0.5)^4 = 0.0625$$

Within a given material, where the atomic number and density are constant, the penetration depends on two factors—photon energy and thickness of the material. This is illustrated in Figure 6. Here the penetration through four different thicknesses of lead is shown for the range of x-ray photon energies normally encountered in diagnostic examinations. The curves break at an energy of 88 keV because of the K edge phenomenon discussed in Chapter IX. Photons with energies of less than 88 keV can interact only with electrons down through the L shell. Above 88 keV, which is the binding energy of the K electrons, more electrons are available for interactions; therefore the penetration is less. For a given thickness, the maximum penetration through lead occurs with photons with energies just below 88 keV. These curves demonstrate the rather dramatic increase of penetration with photon energy. Of special interest is the curve for 0.75 mm of lead thickness which corresponds to the typical lead apron. The penetration ranges from generally negligible values at the lower end of the energy spectrum up to 0.22 (22%) at 88 keV. Because an x-ray beam is made up of a range of photon energies, the effective penetration for the beam will fall somewhere between these two extreme values, depending on the shape of the spectrum. At some points the penetration increases by as much as a factor of 10, when the photon energy is increased by 10 keV or a

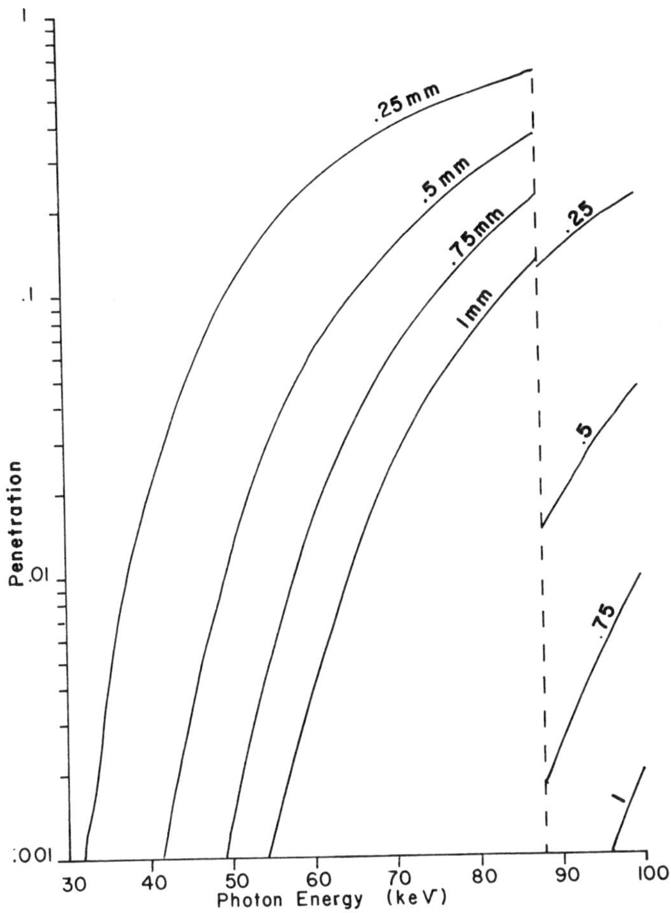

Figure 6. The relationship of penetration to photon energy for various thicknesses of lead.

factor of approximately 1.2. Because of this the photon energy spectrum must be taken into consideration when calculating the thickness of lead necessary to provide a certain amount of shielding.

Figure 7 shows the relationship between penetration of primary radiation and thickness of soft tissue for several different energies. Because a logarithmic or exponential scale is used for penetration the relationship with respect to thickness can be represented by a straight line. Several important factors are illustrated in this graph. As discussed previously the penetration through a given thickness increases with photon energy. Atten-

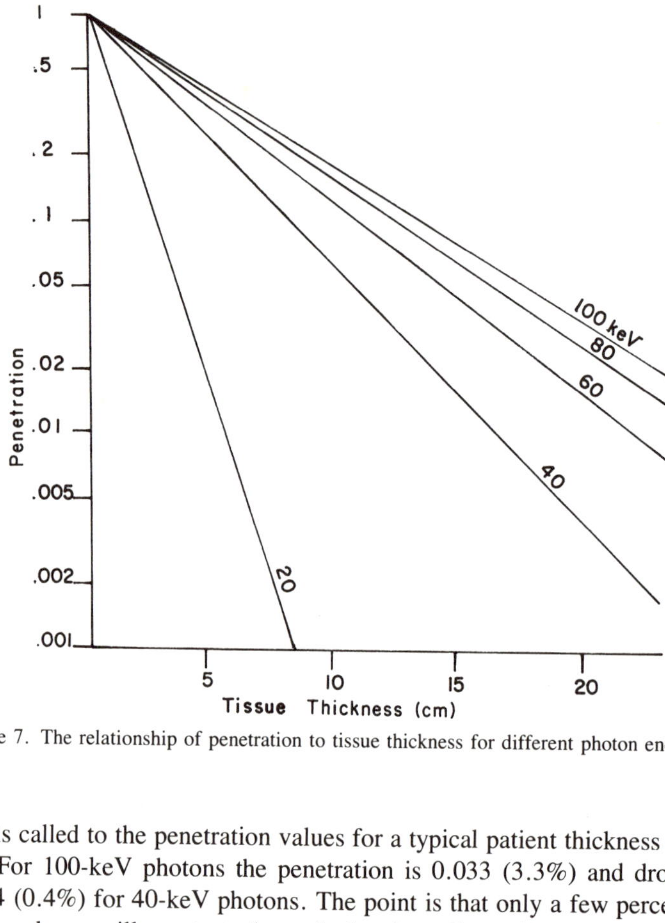

Figure 7. The relationship of penetration to tissue thickness for different photon energies.

tion is called to the penetration values for a typical patient thickness of 20 cm. For 100-keV photons the penetration is 0.033 (3.3%) and drops to 0.004 (0.4%) for 40-keV photons. The point is that only a few percent of an x-ray beam will penetrate the typical patient. Generally speaking, radiation with photon energies below about 40 keV does not have sufficient penetration to significantly contribute to x-ray image formation in the thicker body sections. It should be noticed that the HVL, that is, the tissue thickness which produces 0.5 penetration, is approximately 3.5 to 4.0 cm for the 60 to 100-keV photon energy range.

The relationship between the x-ray penetration, P, of an object and the characteristics of the object and the radiation is summarized in Figure 8. The characteristics of the object material which affect penetration are density, atomic number, and thickness. The penetration (or attenuation) per unit of thickness can be expressed in terms of the attenuation coefficient, penetration factor, or HVL. The values of these factors are functions of object material density and atomic number and the energy of the x-ray

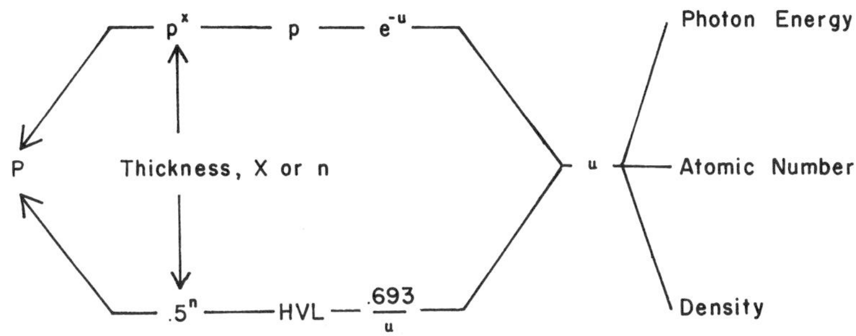

Figure 8. The relationship of penetration to the characteristics of the material and photon energy.

photons. For a given penetration factor, p, or HVL value the total object penetration, P, is exponentially related to object thickness, X.

X-RAY BEAM QUALITY

The general term, quality, refers to an x-ray beam's penetrating ability. It has been shown that, for a given material, the penetrating ability of an x-ray beam depends on the energy of the photons. Up to this point, the discussion has related penetration to specific photon energies, as illustrated in Figures 3 and 6. For x-ray beams which contain a spectrum of photon energies the penetration will be different for each energy. The overall penetration will generally correspond to the penetration of a photon energy located somewhere between the minimum and maximum energies of the spectrum. This energy is designated as the effective energy of the x-ray spectrum. For example, the x-ray spectrum shown in Figure 9, which is produced by a machine operating at a KVP = 70, has a penetrating ability which can be measured relatively easily. If exposure measurements are made before and after the beam passes through a 1-mm thickness of aluminum, the penetration factor will be found to be approximately 0.72. If the HVL is determined, it will be found to have a value of approximately 2.4 mm of aluminum. By referring to the p and HVL curves in Figure 3, it is seen that these values correspond to a photon energy of 24 keV. This spectrum therefore has, with respect to penetrating ability, an effective energy of 24 keV. The effective energy of an x-ray spectrum is the energy of a monoenergetic beam of photons which has the same penetrating ability (p or HVL) as the spectrum of photons.

The effective energy is generally close to 30 or 40% of peak energy, but its exact value depends on the shape of the spectrum. For a given kVp, two factors which can alter the spectrum are the amount of filtration in the beam and the high voltage waveform used to produce the x-rays.

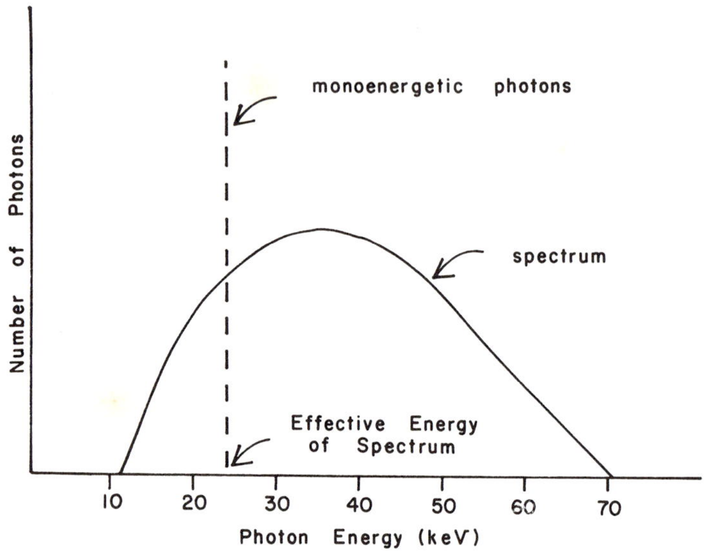

Figure 9. The effective energy of an x-ray spectrum.

Filtration

As an x-ray beam made up of different photon energies passes through many materials, photons of certain energies will penetrate better than others. This selective attenuation of photons, according to their energy, is referred to as filtration. Figure 10 shows the penetration through two different materials of special interest, a 1-cm thickness of muscle and a 1-mm thickness of aluminum. The penetration through the muscle, or soft tissue, will be considered first. For photons with energies less than 10 keV, there is virtually no penetration. All of the photons are attenuated by the tissue. The low penetration in tissue by photons of this energy is due to the high value for the attenuation coefficient. It should be recalled that the high attenuation coefficient value is the result of photoelectric interactions which are highly probable at this energy, as shown in Figure 9 of Chapter IX. In the range of 10 to 25 keV there is a rapid increase in penetration with energy. As photon energy is increased up to about 40 keV, there is an additional increase in penetration, but it is much more gradual. Of special interest is the very low penetrating ability of x-ray photons with energies below approximately 20 keV. At this energy, the penetration through 1 cm of tissue is 0.45 and the penetration through 15 cm of tissue is:

$$P = (0.45)^{15} = 0.0000063$$

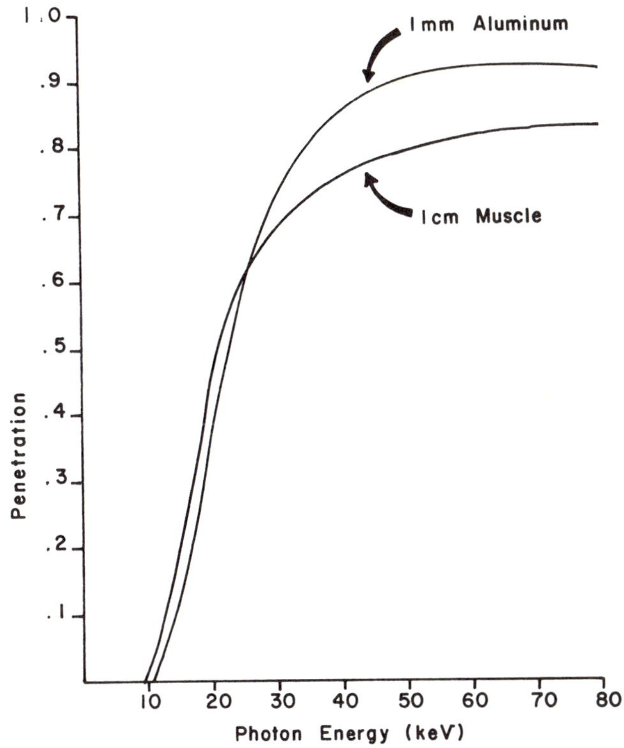

Figure 10. The penetration of soft tissue and aluminum for various photon energies.

On the other hand, the penetration through 15 cm of tissue for photons with an energy of 50 keV is:

$$P = (0.8)^{15} = 0.035$$

A significant portion (3.5%) of photons with an energy near 50 keV will penetrate a 15-cm-thick patient whereas vitrually no photons with energies of 20 keV or less will make it through. This means that low energy photons in an x-ray spectrum do not contribute to image formation; they just contribute to patient exposure. In other words, the tissue of the body selectively filters out the low energy photons.

An obvious solution is to place some material in the x-ray beam, before it enters the patient, to filter out the low energy photons. In diagnostic x-ray equipment, aluminum is normally used for this purpose. Figure 10 also shows the penetration through a 1-mm thickness of aluminum. Typically, most x-ray machines will contain the equivalent of several millimeters of aluminum filtration. This might not always be in the form of actual aluminum because several objects contribute to x-ray beam filtration. These are the x-ray tube window, the x-ray beam collimator mirror, and the table top in fluoroscopic equipment. The total amount of filtration in a given x-ray machine is generlaly specified in terms of an equivalent aluminum thickness.

The addition of filtration significantly alters the shape of the x-ray spectrum, as shown in Figure 11. Since filtration selectively absorbs the lower energy photons, it produces a shift in the effective energy of an x-ray beam. Figure 11 compares an unfiltered spectrum to spectra which have passed through 1-mm and 3-mm aluminum filters. It is apparent that increasing the filtration from 1 to 3 mm of aluminum produces a noticeable decrease in the number of x-ray photons. It should be observed, however,

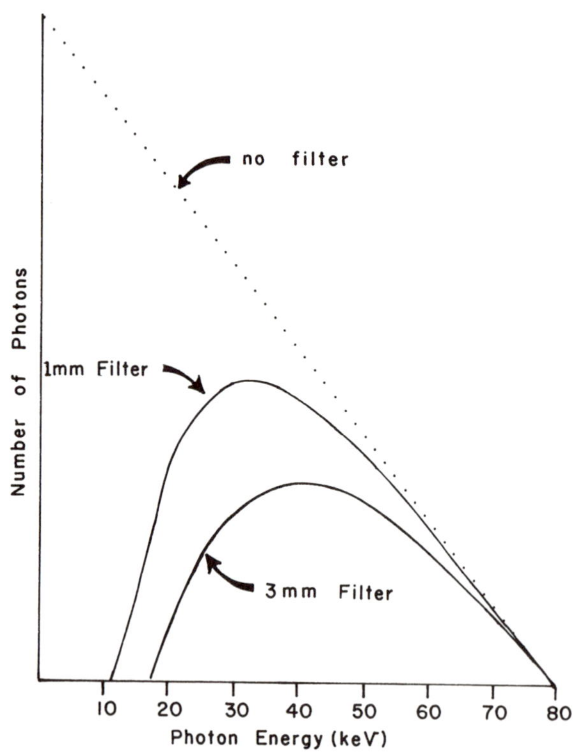

Figure 11. X-ray spectra after filtration.

that most of this decrease is for photons with energies less than approximately 40 keV. It should be recalled that these are the photons which have a low probability of penetrating a typical patient and contributing to image formation. They do, however, contribute to patient exposure.

Adding filtration increases the penetration (p or HVL) of an x-ray beam by removing the low energy photons.

HVL Determinations

Good operating practice and various regulations require adequate amounts of filtration in the x-ray beam. It is desirable to have a method which can be used periodically to confirm the amount of filtration. Direct measurement is not always practical because it would require disassembly of the equipment and also because a significant portion of the filtration is provided by the x-ray tube window, collimator mirror, and other elements whose thickness cannot readily be measured. The accepted method for determining whether an x-ray machine contains adequate filtration is to measure the HVL of the beam when operating at a specified KVP. For a specific KVP and waveform, the penetration (HVL) will be primarily a function of the amount of filtration.

The general procedure for determining the HVL value is illustrated in Figure 12. Two items are required. One is an instrument for measuring radiation exposure, and the second is a set of aluminum absorbers. Typically, the set will include thicknesses of both 0.5 and 1 mm.

The exposure meter is positioned as shown and a reading is made. Aluminum absorbers are then placed in the beam, typically in 0.5- or 1-mm increments, and an exposure reading is made. Dividing each exposure reading by the exposure with no absorber gives the penetration for each thickness of absorber.

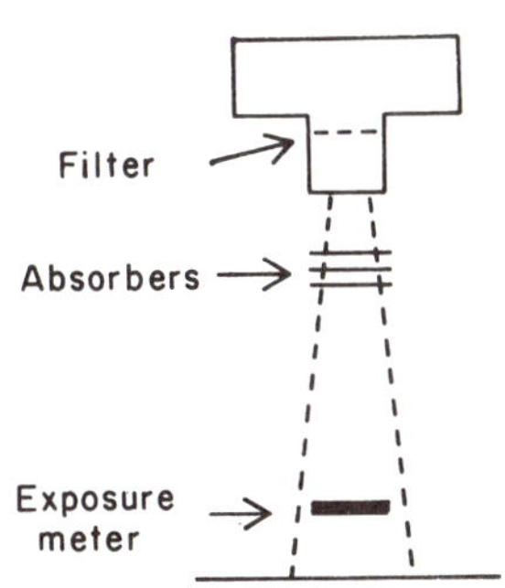

Figure 12. The procedure for determining the HVL of an x-ray beam.

Table 2. Recommended minimum penetration (HVL) for various KVP values

KVP	Minimum penetration (HVL) for aluminum, mm
30	0.3
50	1.2
70	1.5
90	2.5
110	3.0

The penetration values are then plotted as a function of aluminum absorber thickness. The absorber thickness corresponding to a penetration value of 0.5 is the HVL. This value is referred to as the first HVL. The so-called second HVL value is the additional thickness which is required to reduce the penetration to 0.25. Generally, it will be larger than the first value. This is because the first aluminum absorbers added to the beam act as a filter and produce an increase in the equivalent energy and corresponding HVL value. In actual practice, it is usually more desirable to plot the penetration values on a logarithmic scale (by using semilogarithmic graph paper) so that the resulting graph is essentially a straight line.

The HVL values obtained are then used to judge the adequacy of the filtration. Regulations which specify filtration requirements generally state a minimum acceptable HVL value. Typical values are shown in Table 2. It is assumed that if an x-ray beam has the minimum specified HVL value at a stated KVP, the filtration is adequate.

KVP AND PENETRATION

In most x-ray examinations the beam penetration can be controlled to some extent by varying the KVP. It was shown in Figure 7 that the penetration of a body section can be significantly increased by increasing photon energy. It should be noted that the relationships illustrated in Figure 7 are for monoenergetic photons. In the case of an x-ray beam with a spectrum of photon energies this would correspond to the effective energy of the beam. For example, an x-ray machine operating at 100 kV peak energy will have an effective energy of approximately 35 to 40 keV. This means it would have approximately the same penetrating quality as a beam of monoenergetic x-ray photons with that energy.

KVP Measurement

Since there is a relationship between KVP and penetration, the KVP of a machine can be determined indirectly by measuring penetration. This normally is done by using a so-called Adrian-Crooks type cassette. The basic components of this type of cassette are shown in Figure 13. The cassette contains a copper step wedge, an intensifying screen, and a light absorber. The use of this cassette is based on the concept that the thickness of copper required to yield a given penetration value, such as 0.3, is, in general, related to the KVP. To determine the KVP, a film is placed in the cassette and exposed to the x-ray beam. A portion of the x-ray beam exposes the intensifying screen in an area not covered by the step wedge. The light from this area passes through an absorber before reaching the film and reducing an exposure. The penetration through the light absorber remains constant and does not change with KVP. This area of the film, when processed, produces a reference density which corresponds to a known penetration value. Other areas of the film are exposed through the various copper thickness. At a given KVP value, the penetration will depend on copper thickness. The film is then examined to determine which copper thickness, or step, produced the same penetration as the light absorber reference. Calibration data are then used to convert the copper thickness, or step number, into a KVP value. As KVP is increased, the thicker copper steps are required to produce a penetration value equivalent to the reference.

In addition to KVP, the two factors which affect penetration are filtration and waveform. In order to prevent variation in filtration from machine to machine from affecting the step wedge penetration, an additional filter is contained in the cassette. The x-ray beam passes through the filter before reaching the step wedge. The added filter is relatively thick in comparison to the x-ray machine filters, and generally overrides their effect. In other words, since the beam is strongly filtered by the cassette, variations in machine filters have very little effect on the beam which reaches the step wedge. Variation in step wedge penetration produced by waveform dif-

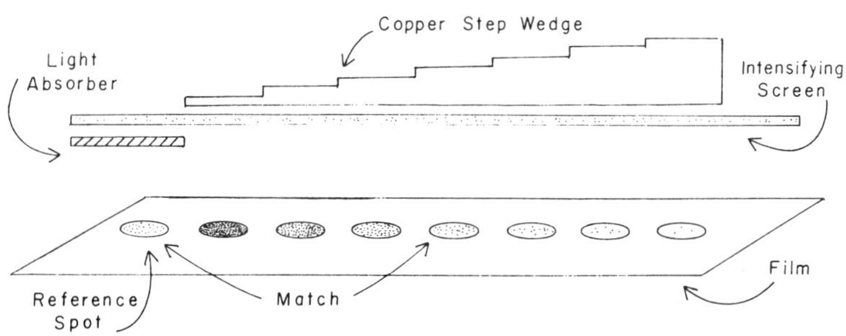

Figure 13. The components of a cassette used to measure x-ray penetration for the purpose of determining KVP.

ferences is compensated for by using different calibration factors for the different waveforms.

PENETRATION WITH SCATTER

Up to this point, it has been considered that the x-ray photons which penetrate an object are those which have escaped both photoelectric and Compton interactions. In situations where there is a significant amount of Compton interactions, it is necessary to modify this concept. This is because some of the radiation which is removed from the primary beam by Compton interactions will be scattered in the forward direction and create the appearance of increased penetration. A prime example of this is an x-ray beam passing through the larger portions of the human body, as illustrated in Figure 14; when significant forward scattered radiation is combining with the penetrated portion of the primary beam, the effective penetration, P_e, is given by:

$$P_e = P \cdot S$$

where S is the scatter factor. Its value ranges from 1 (no scatter) to approximately 6 for conditions encountered in some diagnostic examinations. Several factors contribute to the amount of radiation which is scattered in the forward direction and hence to the value of S.

One of the most significant factors is the x-ray beam area or field size. Since the source of the scattered radiation is the volume of the patient within the primary x-ray beam, the source size is proportional to beam

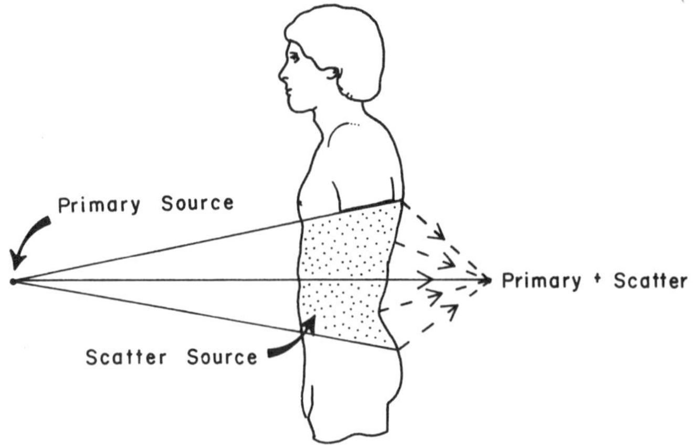

Figure 14. Scattered radiation adds to the primary radiation which penetrates an object.

area. Within limits, the value of S increases from a value of 1 more or less in proportion to field size. Another important factor is body section thickness, which affects the size of the scattered radiation source.

A third significant factor is KVP. As the KVP is increased over the diagnostic range, several changes occur. A greater proportion of the photons which interact with the body are involved in Compton interactions. Also, a greater proportion of the photons created in Compton interactions scatters in the forward direction. Perhaps the most significant factor is that the scattered radiation produced at the higher KVP values is more penetrating. A larger proportion of it will leave the body before being absorbed. When the scattered radiation is more penetrating, there is a larger effective source within the patient. At low KVP values, most of the scattered radiation created near the entrance surface of the x-ray beam will not penetrate the body. However, at higher KVP values, this area makes more of a contribution to the radiation passing through the body.

Chapter XI

Formation of Image Contrast

The typical x-ray image is a rather complex pattern made up of individual images of many different objects within the human body. In a discussion of image formation, it is easier to begin with a simplified situation in which a single object is being imaged. Actually, the typical x-ray image is formed by superimposing the images of the many individual objects. The objects include bones, calcifications, contrast media-filled vessels and cavities, and pockets of air. The major difficulty in producing a high quality image of these various objects is that they are embedded within a larger volume of material, the human body.

An x-ray image differs from a typical photograph of an object in two major respects. First, x-radiation is used rather than light to transfer the image from the object to the receptor. Second, the typical photograph is an image of the light reflected by an object, whereas a radiograph is an image of the x-ray penetration of an object. In this respect, an x-ray image is related to the total object, not just its front surface.

One of the most significant characteristics of an image is contrast. Figure 1 is a radiograph of nine different circular objects. The only difference among the various images is contrast. In developing a concept of image contrast, it is helpful to recognize that the image of a given object is always superimposed on some background. It is generally the appearance of an object's image with respect to the surrounding background that is known as contrast. In Figure 1 the object in the upper left corner has maximum contrast with respect to the background. The contrast gradually decreases and is a minimum for the object in the lower right corner. The contrast in an image on film is generally referred to as radiographic contrast. The actual value of the radiographic contrast of the image of an object is defined as the difference in film density between the object area and the background area. Film density will be defined more precisely in a later

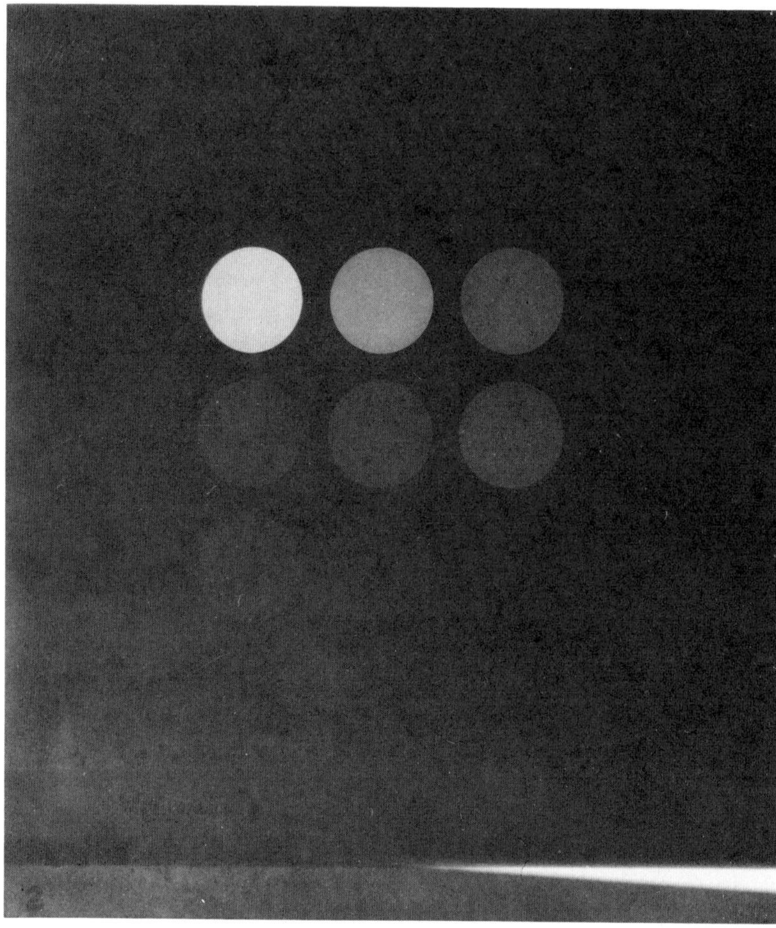

Figure 1. Radiograph of objects with different amounts of contrast.

chapter, but for the present it is necessary only to recognize that the density of some point on a film simply refers to the degree of darkening. It will also be shown later that the density of film can be measured and assigned values which generally range from slightly above 0 to approximately 3 density units. For example, the background area in Figure 1 has a density value of 1.0 and the upper left object area has a density of 0.6. Therefore, the radiographic contrast of this particular object is 0.4. The density of the other objects is progressively less and approaches the density of the background area. As the density of an object area approaches the density of the background area, the contrast decreases and finally a point is reached at which the image of the object is no longer visible. It is generally considered that an object area should differ from background density, that is, that it should have a contrast of at least 0.03 in order to be readily visible.

Since the formation of an x-ray image is a multistep process, it is necessary to consider contrast at several points within the x-ray system. As shown in Figure 2, the contrast which ultimately appears on the film, that is, the radiographic contrast, depends on a number of other factors. Perhaps the most significant factor is the amount of contrast within the x-ray beam when it reaches the receptor. This is known as subject contrast. Another important factor is the contrast characteristics of the film being used. The film, in effect, converts subject contrast to radiographic contrast. This conversion is not the same for all films. Some film and exposure conditions can increase contrast, whereas some may actually reduce contrast. The contrast transfer characteristics of a film depend on 1) the inherent characteristics of the film, 2) film processing, 3) film exposure level. The contrast characteristics of film will be discussed in depth in Chapter XIV.

For large objects, such as those shown in Figure 1, radiographic contrast is determined only by the amount of subject contrast and the characteristics of the film. However, for small objects, another factor may be present which will tend to reduce radiographic contrast. This additional factor is blur, which will be discussed in Chapter XV.

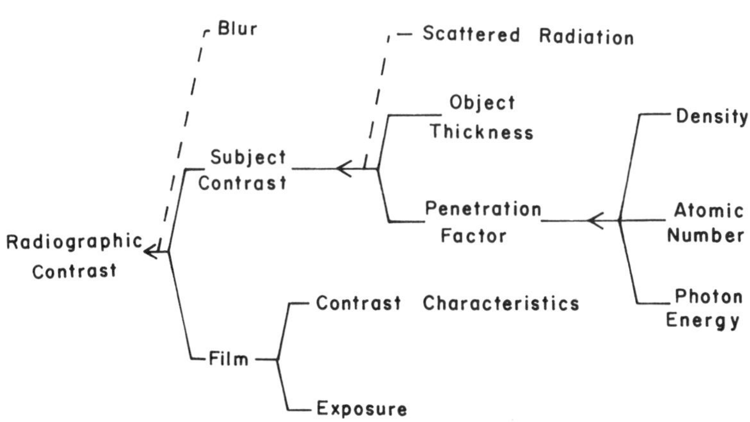

Figure 2. The factors which determine radiographic contrast.

SUBJECT CONTRAST

The concept of subject contrast is illustrated in Figure 3. Here, an x-ray image of a simple object is being formed. The x-ray beam is partially attenuated as it passes through the object, causing a shadow image to be formed on the receptor surface. Subject contrast describes the "strength" of the x-ray shadow. This is determined by the quality of x-ray exposure to the receptor in the object area, that is, in the shadow of the object. More specifically, it is the relationship between the exposure to the background and the object area which determines the amount of subject contrast. The relationship between subject contrast, C_s, and exposure is given by:

$$C_s = \left(\frac{X_{bg} - X_{oa}}{X_{bg}}\right) \cdot 100$$

where X_{oa} is the exposure to the object area of the receptor and X_{bg} is the exposure to the background area surrounding the object. This relationship between subject contrast and receptor exposure is shown by means of an exposure profile in Figure 3. For the purpose of describing contrast, the background area exposure is designated as 100%. The object area exposure is then expressed as a percentage of the background. The difference between the two is the amount of subject contrast. For example, if the object completely attenuates the x-ray beam so that there is no exposure to the

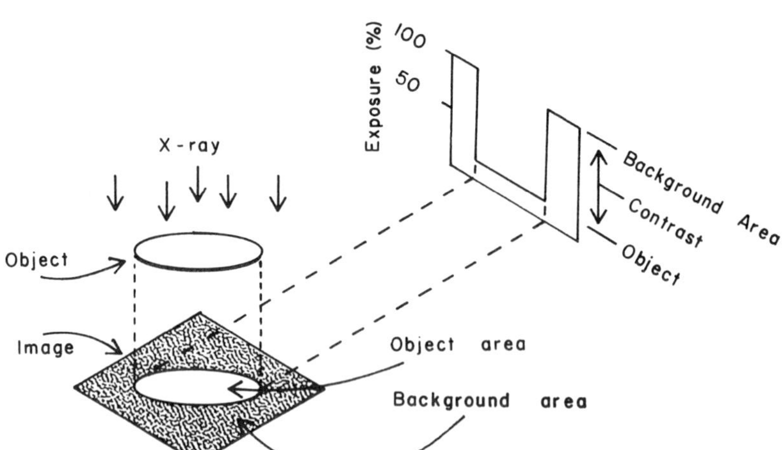

Figure 3. The relationship of subject contrast to exposure.

object area, the subject contrast will be 100%. However, if some x-ray exposure reaches the object area, either by penetrating the object or from scattered radiation, the subject contrast will be reduced. The exposure profile in Figure 3 indicates that the exposure in the object area, that is, the shadow of the object, is approximately 20% of the background area exposure. This will yield a subject contrast of 80%.

In most x-ray examinations the subject contrast for objects within the body is less than 100%. As indicated in Figure 2, there are two major factors which determine the amount of subject contrast. One is exposure arising from radiation which penetrates the object; the second is exposure which reaches the object area by scattering around the object because of Compton interactions. Reduction of contrast by scattered radiation will be discussed in the next chapter.

OBJECT PENETRATION AND CONTRAST

The penetration of x-radiation through an object reduces subject contrast. The relationship between subject contrast and object penetration is given by:

$$C_s = (1 - P_{ot}) \cdot 100$$

where a P_{ot} is the relative penetration through the object. Relative penetration means the penetration value of the object divided by the penetration value of an equal thickness of the tissue which surrounds the object. In many examinations, especially where the object is of relatively high contrast, the penetration through an equal thickness of surrounding tissue has a value of approximately 1, so that the relative object penetration is approximately equal to the actual object penetration. For example, if an object such as a contrast media-filled blood vessel has a penetration value of 0.4, the subject contrast would be 60%. The significant point is that, as the relative penetration through the object increases, the contrast is reduced.

It was shown previously that the penetration of an object, P, is related to the penetration factor of the object material, p, and the object thickness, x, by:

$$P = p^x$$

In the case of relative object penetration, P_{ot}, the relationship becomes:

$$P_{ot} = \left(\frac{p_o}{p_t}\right)^x$$

where p_o is the penetration factor for the object material and p_t is the penetration factor for the adjacent tissue. By substituting this expression for relative object penetration into the relationship given above for subject contrast, the following equation is obtained.

$$C_s = \left[1 - \left(\frac{p_o}{p_t}\right)^x\right] \cdot 100$$

Inspection of this relationship reveals a rather obvious fact. That is, an object can be imaged only if its penetration factor is different from that of the surrounding tissue. Actually, it is the ratio of the penetration factors, rather than the difference, which determines the amount of contrast. This ratio, that is, the relative penetration factor of the object with respect to that of the surrounding tissue, is then enhanced by the object thickness to yield a certain amount of subject contrast. It should be recalled that two different materials will have different penetration factors if they differ either in terms of density or atomic number. As illustrated in Figure 2, the three factors which contribute to the contrast of an object are: 1) object thickness; 2) relative atomic number; 3) density relative to surrounding tissue. The relationship of each of these to subject contrast will now be considered.

Object Thickness

For an object with a given relative penetration factor, subject contrast varies exponentially with object thickness. This makes the relationship between subject contrast and object thickness somewhat difficult to visualize, other than the fact that increasing object thickness does indeed increase subject contrast. A more useful relationship for radiologists is the one between radiographic contrast, C_r, and object thickness, x, which is given by:

$$C_r = 3.32 \cdot G \cdot x \cdot (-\log p_{ot})$$

In this relationship, G is the contrast factor of the film and will generally have a value ranging from 0 to approximately 1 for most x-ray films. The reader should not be unduly concerned over the presence of a logarithmic term in this relationship. For each value of the relative penetration factor, p_{ot}, there is a corresponding value of log p_{ot} which can be obtained from appropriate tables, such as in Appendix I. For the present, the concern is with the relationship between radiographic contrast and object thickness. The above relationship shows that, for specific values of object penetration and film contrast factor, the radiographic contrast is proportional to object thickness. Since radiographic contrast is defined as the difference in film density between an object area and the surrounding background, the above relationship points up another rather significant factor. That is, within certain limits, the film density of an object's image is directly related to its thickness. Since the density of conventional radiographic film increases with film exposure, the density in an object area will decrease with increased object thickness. The most significant limitation of this relationship is that the film contrast factor is not constant over the full film density range. Also, the relative object penetration factor often changes with x-ray photon energy, or KVP.

Another important point to be considered is this: what is the minimum object thickness which will produce a visible image? This is generally referred to as depth resolution in x-ray examinations. It is generally considered that an image of an object must have a radiographic contrast of at least 0.03 in order to be visible on film. If the previous relationship between radiographic contrast and object thickness is rearranged and the minimum value of visible radiographic contrast (0.03) is substituted, the following expression for minimum visible object thickness, x_{min}, is obtained.

$$x_{min} = \frac{0.009}{G(-\log p_{ot})}$$

Here it is seen that the depth resolution, or minimum visible thickness, is related only to the contrast factor of the film and the relative penetration of the object. This relationship does not take into account the effects of scattered radiation. If significant scatter is present, it will have the same effect as increased penetration and will require a greater thickness for visibility. The relationship between depth resolution and penetration factor is not obvious from the above equation. The value of the relative penetration factor, p_{ot}, is always a fraction. The logarithm of a fraction is a negative number which becomes larger as the number, in this case the penetration factor, becomes smaller. Therefore, as p is increased, the term $(-\log p)$ becomes smaller and the minimum thickness for visibility increases. In other words, for a given film contrast factor, as the object penetration factor is increased, by increasing KVP, for instance, the object must be thicker to be detectable on a film.

It should be mentioned, at this point, that depth resolution is not the only factor which can affect the visibility of an object. If the object is relatively small, image blur becomes a significant factor in determining whether an object can be imaged. Also, the presence of image noise can affect visibility. Both of these factors and their relationship to visibility will be discussed in later chapters.

The specific value of the relative penetration factor depends on the relative density and chemical composition (effective atomic number) of the object and the photon energy spectrum. An extremely wide range of pene-

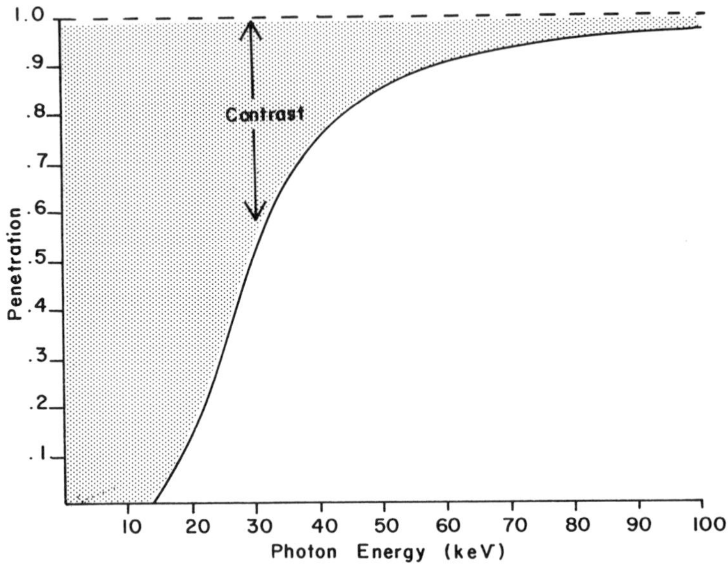

Figure 4. The relationship of calcium penetration and contrast to photon energy. The penetration values are for a 1 mm thickness of calcium.

tration factors is encountered. Object materials which have relatively high densities, or atomic numbers, will generally have relatively low penetration factors and, therefore, very thin objects can be imaged.

A very significant factor is the variation of the penetration factor with photon energy. This is usually most significant for materials such as calcium, bone, and the various contrast media agents (iodine and barium). Figure 4 shows the change in the penetration factor of calcium over the photon energy range normally encountered in x-ray examinations. When using an x-ray beam made up of relatively low energy photons (low KVP), the penetration factor of calcium has a very low value and, therefore, thin calcified objects can be imaged. As the KVP is increased, penetration increases and objects must be thicker in order to produce a visible image. Another important point concerning the imaging of calcified objects is also illustrated in Figure 4. For a 1-mm thick object, the object penetration, P_{ot}, and the penetration factor, p_{ot}, have the same value. By applying the relationships discussed previously, it can be seen that the subject contrast of an object is proportional to $(1 - P_{ot})$. This quantity is illustrated by the arrow in Figure 5. With this in mind, it is easy to see the effect on contrast

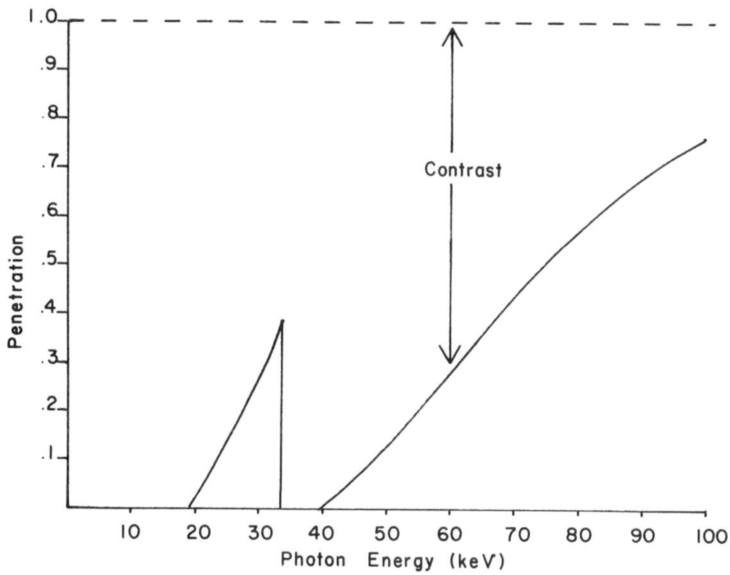

Figure 5. The relationship of iodine penetration and contrast to photon energy. The values shown are for a 1 mm thickness of iodine containing contrast medium.

produced by changing the photon energy spectrum. When imaging calcified objects, maximum subject contrast is obtained by using the lowest possible KVP.

A different situation exists when the object being imaged, such as a blood vessel, is filled with an iodine contrast medium. Because of its relatively high atomic number, the K edge occurs at a photon energy of approximately 33 keV. This produces a large change in penetration, as shown in Figure 5. Photons with energies below this value have an increased chance of penetrating because they cannot interact with the K shell electrons. Except for extremely low energy photons which are generally not present in the typical x-ray beam, maximum contrast is produced by using a monoenergetic beam with an energy of approximately 34 keV. As such a source of x-rays is not available in a form which can be used clinically, the conventional broad x-ray spectrum must be used. The conventional spectrum which will produce maximum contrast is generated by operating the x-ray equipment at a KVP of approximately 60. An increase in KVP above this value will generally increase penetration through the iodine medium and reduce contrast.

CONTRAST RANGE

Up to this point the concept of contrast has been discussed with respect to a single object embedded in a mass of tissue. It was generally assumed that the object penetration was less than that of an equivalent thickness of the surrounding tissue. Most x-ray images cannot be completely described by this simplified model because the total image is made up of many individual objects, some of which have greater penetration than the surrounding tissue. The only difficulty with objects such as bubbles of gas or air which have a higher penetration than the surrounding tissue is a mathematical one. In order to obtain the correct expression for the percentage of subject contrast of such objects in the relationship described earlier it is necessary to interchange the object and background tissue penetration values.

An x-ray image of the chest is an excellent example of a situation in which there is a considerable difference in the penetration of the various areas.

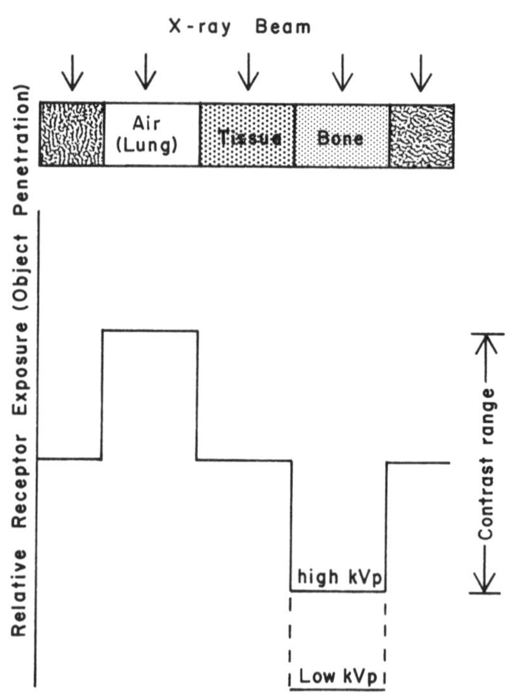

Figure 6. The relationship of subject contrast range to receptor exposure.

The penetration of the lungs is relatively high compared to the mediastinum or bony areas. In a situation such as this the total subject contrast range can have a significant effect on overall image quality. The concept of subject contrast range is illustrated in Figure 6. This illustration shows a much simplified chest area containing lungs, bones, and muscular tissue. Receptor exposure is proportional to the penetration of each area. The relatively high penetration of the lung areas results from the presence of air. The subject contrast range is determined by the minimum and maximum penetration values of the body section. In the case of a chest image the minimum penetration will generally be through the spine and mediastinum and the maximum penetration will be through the lung area. The subject contrast range, R_c, is related to the penetration values by:

$$R_c = \frac{P_{max}}{P_{min}}$$

One of the most significant aspects of contrast range is that if it is too large it might exceed the latitude of the film being used. Film latitude is discussed in Chapter XIV.

For a given body section, such as the chest, the contrast range is determined by the photon energy spectrum. Figure 7 shows the penetration of an arbitrary thickness of air and bone relative to the penetration of soft

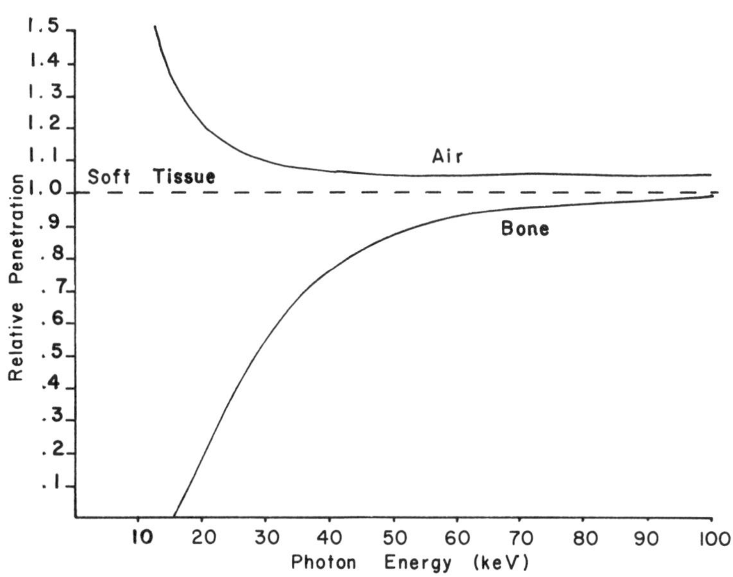

Figure 7. The relationship of relative penetration of several materials to photon energy.

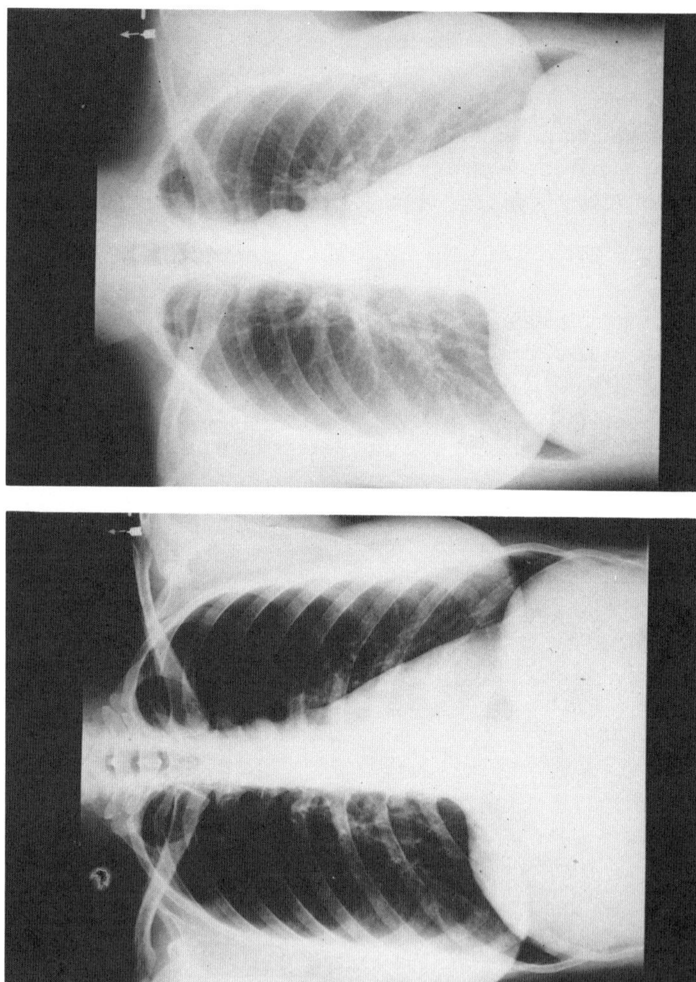

Figure 8. Radiography illustrating a difference in subject contrast range. The film on the left was made at a KVP of 60, that on the right was made at a KVP of 140.

tissue. The reader is cautioned not to misinterpret this illustration. It might appear that the penetration of air decreases with increased photon energy. This is not what happens. Actually the penetration of soft tissue increases with increased photon energy more than the penetration of air does. In other words, it is the penetration of air relative to soft tissue which decreases with increased photon energy. Changes in relative penetration with photon energy occur because of differences in atomic number. The difference in the atomic number of air and soft tissue is quite small. Most of the change in relative penetration is limited to the lower photon energies. Because the atomic number of bone is considerably different from that of soft tissue, a change in relative penetration occurs over a much larger energy range. It should be noticed that in this example changing photon energy from approximately 40 to 200 keV produces relatively little change in air-soft tissue contrast but produces a significant change in bone-soft tissue contrast.

Since KVP can be used to control the photon energy spectrum from an x-ray machine it can be used to control bone penetration and contrast. As indicated in Figure 7, increasing the KVP reduces the subject contrast range primarily by increasing the penetration of bone relative to soft tissue. Figure 8 shows two chest radiographs in which there is a significant difference in contrast range because of different KVP values used.

In x-ray examinations maximum subject contrast is not necessarily always desirable. This is especially true if the total contrast range exceeds the useful latitude of the film.

Chapter XII

Scattered Radiation and Contrast

Subject contrast was previously defined as the exposure to the object area on a film expressed as a percentage of the exposure to the surrounding background. Maximum contrast, i.e., 100%, is obtained when the object area receives no exposure with respect to the background. The previous chapter discussed the reduction of subject contrast because of x-ray penetration through the object being images. This chapter discusses the further reduction of contrast by scattered radiation.

CONTRAST REDUCTION

The basic concept of contrast reduction by scattered radiation is illustrated in Figure 1. For simplicity, it is assumed that the object is not penetrated and, if it were not for scattered radiation, would produce 100% subject contrast. Also, the object in Figure 1 is assumed to be embedded in a larger mass of material, such as the human body, which is producing the scattered radiation. The exposure to the background area of the receptor, or film, is produced by radiation which penetrates the body adjacent to the object plus the scattered radiation. For a given x-ray machine setting, the background area exposure is proportional to PS, the product of the penetration through the patient and the scatter factor. For the same exposure conditions, the exposure to the object area is proportional to P(S − 1). By substituting these expressions for relative background and object area exposure in the previously developed relationship for contrast, it can be shown that the contrast is directly related to the value of the scatter factor,

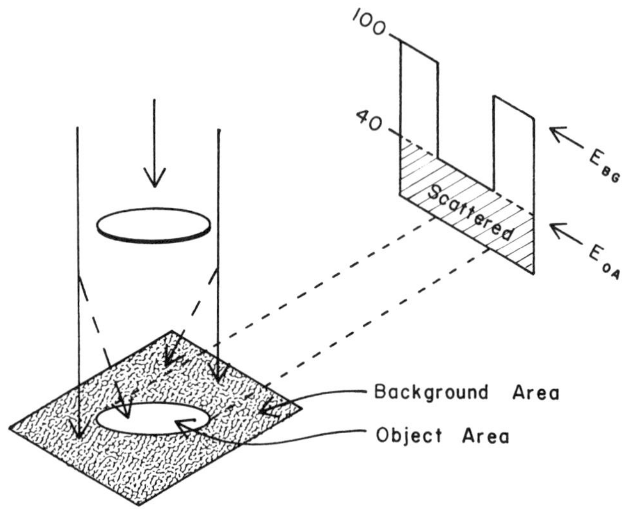

Figure 1. The reduction of contrast by scattered radiation.

as follows:

$$C_s(\%) = \left[1 - \frac{P(S - 1)}{PS}\right] \cdot 100$$

or,

$$C_s(\%) = \frac{100}{S}$$

This relationship shows that, as the proportion of scattered radiation in the x-ray beam increases, contrast will be proportionally decreased. For example, if the scatter factor has a value of 4, the contrast between the object and background areas will be reduced to 25%. Or, in other words, the object area exposure is 75% of the exposure reaching the surrounding background. The contrast can also be determined as follows. The ratio of scattered to primary radiation is always S − 1. For a scatter factor value of 4, the scatter-primary ratio will be 3. The background area exposure would, therefore, be made up of 1 unit of primary and 3 units of scattered radiation. The object area would receive only the 3 units of scattered radiation. This yields an object area exposure of 75% of background and a contrast of 25%.

With respect to image contrast, the scatter factor, S, is also referred to as the contrast reduction factor. For example, if the scatter (contrast reduc-

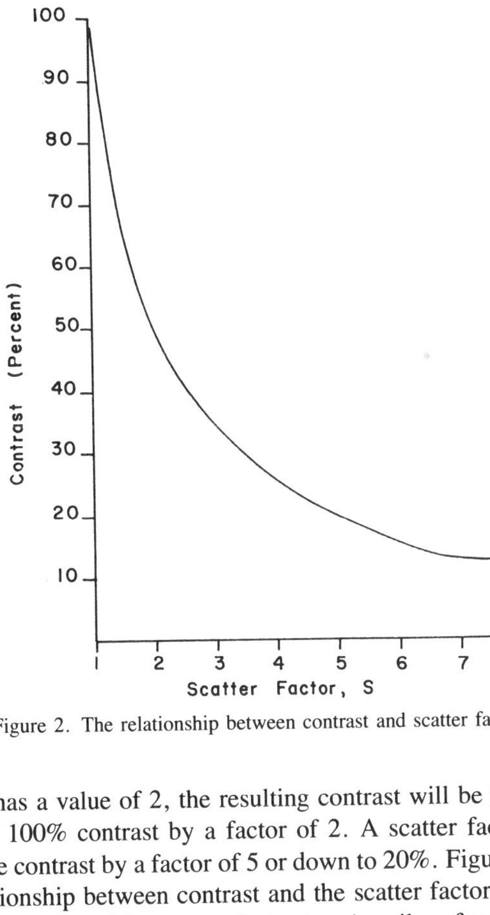

Figure 2. The relationship between contrast and scatter factor.

tion) factor has a value of 2, the resulting contrast will be 50%. This is a reduction of 100% contrast by a factor of 2. A scatter factor value of 5 would reduce contrast by a factor of 5 or down to 20%. Figure 2 shows this general relationship between contrast and the scatter factor. It was shown earlier that the value of the scatter factor is primarily a function of patient thickness, field size, and kVp. In examinations of relatively thick body sections, contrast reduction factors of 5 or 6 are not uncommon.

GRIDS

In most examinations the most effective method of removing a portion of the scattered radiation is to use a grid. The grid is placed between the patient's body and the receptor, as shown in Figure 3. It is constructed of alternate strips of an x-ray absorbing material, such as lead, and a relatively nonabsorbing interspace material, such as fiber or aluminum. Under normal operating conditions the grid strips are aligned with the direction of

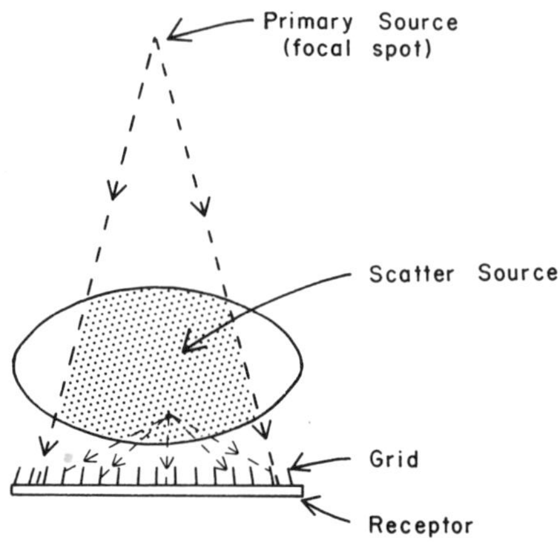

Figure 3. The use of a grid to reduce the amount of scattered radiation reaching the receptor.

the primary x-ray beam. Most grids have the interspaces angled so that they are aligned with a specific point in space. These are designated as focused grids. The focal point of the grid should coincide with the focal spot of the x-ray tube which is the source of the primary radiation. An unfocused grid is one in which the interspaces and strips are parallel to each other and not aligned with a single point in space. Much of the primary radiation passes through the interspaces without encountering the lead strips. Scattered radiation, on the other hand, leaves the patient's body in a direction which is different from that of the primary beam. Since the scattered radiation is not generally lined up with the grid strips, a large portion of this will be absorbed by the grid. The ideal grid would absorb all scattered radiation and allow all primary x-rays to penetrate the receptor. Unfortunately, there is no such thing as an ideal grid, because all such devices absorb some of the primary radiation and allow a portion of the scattered radiation to pass through.

The penetration characteristics of a grid to scattered radiation are largely determined by the dimensions of the lead strips and the interspaces. The significant dimensions are illustrated in Figure 4. The height of the strips, h, is the thickness of the grid. This is typically in the range of 2 to 5 mm. Another significant dimension is the width of the interspace, D. This dimension will vary with grid design, but will generally range from 0.25 to 0.4 mm. With respect to grid performance, the important parameter is the ratio of these two dimensions and is designated as the grid ratio, r. Most grids used in x-ray examinations will have grid ratios ranging from 5:1 up

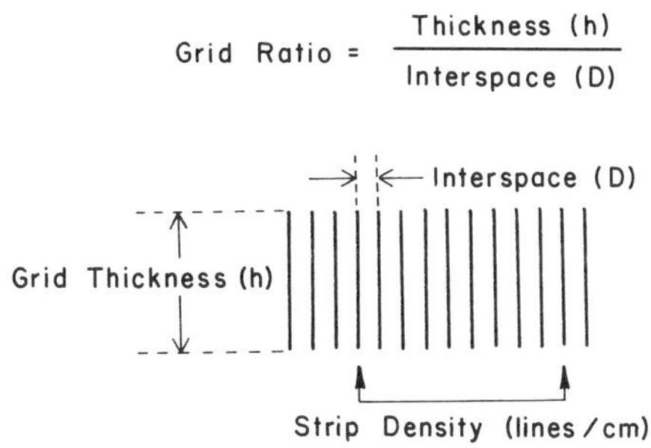

Figure 4. The significant dimensions of a grid.

to 16:1. The selection of the appropriate grid ratio for a given examination involves the consideration of a number of factors. Although the higher grid ratios eliminate more scattered radiation, they tend to increase patient exposure and x-ray tube loading, and also require more precise positioning.

Scatter Radiation Penetration

The relationship between the quantity of scattered radiation which passes through the grid and the grid ratio can be visualized by referring to Figure 5. Consider the exposure which reaches a point on the receptor which is located at the bottom of an interspace. Assuming that no radiation penetrates the lead strips, radiation can reach the point on the receptor only from the directions indicated. Generally speaking, the amount of radiation reaching this point is proportional to the volume of the patient's body which is in direct "view" from this point. As the grid ratio is increased, this volume becomes smaller and the amount of radiation reaching this point is reduced. In effect, with a high ratio grid, each point on the receptor surface is exposed to a smaller portion of the patient's body which is the source of scattered radiation. Using basic geometrical relationships, the theoretical penetration of scattered radiation through grids of various ratios can be determined. This is shown graphically in Figure 6. In actual usage, the relationship can differ from the one shown, especially for certain grid ratio-KVP combinations.

Because of the presence of the lead strips, grids also attenuate part of the primary radiation. The penetration of primary radiation through the grid, P_{gp}, will generally be in the range of 0.6 to 0.7. This value depends on grid design and generally is inversely related to grid ratio. All data presented in this discussion are based on a primary radiation penetration of 0.65.

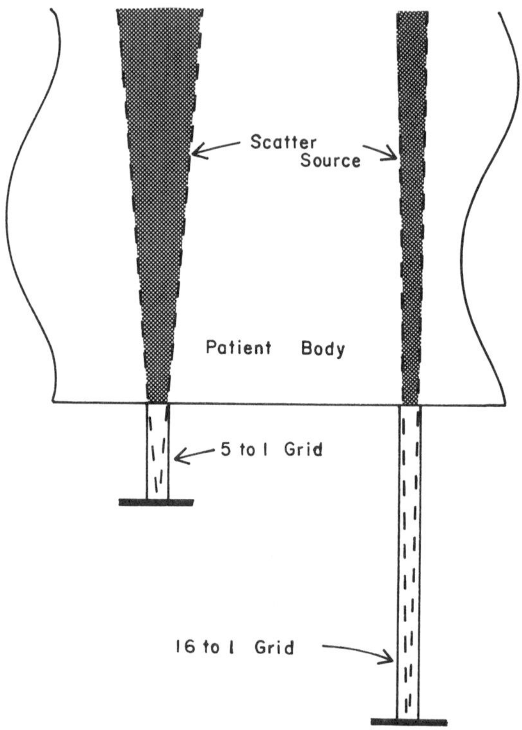

Figure 5. Relationship of receptor exposure to grid ratio.

Contrast Improvement

It has been shown that as the grid ratio is increased a greater proportion of the scattered radiation is removed from the beam. By using the scattered radiation penetration shown in Figure 6 and an average primary penetration of 0.65, it is possible to calculate the expected contrast for various combinations of grid ratio and scatter factors, S.

$$C_s(\%) = \frac{100}{(S\text{-}1)(P_{gs}/P_{gp}) + 1}$$

Some values are shown in Figure 7.

For a grid ratio of 0, that is, no grid, the contrast percentage is equal to 100 divided by S. As the grid ratio is increased and scatter penetration, P_{gs}, decreases, the contrast improves. Several aspects of grid function are illustrated here. For relatively low amounts of scattered radiation, that is, S = 2, a grid ratio of 8:1 restores the contrast to 90%. The additional improve-

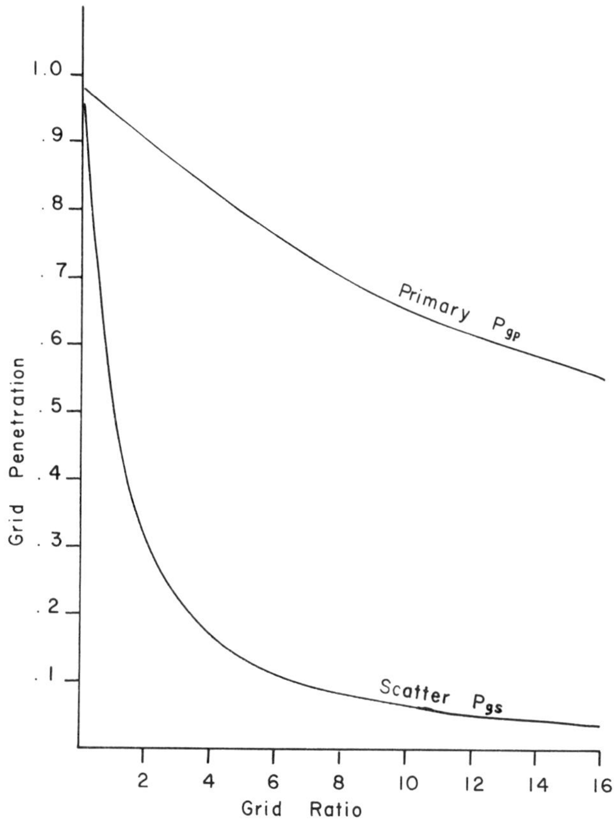

Figure 6. Relationship of grid penetration to grid ratio.

ment in contrast with higher grid ratios is relatively small. It should be noticed, however, that even with the high grid ratios all contrast is not restored. When the proportion of scattered radiation in the beam is higher, for example, when S has a value of 6, the situation is significantly different. At each grid ratio value the contrast is much less than for lower scatter factor values. Also, even with a high ratio grid, such as 16:1, the contrast has been restored to only about 76%. This graph illustrates that contrast is not only a function of grid ratio, but is also determined by the quantity of scattered radiation in the beam, the value of S.

It might appear that the data in Figure 7 indicate that grids do not remove as much scattered radiation when there is a relatively large amount of scattered radiation in the beam, such as for a value of S of 5 or 6. The

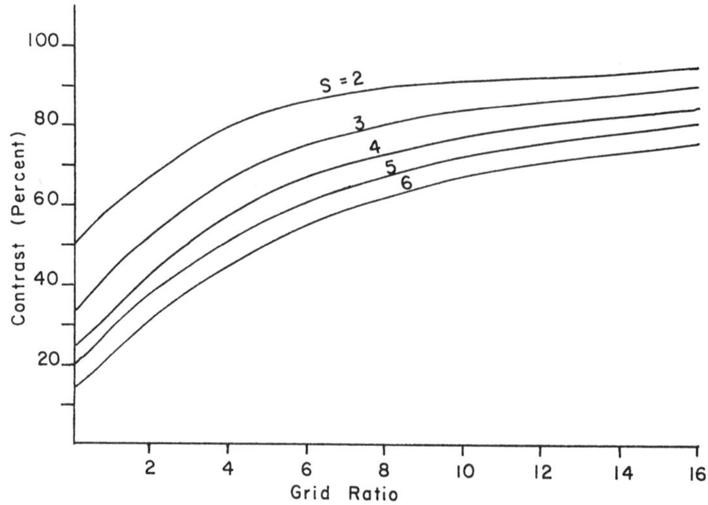

Figure 7. Relationship of contrast to grid ratio and quantity of scattered radiation, S.

relatively lower contrast obtained when large amounts of scattered radiation are present is because of the very low contrast values which are present without the grid. Actually, grids improve contrast by larger factors when the proportion of scattered radiation in the beam is higher. This can be illustrated by observing values of the contrast improvement factor, K. The contrast improvement factor is the ratio of the contrast when a specific grid is used, compared to the contrast without the grid. It is a function of the grid penetration characteristics, P_{gs} and P_{gp}, and the amount of scattered radiation, S. The relationship is:

$$K = \frac{S}{(S-1)(P_{gs}/P_{gp}) + 1}$$

For example, in Figure 7 it is shown that when S has a value of 3 the contrast without a grid is 33.3%. The use of an 8:1 grid raises the contrast to 80%. This is an improvement in contrast by a factor of 80 to 33.3 or 2.4. The value of the contrast improvement factor, K, generally increases both with grid ratio and the quantity of scattered radiation in the beam, S. Although it is true that grids improve contrast by larger factors under conditions of high scattered radiation, one significant fact should not be overlooked. That is, the total restoration of contrast for a given grid is always less for the higher values of scattered radiation. This becomes apparent by comparing the value of the contrast improvement factor to the value of the contrast reduction factor, which is equal to the value of S. This

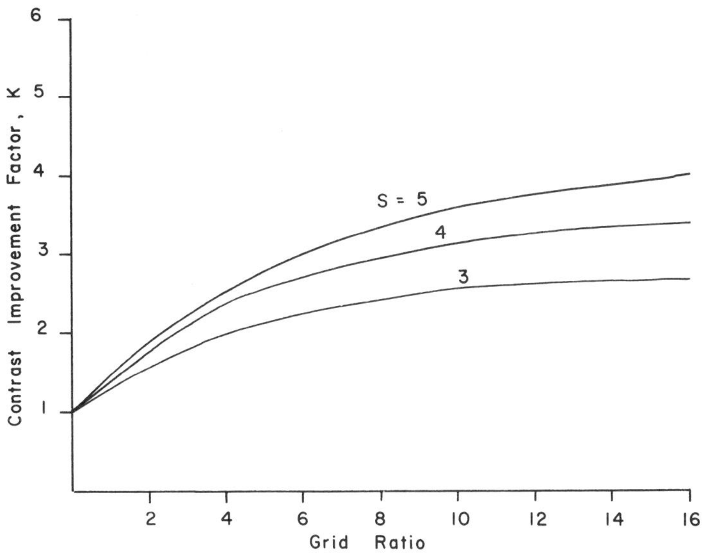

Figure 8. Relationship of contrast improvement factor to grid ratio and scatter factor values.

expresses the ability of a grid under various scatter conditions to recover lost contrast. For example, in Figure 8 it is shown that when S is equal to 5 a 16:1 grid produces a contrast improvement factor of 4. The contrast recovery, therefore, would be four-fifths, or 80%. However, at a lower level of scattered radiation, such as S = 3, the 16:1 grid produces a contrast improvement factor of 2.7, which represents a contrast recovery of 90%.

The relationship between the improvement in contrast and grid ratio is strongly dependent on the proportion of scattered radiation in the beam, emerging from the patient's body. This, in turn, is a function of patient thickness, field size, and kVp. Under conditions which produce high scatter radiation values, a given grid improves contrast by a greater factor, but cannot obtain the same contrast recovery that is possible at lower scattered radiation levels.

GRID PENETRATION

A knowledge of the total penetration of primary and scattered radiation through a grid is necessary in order to properly select appropriate x-ray machine factors. The total grid penetration, P_g, is a function of the scattered radiation penetration, P_{gs}, and the penetration of primary radiation, P_{gp}. The relationship also involves the proportion of scattered radiation in the beam, S. A relationship between the total grid penetration P_g and these three factors is given by:

$$P_t = \frac{P_{gp} + P_{gs}(S-1)}{S}$$

Primary penetration, P_{gp}, does not change with the amount of scattered radiation and changes only slightly with grid ratio. On the other hand, P_{gs} is strongly dependent on grid ratio. Because the typical grid removes more scattered radiation than primary radiation, the total penetration decreases as the scattered radiation content of the beam goes up. The two major factors, therefore, which determine the total grid penetration are the grid ratio and the scatter factor, S.

It has been a common practice to express the grid penetration in terms of the Bucky factor, B. This factor is named after Dr. Gustave Bucky, who constructed the first grid in 1913. The Bucky factor is the reciprocal of the total grid penetration, or:

$$B = \frac{1}{P_g}$$

Grid penetration and Bucky factor values are shown in Figure 9 for various grid ratios and scatter factors. It should be recalled that in most cases there is a correlation between S and KVP. Since high KVP values are

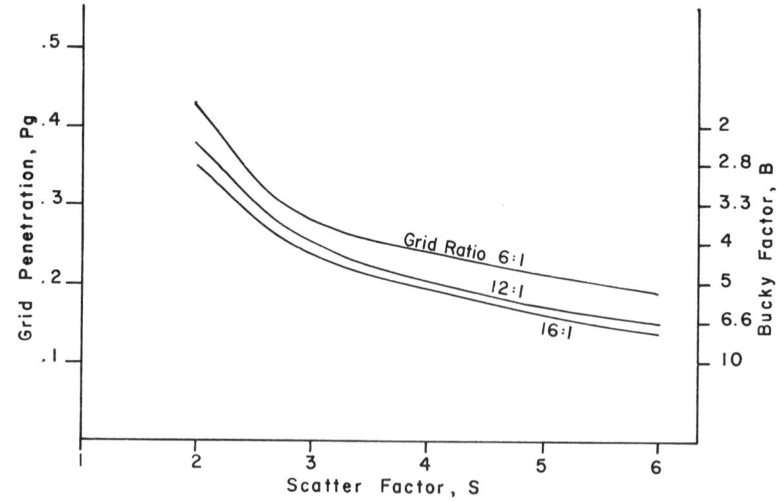

Figure 9. Relationship of grid penetration and Bucky factor to grid ratio and quantity of scattered radiation.

generally used for thick body sections, and both factors increase S, grid penetration appears to decrease as KVP goes up. This is simply because the scatter radiation content at the higher KVP values is generally greater with respect to the primary.

GRID INTERFERENCE

Since the grid is physically located between the patient and the receptor, there is always a possibility that its presence will interfere with the formulation of the image. This interference can be in the form of an image of the grid strips (lines) appearing on the film, or the abnormal attenuation of the radiation in certain portions of the field.

Grid Lines

To some extent the appearance of grid lines on the x-ray film depends on the thickness of the strips and the interspaces. This is usually specified in terms of the number of strips or lines per unit distance. The spacing of lines in grids normally encountered will range from approximately 24 to 44 lines per cm (60 to 110 lines per inch). The grid lines are generally less distracting for the higher spacing densities.

A method which is frequently used to eliminate grid lines in the image is to move the grid during the exposure. The mechanism for accomplishing this was first introduced by Dr. Hollis Potter, and a moving grid system is commonly referred to as a Potter-Bucky diaphragm.

In a Potter-Bucky system the grid moves in a direction which is at right angles to the grid lines. The speed with which the grid moves determines the shortest exposure time which will be free of grid lines.

Grid motion during exposure is also helpful in eliminating image patterns created by the irregular spacing of the grid strips. This type of interference is generally less when grids with aluminum interspaces are used.

Grid Cutoff

The basic characteristic of a grid is to absorb radiation which is moving along a path which is not properly aligned with the grid interspaces. It is desirable that the primary radiation from the x-ray tube focal spot pass through the grid with a minimum of absorption. Maximum grid penetration by the primary radiation can occur only if the x-ray tube focal spot is located at the grid focal point. If these two points are not properly aligned, as shown in Figure 10, the direction of the primary radiation might be such that it does not adequately penetrate certain sections of the grid.

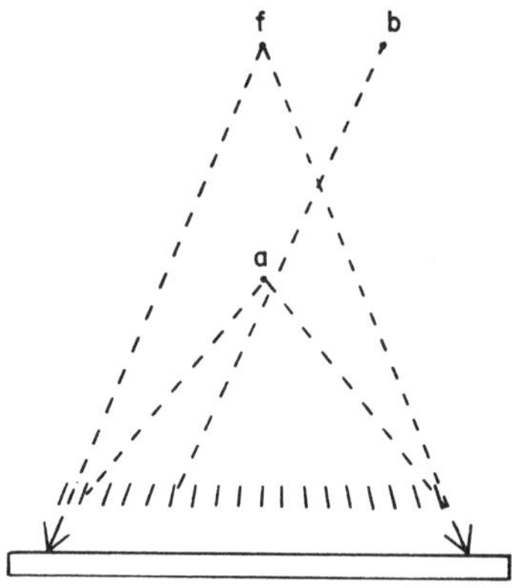

Figure 10. Focal spot locations for different types of misalignment. Location "b" represents lateral misalignment and location "a" represents vertical misalignment.

Misalignment of the x-ray tube focal spot with respect to the focal point of the grid can be either in the lateral or vertical direction, or a combination of both. Lateral misalignment causes the x-ray beam to be misaligned with all interspaces and grid penetration is decreased over the entire beam area. The amount of penetration reduction is related to the amount of misalignment and the grid ratio. Alignment becomes more critical for the higher ratio grids. That is, the loss of grid penetration due to misalignment will be much greater for a high ratio grid.

Vertical misalignment does not alter penetration in the center of the grid. There is, however, decreased penetration near the edges. The loss of penetration is related to the amount of misalignment and the grid ratio. The reduction in penetration for a given amount of misalignment increases with grid ratio. Focused grids are labeled with either a focal distance or a focal range. This should be carefully observed in order to prevent this type of grid cutoff. Cutoff toward the edges of the image area will also occur if a focused grid is turned upside down.

GRID SELECTION

A number of factors must be taken into consideration when selecting a grid for a specific application. In most cases a grid is selected which provides a reasonable compromise between contrast improvement and patient exposure, machine loading, and criticality of positioning.

The advantages of a 5:1 ratio grid are that it is easy to use and does not require critical positioning. Its use must be restricted, however, to situations in which there is a relatively small amount of scattered radiation (thin body section, low kVp) or where maximum image contrast is not necessary. On the other hand, a 16:1 grid produces high contrast recovery but significantly increases patient exposure. With a high ratio grid of this type there is very little latitude in positioning. Many applications are best served by grid ratio values between these two extremes. Such grids are generally compromises between image quality and the other factors discussed above.

Some grids have strips running at right angles to each other. These are generally designated as crossed grids. This design generally increases contrast improvement but cannot be used in examinations in which the x-ray tube is tilted.

In applications where grid lines in the image are undesirable, grids with a high spacing density (lines per centimeter) can be used. An increase in the spacing density will generally require a higher ratio to produce the same contrast improvement.

AIR GAP

The quantity of scattered radiation in an x-ray beam reaching a receptor can be reduced by separating the patient's body and receptor surface. This separation is known as an air gap. Scattered radiation leaving a patient's body is more diverging than the primary x-ray beam. Therefore, the scattered radiation will spread out of the primary beam area. The reduction of the scattered radiation in proportion to the primary radiation increases with the air gap distance. There are several factors however which must be considered when using this method of scatter reduction. Patient exposure is increased because of the inverse-square effect. The use of an air gap introduces magnification. Therefore, a larger receptor size is required in order to obtain the same patient area coverage. If the air gap is obtained by increasing the tube-to-receptor distance the x-ray equipment must be operated at a higher output in order to obtain adequate receptor exposure.

Chapter XIII

Film Density Control

One of the major concerns when conducting an x-ray examination is making sure that the film receives an exposure that will produce the desired densities. The problem can become somewhat complex because there are many factors that can produce variations in film exposure. A properly exposed film is obtained when the two basic x-ray machine parameters, KVP and MAS, are chosen to "match" the various factors associated with the x-ray generator, the patient, and the receptor. This is achieved either manually by the technologist or by means of automatic exposure control circuits within the x-ray system. This chapter will discuss the various factors that relate to film density and how they relate to each other.

FACTORS IN FILM EXPOSURE

Figure 1 shows the basic components within an x-ray system that affect film density. The relationship of the various factors to film density is shown in Figure 2. As stated previously, the object is to select a KVP and MAS value that will produce the correct receptor exposure. The required receptor exposure, in turn, is determined by the sensitivity of the receptor system. Obviously all points on the receptor do not receive the same exposure, or there would be no image, because an x-ray image is produced by a variation in exposure to the film. This discussion assumes that the "correct" exposure is one that will produce a film density near the middle of the useful density range. Therefore, the desired exposure is the median density exposure, X_m, which depends on the sensitivity of the receptor system. The approximate sensitivity of various x-ray receptors is given in Table 1. These are approximate values only because there is a considerable variation in sensitivity for a given type of receptor. Factors which determine the sensitivity of the various receptors, and therefore the amount of

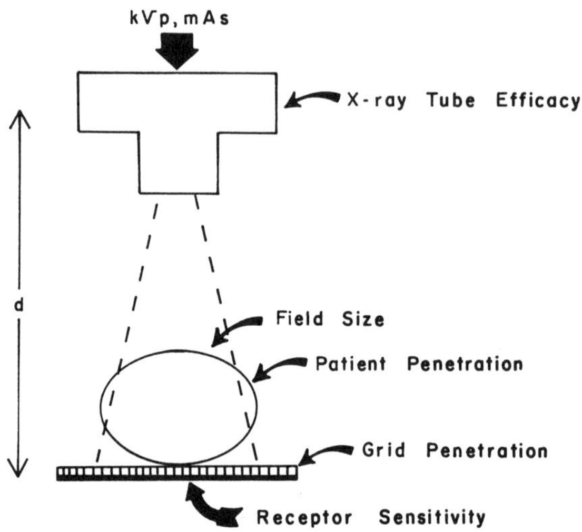

Figure 1. Factors which affect radiographic film density.

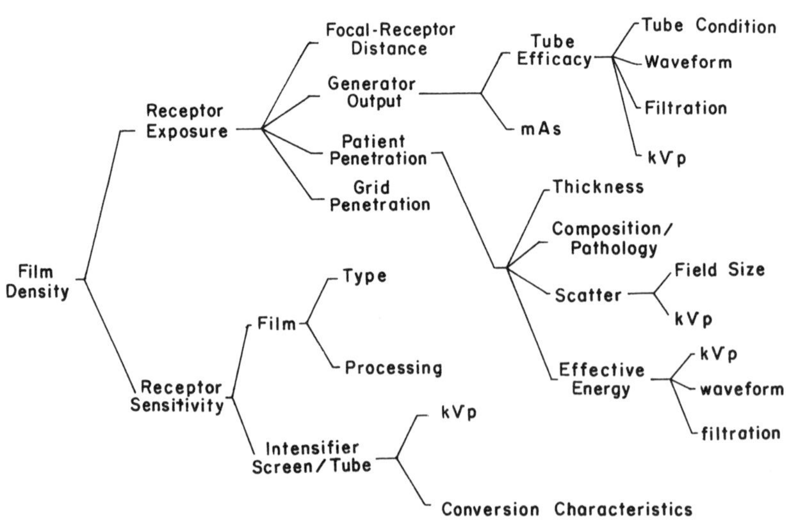

Figure 2. Relationship of film density to other factors.

Table 1. Approximate receptor sensitivity values

Receptor	Sensitivity (mR)
Industrial film (mammography)	500
Xeroradiography	200
Screen type film without screens	50–150
Nonscreen film	20–35
Par speed screens	1.0
High speed screens	0.25–0.5
100-mm film, 10-cm intensifier	0.5
100-mm film, 15-cm intensifier	0.23
100-mm film, 23-cm intensifier	0.1
35-mm film, 23-cm intensifier	0.002

exposure which must be delivered to the receptor, will be discussed in detail in later chapters. As indicated in Figure 2, receptor sensitivity generally depends on the type of film being used, the processing conditions, and the characteristics of either the intensifying screens or intensifier tube.

Receptor Exposure

The exposure which reaches the receptor, X, is given by:

$$X\ (\text{mR}) = \frac{\text{MAS}\cdot E_x\cdot P_p\cdot P_g\cdot S}{d^2}$$

where E_x is the x-ray tube efficacy; MAS is the quantity of electrons passing through the tube; P_p is patient penetration; S is the scatter factor; P_g is the grid penetration; and d is the focal receptor distance (frd). This relationship is based on principles discussed previously. The x-ray tube efficacy, E_x, expresses the exposure produced at a distance of 1 m per mAs. Multiplying the efficacy value by the total MAS gives the exposure which would be produced at a distance of 1 m from the focal spot if there were no attenuating objects (patient or grid) in the beam. The exposure which will pass through the patient's body is determined by multiplying the unattenuated exposure value by the patient penetration, P_p, and the scatter factor. Multiplying this quantity by the grid penetration, P_g, is necessary in order to correct for the attenuation produced by the grid. If the focal-receptor distance, d, is other than 1 m, it is necessary to divide by d^2 because of the inverse square effect.

When conducting an x-ray examination the question generally is not how much exposure the receptor will receive, but rather what factors must be used in order to deliver a certain exposure to the receptor. Assuming that the desired receptor exposure is the median density exposure, X_m, the relationship given above can be rearranged to give an expression for the required MAS as follows:

$$MAS = \frac{X_m \cdot d^2}{E_x \cdot P_p \cdot P_g \cdot S}$$

For those who are familiar with x-ray procedures, it is perhaps surprising that KVP does not appear in the above relationship. This does not mean that the KVP value has no effect on receptor exposure or that it cannot be used as one of the adjustable factors in setting proper exposure. The fact is that all of the factors on the right-hand side of the above equation, with the exception of distance, depend to some degree on KVP. The relationship between x-ray tube efficacy, E_x, and KVP was discussed earlier and is shown graphically in Figure 7 of Chapter VI. It was also shown earlier (Chapter X, Figure 7) that patient penetration, P_p, increases with photon energy or KVP. Likewise, the value of the scatter factor, S, generally increases with KVP. Grid penetration, P_g, which is dependent on the quantity of scattered radiation leaving the patient, S, will therefore also change with KVP. The relationship between receptor sensitivity, X_m, and KVP is generally not as predictable as the other factors. It varies from one type of receptor to another and the sensitivity might either increase or decrease with KVP. Generally speaking, the change in receptor sensitivity with KVP is not nearly as significant as the changes in tube efficacy, patient penetration, and the quantity of scattered radiation. Since the four factors which generally increase with KVP are in the denominator of the above equation there is an inverse relationship between required MAS and KVP. In other words, if KVP is increased, the same film density can be produced with a lower value of MAS because of increases in tube efficacy, patient penetration, and, perhaps, receptor sensitivity.

KVP AND MAS

For a given x-ray system and patient there are many combinations of KVP and MAS which will give essentially the same film density. The approximate relationship between KVP and MAS for a constant film exposure is shown in Figure 3. This relationship is generally known as the "15% rule." It is designated as that because within limits a 15% change in KVP is approximately equivalent to changing the MAS by a factor of 2. This relationship is used to find a KVP change which is equivalent to a given MAS change or vice versa. For example, suppose 70 kVp and 50 MAS produce a good film exposure in a specific examination. For some reason

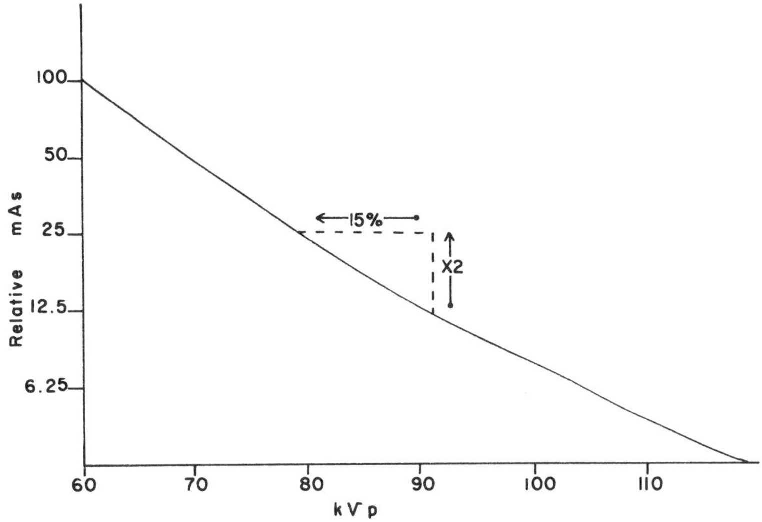

Figure 3. Approximate relationship between relative MAS and kVp for equal film exposure.

it might be desirable to reduce the MAS by a factor of 2 down to 25. The question is, what KVP will give the same film exposure? Assuming that the 15% rule is valid for the particular conditions of the examination the new KVP would be 70 plus 15% (10.5 KVP) or 80.5 KVP. Another situation might be when a given set of factors produces an underexposed film. If it is decided to double the film exposure this can be accomplished by either doubling the MAS or increasing the KVP by approximately 15%.

It should be emphasized that the 15% rule is only an approximation which lumps together a number of factors which change with KVP.

The KVP-MAS factors for good film exposure will vary from examination to examination because of differences in patient and also from one x-ray room to another because of differences in equipment. For a given x-ray system the basic technique factors, KVP and MAS, are determined by experimentation and then various known relationships are used to find the correct factors for different patients or x-ray systems configurations.

There are two general approaches to setting an x-ray machine to compensate for differences among patients. One method is to use a fixed MAS value for a particular type of examination and to adjust KVP to compensate for patient variations. Another method is to use a fixed KVP and then to make adjustments by changing the MAS. There are advantages and disadvantages to both methods. A variable KVP technique produces a change in patient penetration in addition to the change in x-ray tube output.

This has some advantages, especially with thick body sections, in that it can reduce patient exposure and x-ray tube loading when compared to a variable MAS technique. A disadvantage of the variable KVP technique is that it can produce a significant change in image contrast. In many types of examinations a combination of the two approaches gives good results. This method typically consists of three steps.

1. Select a KVP value which will give adequate body penetration with a reasonable level of contrast.
2. Use MAS adjustments to compensate for patient variations within certain established limits.
3. Readjust KVP to compensate for relatively large patient differences.

Patient Penetration

For a given type of examination the factor which is subject to the greatest variation from patient to patient is the penetration of the body section. For a given x-ray beam quality, or KVP, the penetration depends on the thickness of the body part being examined and the composition of the body section. Changes in body thickness from one patient to another can be compensated for by changing either KVP or MAS. An approximate relationship between KVP and body thickness, t, is given by:

$$\text{KVP} = 50 + 2t(\text{cm})$$

For example, a 15-cm thickness would require a KVP of approximately 80 whereas a 20-cm thickness would require a KVP of 90.

When a change in patient thickness is compensated for by changing MAS, a factor-of-2 change is generally required for a thickness difference of approximately 5 cm. This varies, however, with the KVP being used. A given thickness difference requires a smaller MAS change when higher KVP values are used.

The presence of various pathological conditions can also alter body penetration and require appropriate exposure adjustments. Muscular patients generally require an additional increase in exposure factors whereas elderly patients require a reduction.

Field Size

As the area covered by the x-ray beam or field size is increased more scattered radiation is produced and contributes to film exposure. Although much of the scattered radiation is removed by the grid, it is often necessary to change exposure factors in order to get the same density with different field sizes. Approximate correction factors for field size changes are given

Table 2. Approximate MAS conversion factors for different field sizes (field dimensions are in centimeters)

From \ To	13 × 18	20 × 25	25 × 30	36 × 43
13 × 18	1	0.8	0.7	0.6
20 × 25	1.1	1	0.8	0.7
25 × 30	1.2	1.2	1	0.8
36 × 43	1.6	1.5	1.3	1

in Table 2. The MAS for the old field size is multiplied by the factors given to arrive at an MAS value for the new field size.

CHANGES IN X-RAY SYSTEM

It is often necessary to change a component or factor within the x-ray system, which will in turn require a change in exposure factors in order to maintain proper film density. Several of these are now considered along with the necessary changes in exposure factors.

Distance

Because of the inverse square effect the exposure which reaches the receptor is related to the focal spot-receptor distance, d. If this distance is changed the new MAS value to obtain the same film exposure is given by:

$$\text{MAS(new)} = \text{MAS(old)} \left(\frac{d_{new}}{d_{old}}\right)^2$$

A characteristic of this relationship is that if the distance is doubled the required MAS increases by a factor of 4. Long focal spot-receptor distances generally decrease image blur, patient exposure, and distortion; however, a significantly higher MAS is required.

Grids

When a grid is changed the exposure factors must be changed. An approximate relationship between the old and new MAS values depends on the Bucky factors, B, or penetration, P_g, of the grids and is:

$$\text{MAS(new)} = \text{MAS(old)} \frac{B_{new}}{B_{old}}$$

or

$$\text{MAS(new)} = \text{MAS(old)}\,\frac{P_g(\text{old})}{P_g(\text{new})}$$

where P_g is the grid penetration which is the reciprocal of the Bucky factor. If one of the conditions being considered is without a grid then the value of the Bucky factor or grid penetration is 1. The value of these factors generally depends on grid ratio and the quantity of scattered radiation in the beam, as discussed in Chapter XII. Values of grid penetration, P_g, range from 1 (no grid) to approximately 0.2 for a high ratio grid. Changing from an examination condition without a grid to one with a grid penetration, P_g, of 0.2 (Bucky factor of 5) requires that the MAS be increased by a factor of 5. Approximate grid penetration and Bucky factor values for different grids are given in Figure 9 of Chapter XII.

Receptor Sensitivity

In conventional radiography the receptor sensitivity is changed either by changing the intensifying screens or the film. In some cases the change might be produced by going between screens and nonscreen techniques. The MAS value required to give equivalent film density is given by:

$$\text{MAS(new)} = \text{MAS(old)}\,\frac{X_m(\text{new})}{X_m(\text{old})}$$

where X_m is the receptor sensitivity expressed in terms of the median density exposure. Typical values are given in Table 1.

X-Ray Generator Output

It is not unusual for two different x-ray systems to require different exposure factors (MAS and KVP) even when such things as receptors, distances, grids, etc., are the same. This is usually attributed to a difference in x-ray tube efficacy between the two x-ray machines. For example, a three-phase machine might require approximately one-half of the milliampere-seconds that would be needed with single-phase equipment. This is because three-phase operation increases both the x-ray tube efficacy and patient penetration. A difference in the amount of filtration can also produce a significant difference in tube efficacy and require different exposure factors.

Chapter XIV Film Characteristics

Radiographic images are recorded on several types of film or paper. Most films are of the transparent type and the image is viewed by illuminating it from the rear on a viewbox. The image then appears as a pattern consisting of areas with different levels of brightness as shown in Figure 1.

DENSITY

The brightness of a specific point on a film is determined by the density of the film at that point. Density is a quantity that is used to describe the degree of opacity of a film. The density value is defined in terms of the fraction of light that penetrates the film. The relationship between the optical density, D, and the light penetration, P, is given by:

$$D = -\log P$$

or

$$P = 10^{-D}$$

The relationship between these two quantities is of the logarithmic or exponential type. The significance of this is that a small change in density produces a relatively large change in light penetration and relative brightness. This can be shown by substituting several values in the second relationship shown above. If a film has a density of 1 unit, the light penetration will be:

$$P = 10^{-1} = 0.1\ (10\%)$$

However, if the film has a density of two, the light penetration will be:

$$P = 10^{-2} = 0.01\ (1\%)$$

It is seen that changing film density by 1 unit produces a change in light penetration (and brightness) by a factor of 10. The characteristic of this relationship is that each density unit reduces light penetration by a factor of

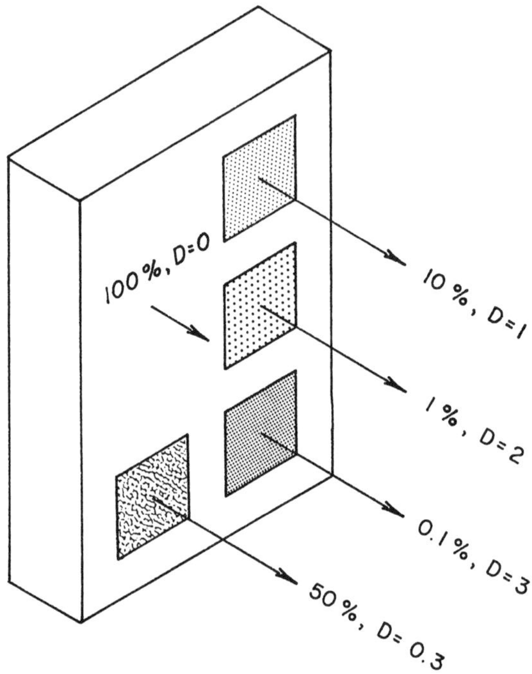

Figure 1. The relationship of viewbox light penetration of film density.

10. This is seen by considering the values shown in Table 1. A density of 0 means that the film is completely clear and all light (100%) penetrates. The light coming through the film is reduced by a factor of 10 for each density unit.

Radiographic films generally have densities ranging from approximately 0.2 to greater than 3. The higher density values do not permit adequate penetration of viewbox light for normal viewing. The range of

Table 1. Relationship of film density and light penetration (relative brightness)

Film density	Light penetration, %
0	100
1	10
2	1
3	0.1

density values which can be viewed on a viewbox are from approximately 0.2 to 2.5.

Photographic Process

The recording media for most x-ray images is a film which contains many small silver halide crystals suspended in a gelatin emulsion. Various metallic salt compounds are photosensitive; however, photographic film is comprised primarily of silver bronite and a smaller concentration of silver iodide. The formation of an image on a silver halide film is a multistep process as illustrated in Figure 2.

The silver halide molecules are grouped together in small crystals which are usually referred to as grains. Grain sizes are on the order of 0.001 mm. Large grains cause the film to be more sensitive or faster but can also contribute to a grainy appearance (noise) in the final image, especially with enlargement. As the silver halide grains absorb light or x-ray photons, free silver atoms are caused to collect and form latent image centers. The absorption of radiation by the silver halide grains does not form a visible image. This latent image requires chemical development before it becomes visible. The development of x-ray films is essentially a three-step process and is usually accomplished in automated processes in a matter of minutes.

The first chemical step is to immerse the exposed film into the developer solution. The basic action of the developer is to free the silver atoms in those grains which have received sufficient exposure and contain latent image centers. The silver atoms within a grain combine to form an opaque speck. In effect, the developing process causes the few silver atoms which constituted the initial latent image center to multiply by a factor of

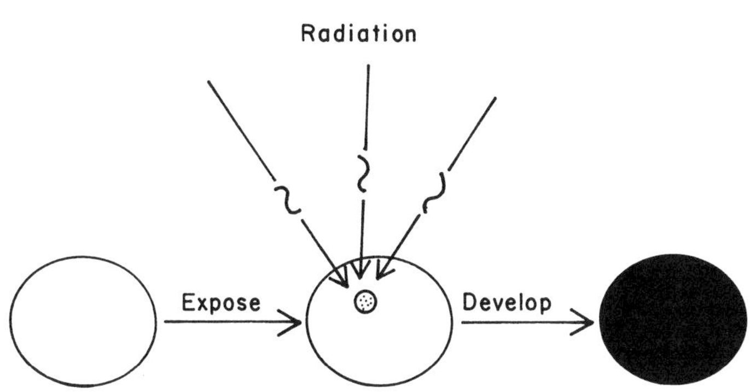

Figure 2. A silver halide grain in three stages; unexposed, exposed, and developed.

10^8 or so. The number of grains which contain latent image centers depends on the exposure delivered to the film whereas the number of latent image centers which become fully developed depends on the degree of development. Factors which alter the degree of film development are discussed below. Overdevelopment will cause some of the grains without latent image centers to break down as if they were exposed. The overall effect of this is that areas on the film which have received no exposure will develop some density, which is generally referred to as fog.

The second step in film processing is fixing. The fixing solution contains several different chemicals and performs several specific functions. One purpose of the fixer is to neutralize the developer on the film and stop the developing action. It also contains a hardening agent which will harden the emulsion and prevent its softening or swelling when the film is washed. Another important function of the fixing solution is to dissolve the undeveloped silver halide crystals and remove them from the emulsion.

After fixing the film must be thoroughly washed in running water to remove the fixing chemicals and dissolved silver halides. If the film is not adequately washed it will contain stains or will become discolored with age.

In some imaging systems the radiographic image is recorded on nontransparent film, or paper. The various areas of such an image exhibit different levels of gray, rather than different density values.

SENSITIVITY

The density of a film is determined by two factors, the quantity of radiation exposure reaching the film and the sensitivity of the film. Some films are more sensitive than others and will produce a given density with less exposure. Film sensitivity is often referred to as film speed. The idea is that a more sensitive film will acquire a given density in a shorter exposure time. It, therefore, has the appearance of responding faster to radiation than a less sensitive film. The sensitivity of a film is normally expressed in terms of the quantity of radiation exposure required to produce a certain density. For radiographic applications, it is desirable to express the sensitivity of the film in terms of the exposure required to produce a density that is near the middle, or median, of the useful density range. This is designated as the median density exposure, X_m. By convention, a density of 1 unit above the base-plus-fog density is used as the reference density for expressing film sensitivity. In other words, the sensitivity of a film is expressed in terms of the exposure required to produce a density of 1 plus base-plus-fog density, which is approximately the median of the useful radiographic density range.

At this point, a distinction must be made between film sensitivity and receptor sensitivity. In most x-ray systems the film is not exposed directly to x-radiation. The x-radiation is converted into light by either intensifying screens or image intensifier tubes. Receptor sensitivity is expressed in terms of x-radiation exposure units, such as milliroentgens. When film is used in direct exposure techniques, the receptor sensitivity is the same as the film sensitivity expressed in x-ray units. Typical values are shown in Table 1 in Chapter XIII.

The sensitivity of film to light exposure is expressed in two different units, depending on the general type of film. Film that is used with intensifying screens will generally have a sensitivity value that is the median density exposure, E_m, expressed in ergs per cm^2 of light. The median density exposure, E_m, for film used in conjunction with image intensifiers is generally expressed in the light units of lux-seconds. This is a unit of illumination which is compatible with the units of nits (cd per m^2) which are used to express the output luminance (brightness) of image intensifiers. The sensitivity (or speed) of this type of film is often expressed by ASA values. The approximate relationship between the median density exposure, E_m, and the ASA rating of a film is given by:

$$E_m(\text{lux} \cdot \text{sec}) = \frac{8}{\text{ASA number}}$$

For example, if a film has an ASA rating of 100, a light exposure of 0.08 lux·sec would be required to produce a density near the middle of the useful density range.

The sensitivity of film, as defined above, is determined by two factors. One factor is the inherent sensitivity, which is related to the composition of the film and the exposure conditions. The other factor which can alter film sensitivity is processing. Additional details of these will be given later.

Spectral Sensitivity

All light detectors such as the human eye, television cameras, and film are more sensitive to certain light wavelengths, or colors, than to others. This relationship between detector response and wavelength is referred to as spectral sensitivity. Films used in radiography are exposed by light from either intensifying screens or image intensifiers. For maximum sensitivity the film should have its maximum response to the wavelength or colors emitted by the screen or intensifier. For many years the most common material used in intensifying screens was calcium tungstate. In recent years, however, a number of new phosphors have been used which emit different light wavelengths. Calcium tungstate and several other phosphors emit essentially a blue spectrum. Some of the rare earth phosphors and image intensifier tubes emit green light.

Silver halide emulsions have an inherent sensitivity to light with wavelengths up to approximately 500 nm. This includes the blue and near ultraviolet which is emitted by several intensifying screen phosphors. The somewhat limited spectral response makes it possible to work with these films in dark rooms equipped with relatively bright yellow safe lights. By adding certain dyes to the emulsion it is possible to extend the sensitivity to include the green portion of the spectrum. This is the so-called orthochromatic type of film. Safe lights for use with orthochromatic film must emit light in the red portion of the spectrum. The sensitivity in panchromatic films covers approximately the same spectral range as the human eye. For that reason it is not possible to work with this film under any safe light which would be visible to the user. Panchromatic films are commonly used in black and white photography and in some intensified radiographic applications.

Reciprocity Failure

In radiography it is usually possible to deliver a given exposure to the film by using many different combinations of radiation intensity (exposure rate) and exposure time. Since radiation intensity is proportional to x-ray tube MA this is equivalent to saying that a given exposure (in milliamperes-seconds) can be produced with many different combinations of MA and time. This is known as the law of reciprocity. In effect, it means that it is possible to swap radiation intensity (in milliamperes) for exposure time and still get the same film exposure. When a film is exposed directly to x-radiation the reciprocity law holds true. That is, 100 mAs will produce the same film density whether it is exposed at 1,000 mA and 0.1 sec or 10 mA and 10 sec. However, when a film is exposed by light, such as from intensifying screens or image intensifiers, the reciprocity law is not completely valid. Light exposure, as opposed to direct x-ray interactions, requires the absorption of more than 1 photon in a single silver halide grain before it becomes a developable grain and can contribute to the image density. This causes the sensitivity of the film to be somewhat dependent on the intensity of the exposing light. This loss of sensitivity varies to some extent from one type of x-ray film to another. Figure 3 shows this variation in film sensitivity as a function of exposure time. For this particular film the maximum sensitivity occurs for the light intensity which produces the

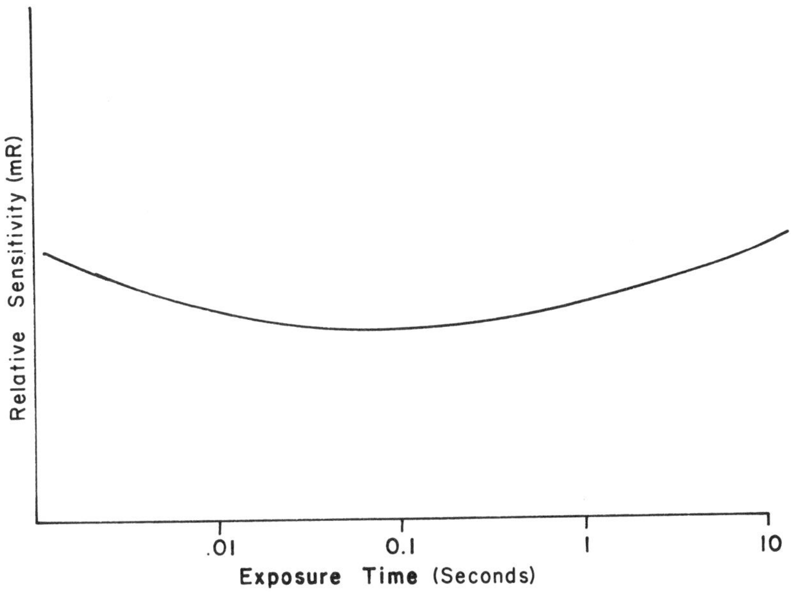

Figure 3. The variation in film sensitivity with exposure time because of reciprocity failure.

desired film exposure in approximately 0.1 sec. If an attempt is made to deliver the same exposure by combining a lower intensity and a longer exposure time the sensitivity is much less as indicated.

CONTRAST TRANSFER CHARACTERISTICS

The film is the element within the x-ray system which converts an x-ray, or light, image into various densities or shades of gray. This is, in effect, converting subject contrast into radiographic contrast. An important characteristic of a film is the amount of radiographic contrast which will be produced for a certain amount of subject contrast. It is helpful, at this point, to recall that subject contrast is the ratio of exposure to two points in an image, usually a background and object area, expressed as a percentage. Radiographic contrast is the difference in film density between the two film areas (background and object area). The relationship between the two types of contrast, subject and radiographic, is best visualized by referring to Figure 4. This graph shows the basic relationship between film density and the exposure which produces the density.

The exposure scale shows exposure values relative to the median

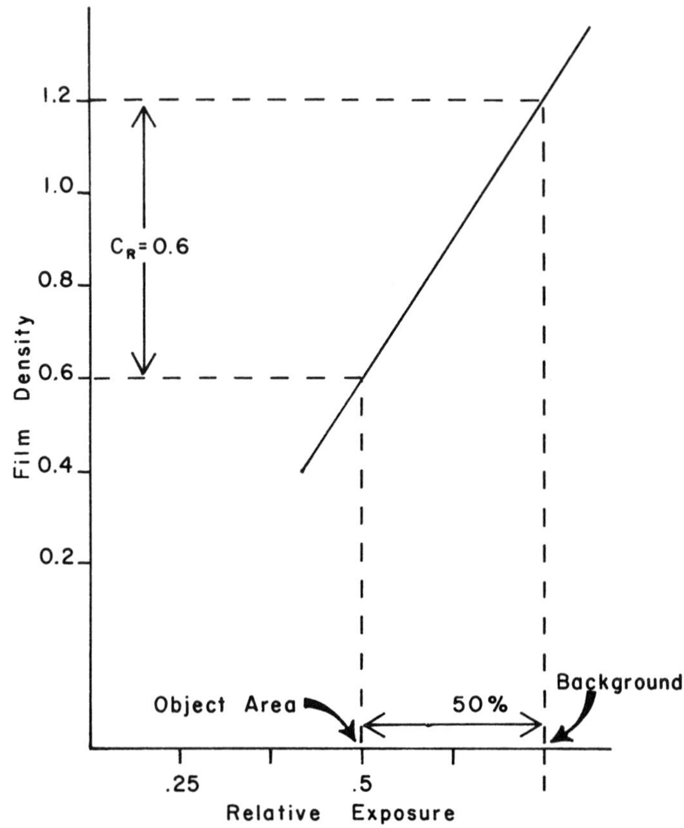

Figure 4. The relationship between radiographic contrast and subject contrast.

density exposure which is assigned a value of 1. It is convenient to use a logarithmic scale for the exposure values. On a logarithmic scale a given distance between two points represents a specific ratio of values. Therefore, on the film exposure scale a certain amount of subject contrast is represented by a specific distance along the scale. For example, the arrow shown has a length which represents 50% subject contrast, regardless of where it is located along the scale.

Since radiographic contrast is the difference in film density between the two image areas it is represented by the distance between the two respective points on the density scale. The density scale is of the linear type where the distance between two points represents a difference, rather than a ratio, as on the logarithmic exposure scale.

From the graph it can be seen that the relationship between subject contrast and radiographic contrast depends on the slope of the line which represents the basic relationship between density and exposure. The slope of the line is expressed in terms of the contrast factor, G. The contrast factor is defined as the difference in density between two areas on a film which have received exposures which differ by a factor of 2. Two film areas which have an exposure ratio of 2:1 will have a subject contrast of 50%. Therefore, the contrast factor of the film is equivalent to the amount of radiographic contrast resulting from 50% subject contrast. A film with a steep slope will yield more radiographic contrast for the same subject contrast than a film with a more gradual slope. This is illustrated in Figure 5. The background areas of both films have been exposed to a density of 1.2. In both cases the exposure to the object area is one-half of that to the background which yields a subject contrast of 50%. When imaged with film A the object area density has a value of 0.9 which is a radiographic contrast of 0.3. Film B, which has a steeper slope, produces an object area density of 0.6 which is a radiographic contrast value of 0.6. It should be observed that the contrast factor values for films A and B are 0.3 and 0.6, respectively.

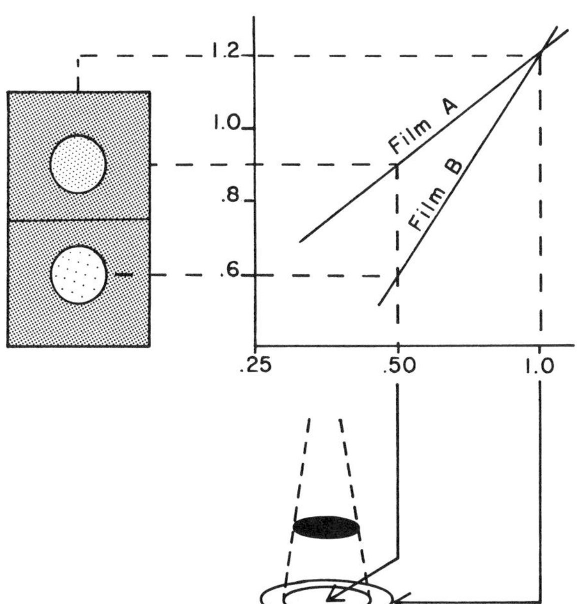

Figure 5. The radiographic contrast produced by 50% subject contrast and two different films.

The relationship between radiographic contrast and subject contrast for various values of the film contrast factor is shown graphically in figure 6. From this it can be seen that a given amount of radiographic contrast can be obtained from many different combinations of subject contrast and film contrast factor values. In examinations where subject contrast might be relatively low because of object penetration or scattered radiation a film with a high contrast factor value can be used to increase radiographic contrast. The actual relationship of subject contrast, C_s, radiographic contrast, C_r, and film contrast factor, G, is given by:

$$C_r = G\,(6.64 - 3.32 \log(100 - C_s))$$

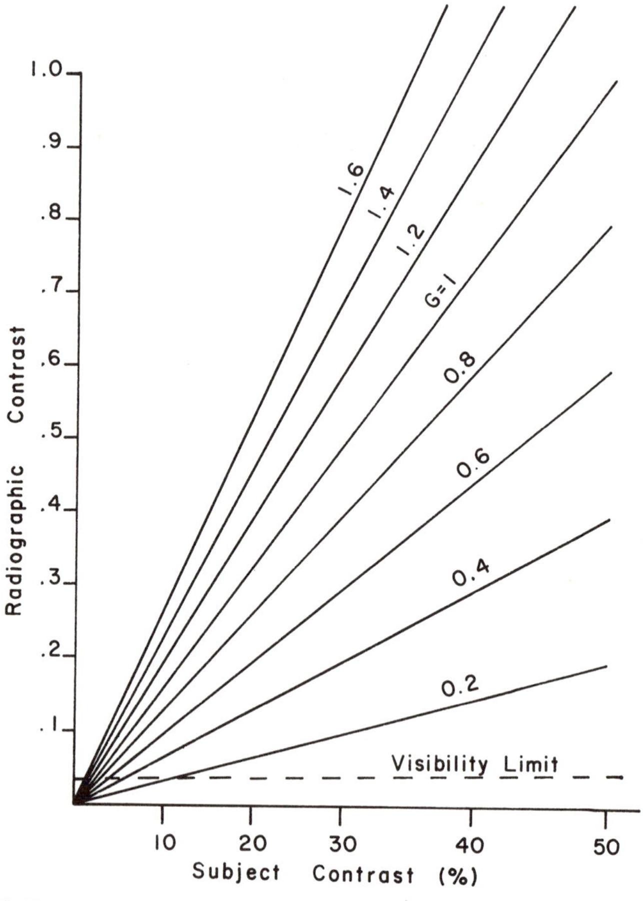

Figure 6. The relationship of radiographic contrast to subject contrast for different film contrast factors.

Although this relationship appears to be somewhat complex it can be easily evaluated by using the logarithm table in Appendix I or a calculator which has a logarithm function.

The contrast factor of a film is generally determined by three things: 1) the composition of the film emulsion, 2) the processing, and 3) the amount of exposure.

Characteristic Curve

Up to this point the relationship between film density and exposure has been represented by a straight line. Although this is generally correct within a certain range of exposures it does not hold true over the total film density range. The relationship between density and exposure for a typical x-ray film is shown in Figure 7. This graph is known as the characteristic or Hurter and Driffield (H and D) curve of the film. The typical characteristic curve has three more or less distinct sections. The midportion is essentially a straight line and is generally referred to as such. This is the region with maximum slope which yields the maximum transfer of contrast. At lower exposure values the slope becomes progressively less and finally becomes 0. This region is designated as the toe of the curve. The horizontal portion of the curve extending from the toe represents the film density value which is present even when the film receives no appreciable exposure. This density results from the inherent density of the film base material in addition to a slight amount of fog in the emulsion.

Toward the upper end of the exposure range the slope again decreases and finally becomes 0. This region is known as the shoulder of the curve. The point where the curve becomes horizontal represents the maximum density which the film can produce.

Because of the changing slope of the characteristic curve the contrast factor of a film depends on the amount of exposure. In addition to the characteristic (density) curve Figure 7 also contains a graph of the contrast factor. The values of the contrast factor are read from the same scale. The contrast factor has a maximum value over the exposure range which corresponds to the straight line portion of the characteristic curve. However, in both the toe and shoulder regions the contrast factor decreases in value as indicated. The important point is that maximum contrast is obtained by adjusting the exposure so that the object and background area exposures fall along the straight line portion of the characteristic curve.

The contrast transfer characteristics of a film over its total exposure range can be described only by using a characteristic curve or contrast factor curve as shown in Figure 7. There are many occasions, however, when it would be desirable to use a single value to describe a film's

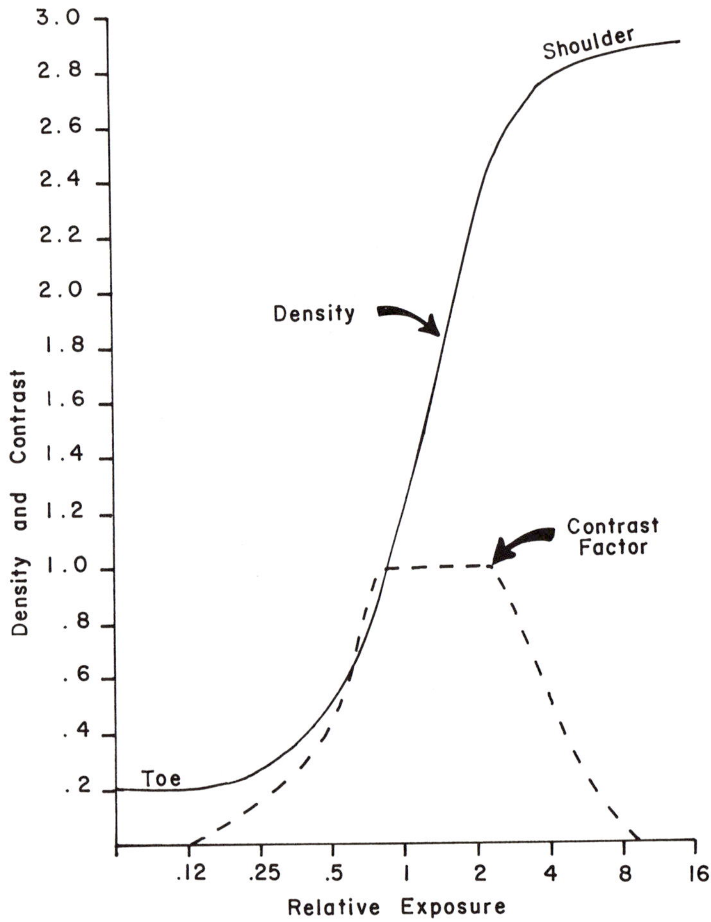

Figure 7. A characteristic curve which shows the relationship of film density and contrast to relative exposure values.

contrast characteristics. Although one number cannot describe the variation in contrast with exposure, it can be used for the purpose of comparing the various types of film and processing. Two parameters which are used for this purpose are the gamma value and the average gradient.

The gamma value of a film is the maximum slope of the characteristic curve. By tradition, the gamma value is the slope expressed in terms of the density difference associated with an exposure ratio of 10:1. The relationship between the film gamma value and the maximum contrast factor is given by:

$$\text{Gamma} = 3.32\ G\ (\text{maximum})$$

The factor of 3.32 converts a slope based on an exposure ratio of 2:1 to a slope expressed with respect to a 10:1 exposure ratio.

The average gradient is the average slope between two designated density values as illustrated in Figure 8. For medical x-ray film the density values of 0.25 and 2.0 above the base plus fog density are used for the determination of average gradient. Average gradient values, like gamma values, are based on an exposure ratio of 10:1. Therefore, the relationship between average gradient and average contrast factor is given by:

$$\text{Average gradient} = 3.32\ G\ (\text{average})$$

The net density is the density of a film area from which the base plus fog density has been subtracted. Most x-ray films will have base plug fog

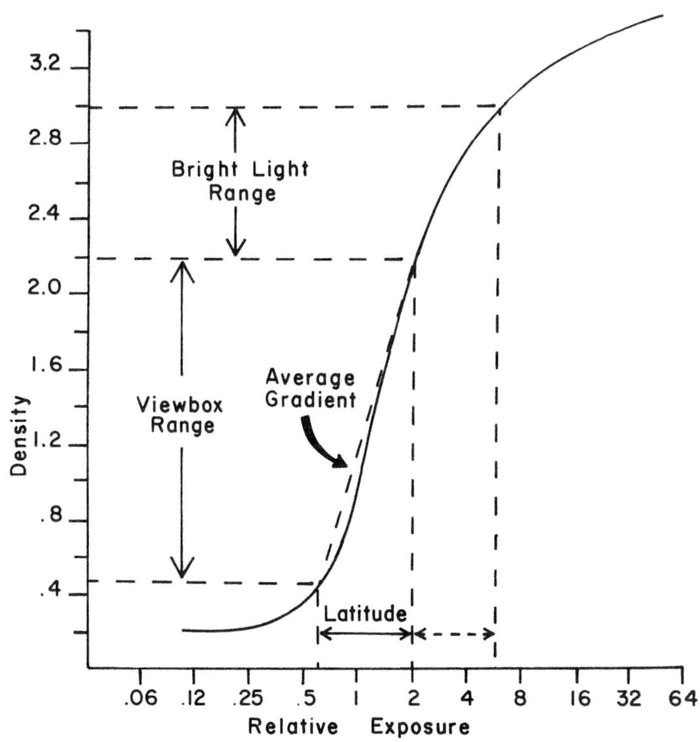

Figure 8. The relationship of film latitude to the useful density range.

densities in the range of 0.15 to 0.2. The net density range of 0.25 to 2.0 is generally considered to be the useful film density range for normal viewbox viewing. However, a small bright light can be used to extend the useful density range up to a value of approximately 3.0 for most x-ray films. The range of densities which can be viewed in turn establishes the range of exposure values which are useful in forming the image. The exposure range is more commonly known as the latitude of the film. As shown in Figure 8 the latitude is the range of exposure values corresponding to the useful density range. The latitude value is the ratio of the maximum and minimum useful exposures. The significance of the latitude

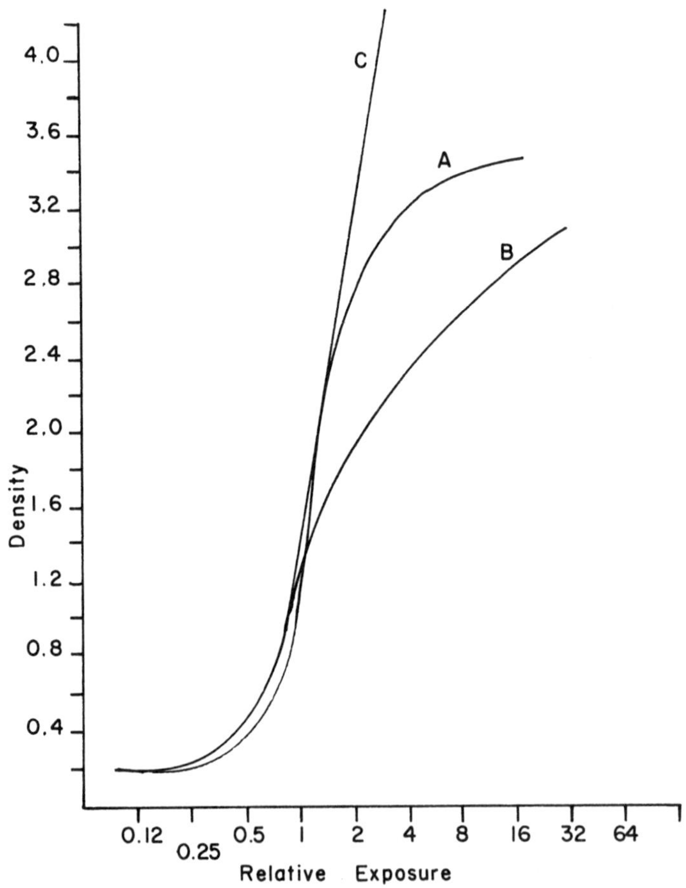

Figure 9. Characteristic curves of a high contrast film (A), a wide latitude film (B), and a nonscreen film (C).

is that it specifies the range of exposure values within an image which will confine the resulting densities values to the useful range. In general, it is usually desirable for the film latitude to be approximately equal to the subject contrast range. This will yield the maximum contrast without having some film areas with densities out of the useful range. The latitude of a film is inversely related to the slope of the characteristic curve. A film that has a high contrast transfer will have a low latitude and vice versa.

Films can be selected which have the most desirable latitude and contrast characteristics for a particular type of examination. Figure 9 shows several different characteristic curves. Films A and B are characteristic of the types used with intensifying screens and film C is a typical nonscreen film. The significant difference between films A and B is the slope of their characteristic curve. Film A would be described as a high contrast film. It would yield more radiographic contrast than film B but has the limitation of a lower latitude value. Film C illustrates a special characteristic of directly exposed (nonscreen) film. When film is exposed by x-radiation as opposed to light the straight line portion extends to much higher density values.

Both the sensitivity and contrast characteristics of a given film type depend on the processing. The degree of processing received by film generally depends on three factors: 1) the chemical activity of the developer solution, 2) the temperature of the developer, and 3) the time of immersion in the developer. In most x-ray applications it is usually desirable to maintain a constant developer activity by replenishment and to control the degree of development by varying the temperature or, in some cases, the development time.

The general effects of changing the degree of development are illustrated in Figure 10. Varying the amount of development by changing either the chemical activity, time, or temperature will produce a shift in the characteristic curve. Increasing development will cause the curve to shift to the left with a rise in the toe. The movement of the curve to the left indicates an increase in sensitivity because a given density value is produced with a lower exposure. As the toe of the curve rises, the general slope of the curve decreases, which results in less contrast. Also, the increased density value of the toe results from an increased fog level. This fog density results from more of the unexposed silver grains becoming developed by the excess processing.

Underprocessing causes the curve to shift to the right, indicating a decrease in sensitivity. Also, the shoulder begins to drop and there is a general decrease in the slope of a curve. This results in less contrast.

The optimum performance of most film types is obtained by using the recommended degree of development. Deviation in either direction will

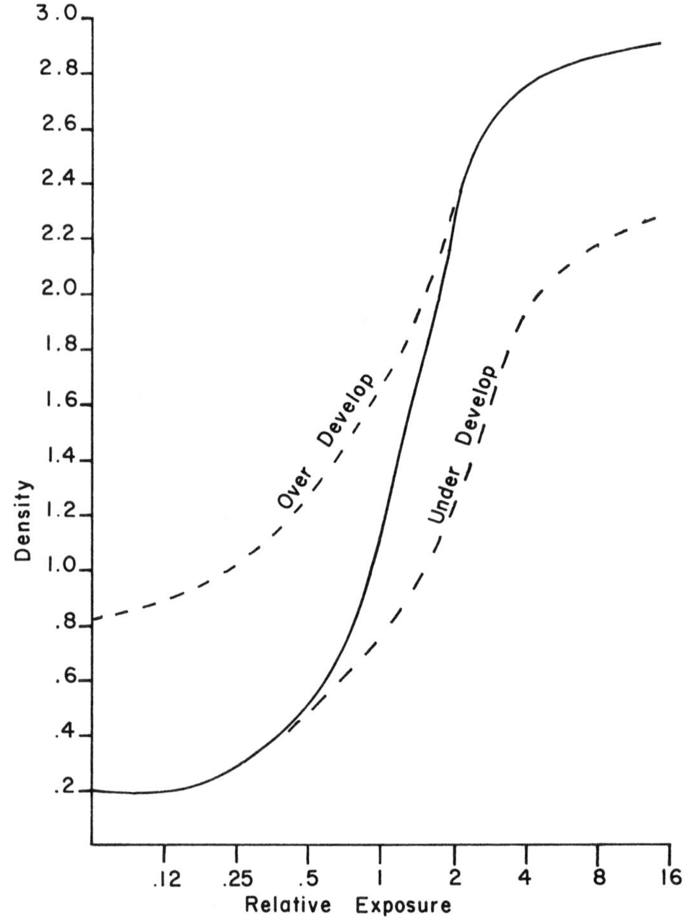

Figure 10. Changes in film characteristics produced by altering development.

generally result in a loss of contrast. Although it is usually possible to increase the sensitivity of film by overdeveloping, this is usually accompanied by an increase in undesirable fog.

SENSITOMETRY

The study of the relationship between film response (density) and exposure is known as sensitometry. This is usually performed by exposing a film to known radiation quantities and measuring the resulting density. The device

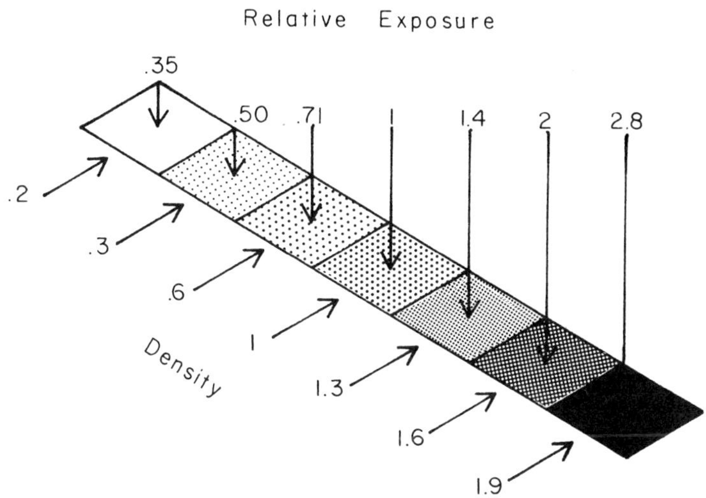

Figure 11. A strip of film exposed in a sensitometer.

which is used to expose the film is known as a sensitometer. A sensitometer can use either x-rays or light to expose the film. Since most x-ray films are actually exposed by light from intensifying screens or image intensifier tubes it is appropriate to use light to study their sensitometric properties.

Most sensitometers will expose a film to a series of exposure values, or steps, as shown in Figure 11. The exposure to two adjacent areas will usually differ by a specific factor. An exposure ratio between steps of 1.4 is used in many sensitometers. Areas on the film located two steps apart will differ in exposure by a factor of 2 ($1.4 \times 1.4 = 2$).

The density of film is measured with a densitometer. The densitometer determines film density by passing light through the film and measuring relative penetration.

The contrast characteristics of a film can be determined by comparing the densities of the various steps. For example, the difference in density between areas which are two steps apart will be the value of the average contrast factor for that particular density range. If the sensitometer produces enough exposure steps the exposure and density values can be used to plot a characteristic curve.

Chapter XV

Image Blur and Resolution

As an x-ray beam passes through a section of the body, it forms an image on the film that generally represents the level of penetration through each point of the body section or objects within. In most types of examinations, it would be desirable for the penetration through each small point of the object to be represented by a film density also confined to an equally small point. In most x-ray systems, however, the x-rays that pass through a small object point form an image that is spread over a larger area on the film. This is illustrated in Figure 1 for several points located on a simple flat object. The spreading of the image of a point is referred to as blurring. An exposure profile of a single point in Figure 1 shows the general effect of blurring in film exposure. If there is no blurring present, the ideal condition, the exposure profile is a single thin line, as indicated. Blurring, in the actual situation, spreads the exposure over a larger area of the film. With respect to the image of a single point within the object, blurring introduces two generally undesirable effects. It spreads the image of the point into surrounding areas on the film, and it reduces contrast.

The exposure profile produced by blurring of a single object point is often referred to as a point-spread function, PSF. The exposure profile, or PSF, shows how the radiation passing through a single small point in the object is spread over the surface of the film. Point exposure profiles have different shapes, depending on the source of the blur. Two common blur profiles, that is, point-spread functions, are shown in Figure 2. The one at the bottom of the illustration has a rectangular shape that is characteristic of blur produced by motion and certain types of focal spots. The blur profile at the top is generally characteristic of blur produced in receptors. Mathematically, the shape of the profile at the top is classified as a Gaussian function. Because the Gaussian shape profile has no single dimension, it is necessary to define an equivalent blur dimension, as shown in Figure

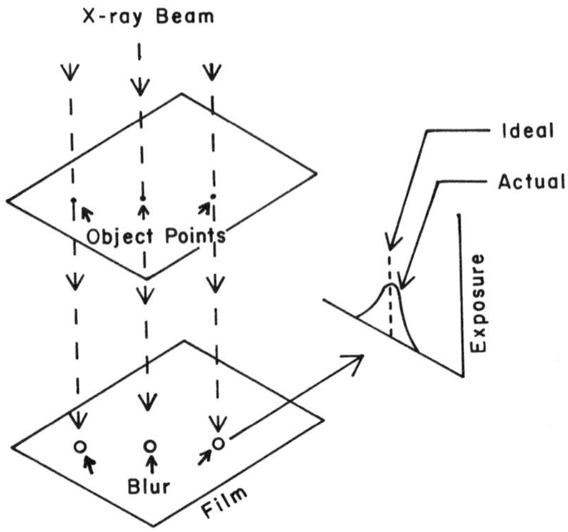

Figure 1. Blur in the image of small object points.

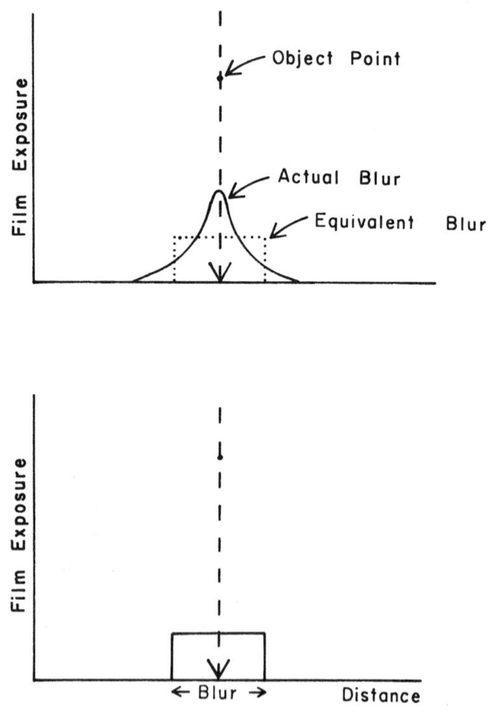

Figure 2. Two types of blur profiles or point-spread functions.

2. The equivalent blur for a Gaussian exposure profile is defined as the dimension of a rectangular profile that will produce the same image quality. The equivalent blur of a Gaussian-shaped blur is approximately 0.6 of the actual dimension.

In most cases the blur is actually in two dimensions or directions on the surface of the film. However, for simplicity, only one dimension is considered in the discussion.

EFFECTS OF BLUR ON IMAGE QUALITY

A number of different descriptive terms are used to describe the effects of blur on image quality. The relationship of several of these qualities to blur is illustrated in Figure 3. In this illustration three different objects are shown, along with the resulting film exposure profiles. In each case the profile in the absence of blur is indicated by a dotted line.

Unsharpness

The presence of significant blur gives an image an appearance that is often described as being unsharp. Although this is more or less a subjective characteristic with respect to a total image, it can be quantitated with respect to the image of a sharp edge, as shown to the left of Figure 3. The image of the edge, as it appears on the film, would not be distinct, but would show a gradual change from the light to the dark areas on each side. The width of this zone of varying exposure, or density, is used as specifica-

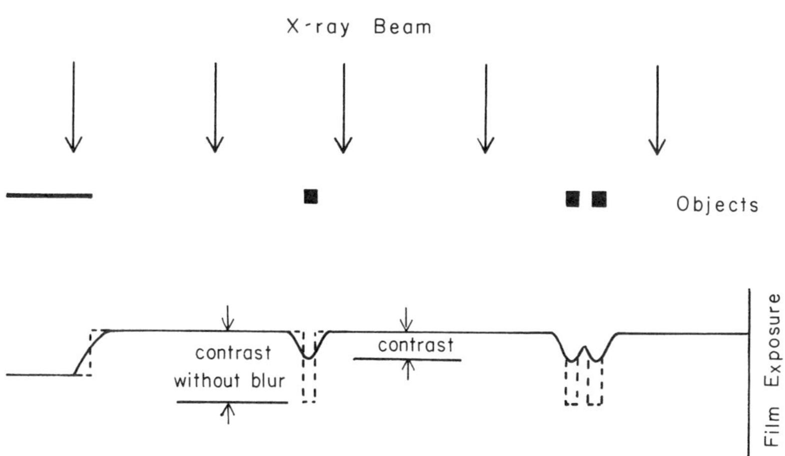

Figure 3. The effect of blur on image quality.

tion of the amount of unsharpness. The classical name for the zone of blur, or unsharpness, that occurs at the edge of a shadow image is penumbra. In x-ray imaging, the amount of unsharpness is equal to the blur. The two terms are essentially synonymous. Unsharpness expresses a characteristic of the image that is produced by the blurring within the imaging system; or, in other words, the blurring process produces unsharp images.

Detail

Detail is an essentially subjective characteristic of an image which describes its ability to show small objects or structural features. The detail in an image is generally dependent on the three more quantitative factors—contrast, blur, and noise. The effect of blur on the detail of the image of a small object is illustrated in the center of Figure 3. In the absence of blur, the film exposure profile is described by the dotted line. The image of the object is well defined and sharp, and the contrast is maximum with respect to the surrounding background. Blurring spreads the image and reduces the contrast, as shown. The small object becomes less visible in the image. Detail is reduced by blur.

Resolution

Resolution describes the ability of an imaging system to form a distinct image of two or more objects located close together. As two objects are brought closer together, the blurred images begin to overlap and merge into one. The resolving ability of the imaging system is generally specified in terms of the minimum distance between objects at which they are detectable as separate objects in the image. For small pointlike objects, the minimum resolving distance is approximately equal to the blur width. The system with the least blur is said to have the best resolution. This is because it can resolve small objects that are located closer together. Resolution is inversely related to blur. Increasing the blur in a system decreases its resolution or resolving ability.

Blur is difficult to measure directly in an x-ray imaging system, and is usually determined by first measuring the resolution. This can be done by making a radiograph of an object that consists of sets of lead strips. Such an object and the resulting radiograph are shown in Figure 4. Each set of strips within the object is characterized by a specific separation distance or spacing frequency. This is generally specified in terms of the number of line pairs per millimeter. A line pair consists of one lead strip and one adjacent space. The resolution of a given system is specified in terms of the maximum spatial frequency or number of line pairs per millimeter that can be imaged. The major problem with this approach is that, in a given image,

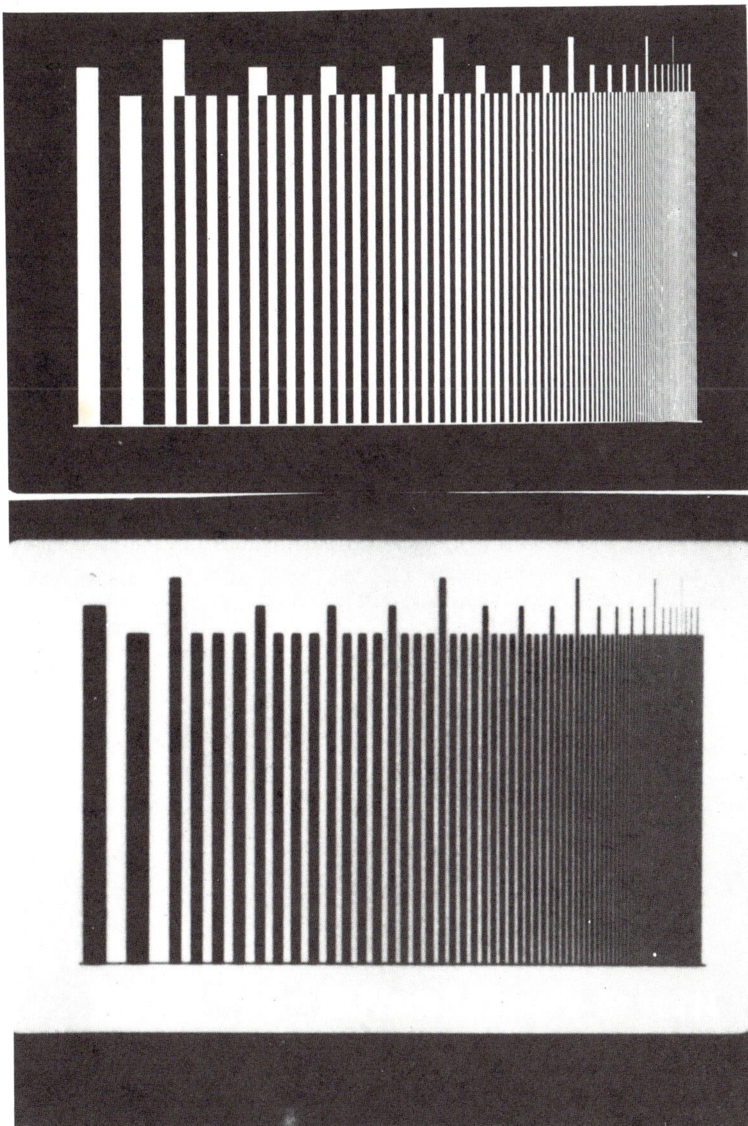

Figure 4. A test object for determining x-ray system resolution and the resulting radiograph. Notice the decrease in contrast between strips and spaces at the higher spacing frequencies.

it is not always possible to determine the exact point at which the lines are no longer visible. This is because the contrast between the strips and spaces gradually decreases with increased spacing frequency. A graph of contrast (between strips and spaces) with respect to spacing frequency is shown in Figure 5. A graph of this relationship between contrast and spacing frequency is known as the contrast transfer function, CTF, of the imaging system. The shape of the curve depends, to some extent, on the major source of blur within the system. For example, the typical CTF curve associated with focal spot blur usually has a specific point at which the contrast becomes 0. This is commonly referred to as the disappearance frequency. This point would represent the resolution limit or resolving ability of the system. When the major source of blur is the receptor, i.e., the intensifying screen or image intensifier tube, the curve might not show a distinct 0 contrast point. Some criteria must be established for defining the maximum resolution point. It is common practice to specify the resolution of such a system as the spacing frequency in line pairs per millimeter, at which the contrast falls to some relatively low value, typically 3%. When comparing resolution values of different systems this should be taken into consideration. For example, if one manufacturer arbitrarily uses a 3% contrast, the resolution values will be higher than those from a company that uses 10%, even if the systems are identical.

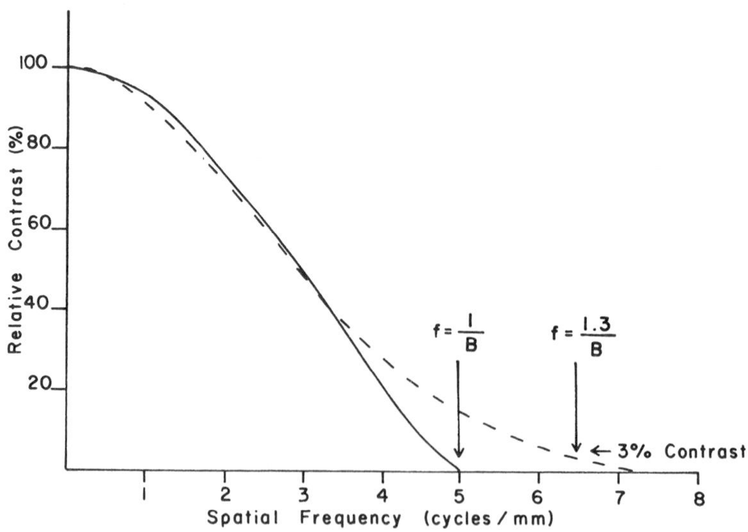

Figure 5. The contrast transfer function associated with two types of blur. The solid line (——) is characteristic of motion and focal spot blur. The dotted line (– – –) is generally characteristic of receptor blur.

The relationship between blur and resolution for a test object of the type shown in Figure 4 is illustrated in Figure 6. A film density (exposure) profile is shown for several sections of the test object. The distance scale is marked in units of blur width. The actual value of the blur width is determined by characteristics of the imaging system and is discussed later. The point here is to establish the relationship between blur width, whatever its value might be, and resolution in line pairs. In the first section the test object line spacing is 0.25 line pairs per blur width. In the density profile it is noted that at point A, which is in the middle of a space, the density is unaffected by blur. A similar situation exists for point B, which is located in the shadow of a strip. The contrast is related to the ratio of the densities at points B and A. The effect of blur is apparent at the strip edges. On the film this represents a gradual change in density from the low value of the strip area to the maximum value in the space area at point A. For this particular line spacing, the blur zones do not overlap and the contrast between the middles of the strip and space areas is unaffected. However, if the average density is considered in each segment, blur must be taken into account. In segment A the average density is reduced by blur at the edges, which produces a corresponding increase in the density of segment B. This produces a decrease in the average contrast between these adjacent line and space areas.

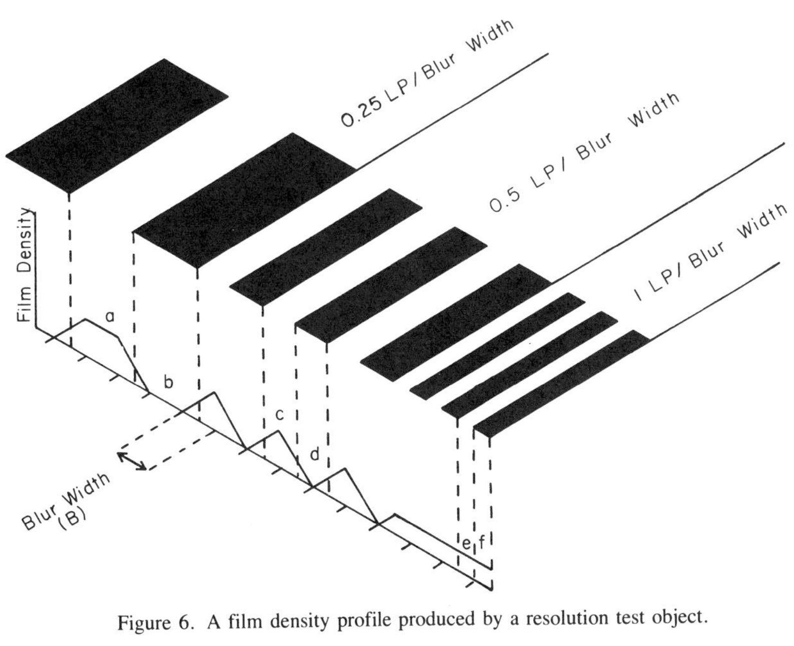

Figure 6. A film density profile produced by a resolution test object.

Where the line spacing is 0.5 line pairs per width, the blur zones meet, but do not overlap. This produces additional reduction in the average contrast between the line and space areas. However, there would normally be sufficient contrast to permit distinction between the lines and spaces in this set.

When the line spacing frequency is increased to 1 line pair per blur width, the blur zones overlap in such a way that there is no contrast between adjacent line and space segments, such as at points E and F. This line spacing, or frequency, is the upper resolution limit. It is also referred to as the disappearance frequency because the lines are no longer visible in the image. This illustration shows that, as the line pair frequency of a test object increases with respect to the x-ray systems blur width, the contrast gradually decreases and finally disappears, as shown graphically in Figure 5. Since the resolution limit is one line pair per blur width, the resolution limit in line pairs (lp) per millimeter is:

$$\text{Resolution (lp per mm)} = 1/\text{blur (mm)}$$

This relationship applies specifically to blur, which has a rectangular exposure profile, which is normally produced by motion and most focal spots. This type of blur produces a CTF that has a definite 0 contrast frequency. As shown in Figure 5, the CTF of most receptor blur does not have a distinct upper limit, but approaches 0 contrast very gradually. The limiting resolution is generally considered to be the spatial frequency at which the contrast transfer has dropped to some designated value, such as 3%. The approximate relationship between equivalent blur and resolution limit for this type of blur is given by:

$$\text{Resolution (lp/mm)} = \frac{1.3}{\text{equivalent blur (mm)}}$$

Blur and Contrast

Perhaps the best description of the image blurring process is that it spreads the image of each point within the patient into the surrounding image area. Since this occurs for all points within an image, the exposure through one object point mixes with the exposure through adjacent points. If the exposures are the same, such as for points within a large uniform object, blurring has no effect on the image. Near the edge of an object, however, blurring mixes the exposure from the object and background, which produces the appearance of an unsharp edge to the object. For most large objects more than a few millimeters wide, blurring of the edges does not

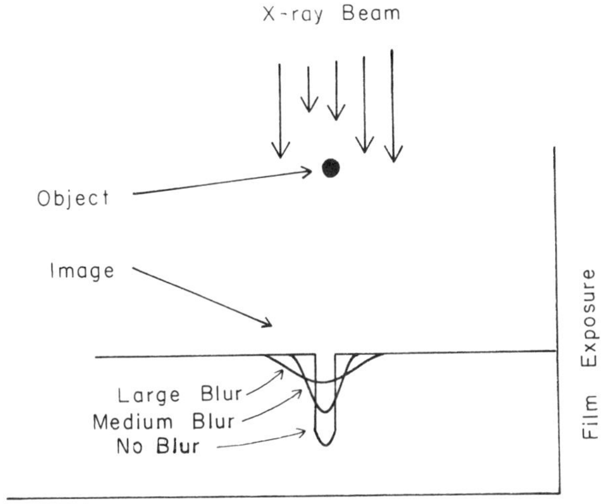

Figure 7. The reduction in contrast of small object images because of blur.

significantly affect the diagnostic quality of an image. Blurring is significant, however, in the imaging of small objects or structural features. As indicated earlier, the basic effect of blur is to reduce the contrast of the object by spreading the image into the surrounding background area, as seen in Figure 7. Objects, such as small calcifications, media-filled vessels, etc., generally produce low subject contrast because of object penetration. Blurring can further reduce the contrast and cause small objects to become undetectable.

SOURCES OF BLUR

In the typical x-ray imaging system there are three potential sources of blur. As indicated earlier, these are the receptor, the focal spot, and motion during the time of exposure. By knowing the factor that determines the amount of blurring, it is often possible to adjust operating conditions or to select system components that will reduce the blur to an acceptable level.

Before proceeding with a discussion of the various types of blur, it is necessary to establish the relationship of several distances within the imaging system. Figure 8 shows the three basic distances. The focal spot-to-receptor distance, frd, is always the sum of the focal spot-to-object distance, fod, and the object-to-receptor distance, ord. With respect to image formation and image quality, the significant parameters are not the actual distances, but certain distance ratios.

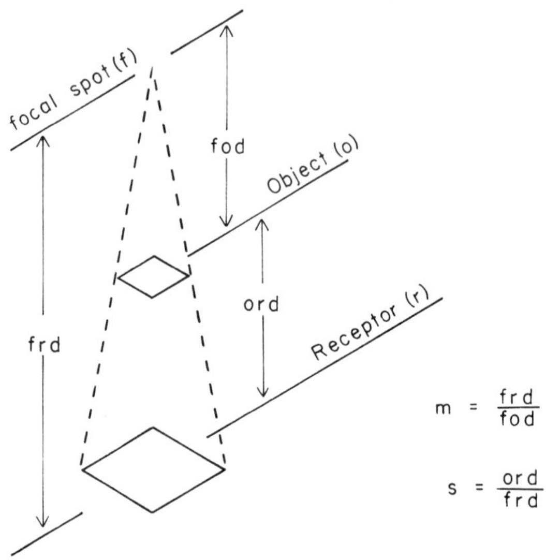

Figure 8. Distances and distance ratios in an x-ray imaging system.

In the formation of an x-ray image, the image will always be larger than the object if the object is separated from the receptor. The amount of enlargement, or magnification, is equal to the ratio of the frd to fod. Magnification, m, is increased by either increasing the frd or bringing the object closer to the x-ray tube, which decreases the fod.

Another useful relationship is the ratio of the ord to the frd. This quantity, s, is used to specify the distance between the object and receptor, ord, in relationship to the total distance between focal spot and receptor. It is helpful to think of a scale running from the receptor to the focal spot. The receptor would be located at the zero-end and the focal spot at the other end, which has a value of 1. The position of the object being radiographed can now be specified with respect to this scale. For example, if it is located at s 0.2 on the scale, the ord is 20% of the frd. It will be shown below that for certain types of blurring the blur value is dependent on s, rather than the actual distance between object and receptor.

When blur is given a specific value, the location within the imaging system must be specified. Blur is enlarged just like the image of an object. The two locations where blur values are generally specified are at the receptor input surface (plane) or at the location of the object being radiographed. For example, if an x-ray system has a blur value of 0.3 mm when measured in the object plane, and a magnification factor of 1.2, the image

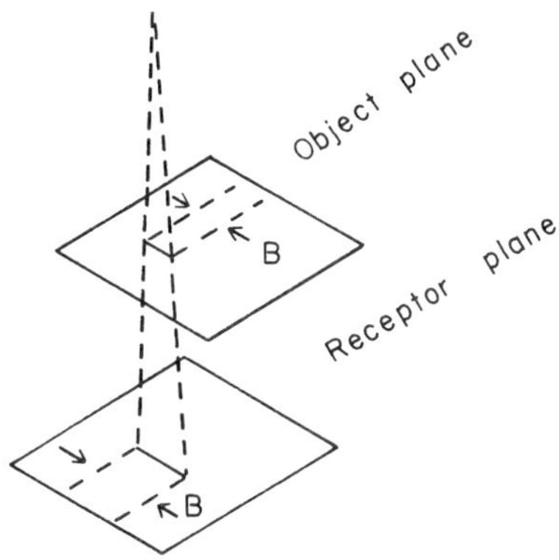

Figure 9. Relationship of blur in the object and receptor planes.

at the receptor location will have a blur value of 0.3 × 1.2 or 0.36 mm. This can also be considered in the other direction. If an imaging system has a blur value specified at the receptor, the amount of blur with respect to the object size is found by dividing by the magnification factor. In all cases, as shown in Figure 9, the relationship between the blur with respect to the size of the object, and as measured at the receptor surface, is just the magnification, m.

Motion Blur

Blurring will occur if the object being imaged moves during the exposure. The amount of blur in the object plane is equal to the distance moved during the exposure, d. As shown in Figure 10, the blur value at the receptor is larger and is in proportion to the magnification factor, m. The effect of motion on each point within the object is to reduce contrast and spread the image over a larger area, as indicated in Figure 10.

In cases where motion of body parts cannot be temporarily halted, motion blur is minimized by reducing exposure time.

One general misconception regarding motion blur is that it is increased by magnification. Although it is true that the blur at the receptor surface is increased, the image quality generally depends on the amount of blur with respect to the object size. This value is not affected by magnification.

Receptor Blur

If the receptor input surface that absorbs the x-ray beam has significant thickness, blur will be introduced as this point. Blurring of this type gener-

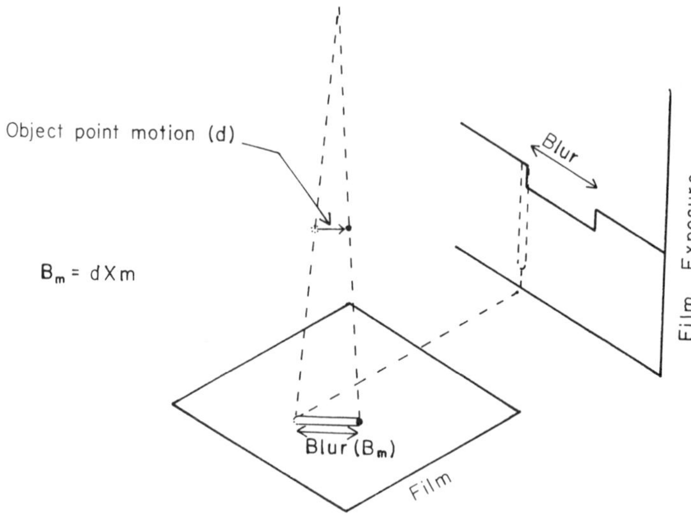

Figure 10. Motion blur.

ally occurs in significant quantities in the input phosphor layers of intensifying screens and image intensifiers. The mechanism for blur production is illustrated in Figure 11. X-ray photons which pass through a point within the object are absorbed by the phosphor layer and converted into light. The light which is created along the x-ray "path" spreads into the surrounding portion of the phosphor layer. When the light emerges from the phosphor it might cover an area that is larger than the object point. In other words, the x-rays that pass through each point within an object will form an image which is blurred into the surrounding area. Because this type of blur is caused by the spreading or "diffusing" of light, the blur profile will generally have a shape different from that of motion blur. In most cases the blur profile will be "bell-shaped" or Gaussian in nature. Because it is somewhat difficult to specify an exact blur dimension, receptor blur is more appropriately described in terms of an effective blur value. The amount of blur is primarily dependent on the thickness of the phosphor layer. In a given imaging system, the blur value with respect to the size of the object can be decreased by introducing magnification. This is illustrated in Figure 12. Here a small round object is being imaged. The presence of receptor blur produces a zone of unsharpness around the periphery. As mentioned previously, the actual blur dimension, or width of the unsharpness zone, at the receptor surface is fixed by the receptor characteris-

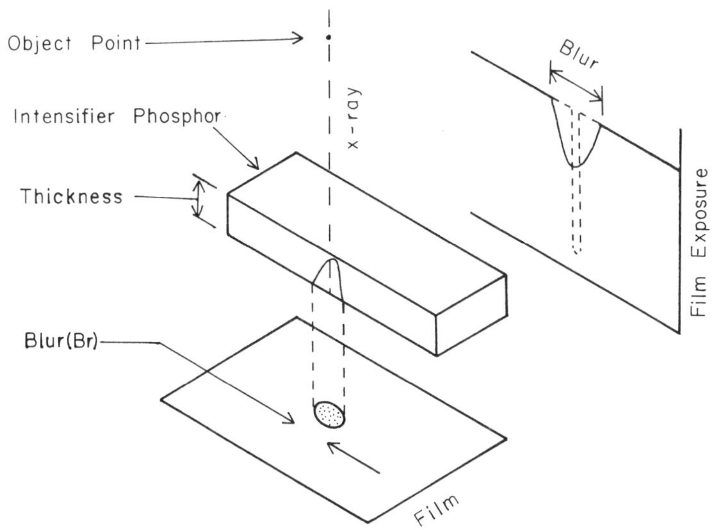

Figure 11. Blur produced in receptors.

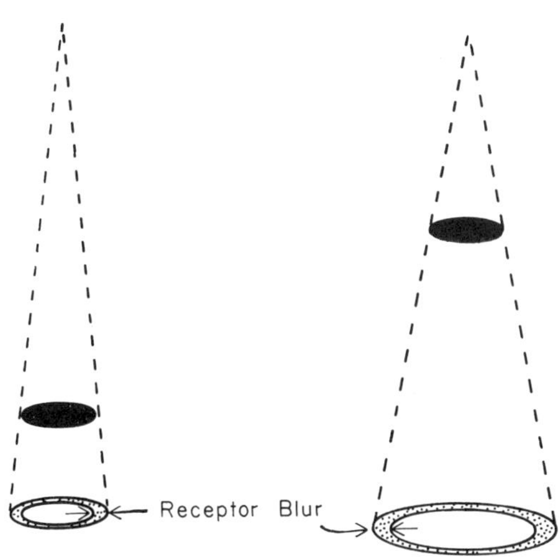

Figure 12. Relationship of receptor blur to image size for two different magnification values.

tics and is unaffected by magnification. In the left portion of the illustration, where magnification is relatively small, the blur covers approximately one-third of the image. When magnification is increased, as shown at the right, the relative blur-to-image size is decreased. Receptor blur in the object plane, B_r, is related to the position of the object, s, by

$$B_r = B_{ro} (1 - s)$$

where B_{ro} is the equivalent blur value of the receptor measured at the receptor surface. Although magnification can be used to reduce receptor blur with respect to object size, it must be approached with caution. There is another type of blur which is discussed below that increases with magnification.

Focal Spot Blur

All x-ray tube focal spots have some finite size, and this contributes to image blur. Consider the example shown in Figure 13. X-rays through each point of the object from the focal spot will diverge and form a blurred

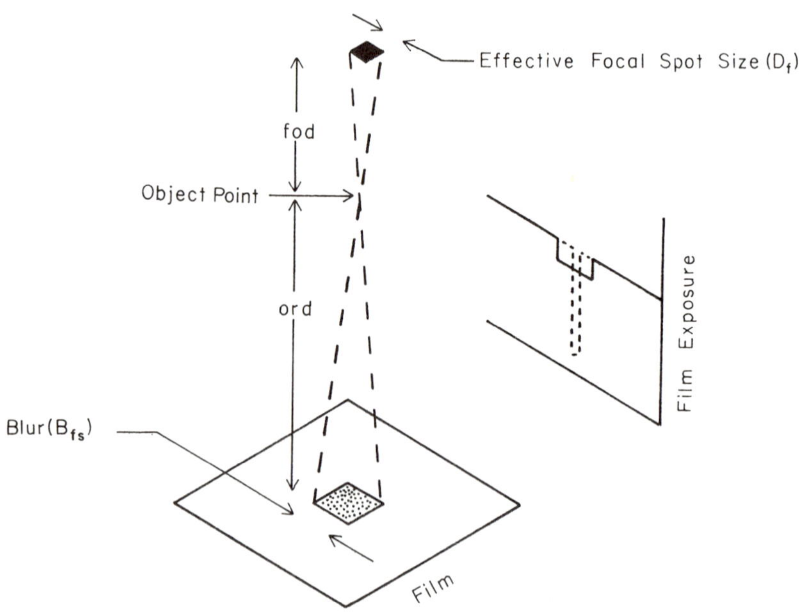

Figure 13. Blur produced by the finite size of a focal spot.

image of the object point. The blur value, with respect to the object size, is given by

$$B_f = F \cdot s$$

where F is the dimension of the focal spot. It should be noted that the value of focal spot blur, for a given focal spot size, is directly related to the position of the object on the s scale. If the object is in direct contact with receptor (s = 0), focal spot blur vanishes. As the object is moved away from the receptor, the blur increases in direct proportion to the value of s. The significance of this is illustrated in Figure 14. In the left portion of the illustration, where the value of s is approximately 0.2, the focal spot blur is relatively small in comparison to the size of the image. When the object is moved away from the receptor, as shown in the right-hand portion, two things happen. Both the image and blur are magnified. The blur value is increased in proportion to the image size, causing a deterioration in image quality.

A distinction must be made between the focal spot dimension, which determines its blur characteristics, and the focal spot size, as specified by tube manufacturers. In a later chapter it will be shown that because of several factors there is a significant difference between the generally stated size of a focal spot and its "blur-producing" size. Blur is related to

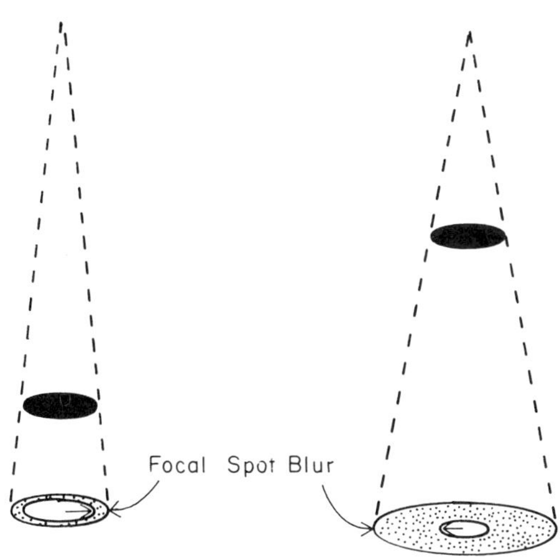

Figure 14. Relationship of focal spot blur to image size for two different magnification values.

the equivalent size of a focal spot, rather than its actual dimensions. The equivalent size is defined as the size of a rectangular focal spot with uniform x-ray emission over its surface which will produce the same blur as the focal spot in question.

COMPOSITE BLUR

It has been shown above that the three potential sources of blur in an x-ray imaging system are: 1) motion; 2) receptor; 3) focal spot. The total blur in an image is a composite of the three different types of blur. In some situations one source of blur, for example, the focal spot, might be much more predominant than the others. When this occurs, the total blur is essentially equal to the largest blur value.

In order to determine the total or composite blur in a system, it is necessary to properly combine the three blur values. Although the exact relationship may vary, depending on conditions, it is generally accepted that the total blur value is given by

$$B_t = \sqrt{B_r^2 + B_f^2 + B_m^2}$$

For example, if: receptor blur, B_r, = 0.3 mm; focal spot blur, B_f, = 0.2 mm; and motion blur, B_m, = 0.2mm; the total blur, B_t, would be found by substituting in the above equation as follows:

$$B_t = \sqrt{(0.3)^2 + (0.2)^2 + (0.2)^2} = 0.41\text{mm}$$

Blur Along s Scale

It was shown earlier that blur from two sources, the receptor and the focal spot, depends on the position of the object with respect to the s scale. As an object is moved away from the receptor, focal spot blur increases and receptor blur decreases. This means that the position of the object on the s scale as shown in Figure 15 should be taken into account when considering the blur characteristics of an x-ray system. Another important aspect of this is that, for most x-ray imaging systems, there is some object position on the s scale which will produce minimum blur. Moving the object in either direction, toward or away from the receptor, will cause the blur to increase.

The relationship between blur and object position is easy to visualize by using a blur nomograph as shown in Figure 16. The nomograph has three scales: one is blur; one is focal spot size; and the third is the position of the object, or s scale. The lines representing the blur from the three different sources are drawn on the diagram according to the following simple rules.

The line representing receptor blur is drawn between a point on the

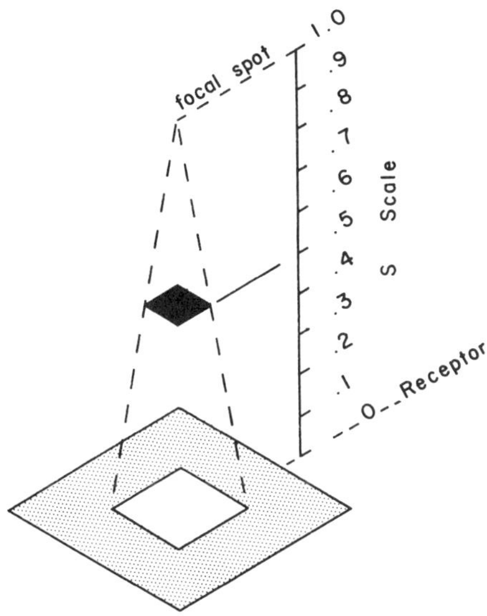

Figure 15. Object position on the s scale.

blur scale which represents the equivalent blur of the particular receptor being used and a point located at a value of 1 on the s scale.

The line representing focal spot blur is drawn between the point at which the blur and s scales intersect and a point on the focal spot scale which corresponds to the size of the focal spot.

The line for motion blur is drawn horizontally and intersects the blur scale at a value which is equal to the distance the object moved during the exposure interval.

The three lines represent the blur of an object from three different blur sources. The composite, or total blur, is found for any point on the s scale by combining the three blur values using the equation discussed above. It is of special significance that the total system blur usually has a minimum value at some point on the s scale. One exception to this is when the major source of blur is motion, in which case the total blur is essentially the same at any point along the s scale. However, when most of the blur arises from the receptor and the focal spot, a distinct minimum point is usually present. The position of the minimum blur point along the s scale depends on the characteristics of the receptor and the focal spot. If the receptor has a relatively low characteristic blur value, the minimum point will be located in the lower portion of the s scale which represents a position close to the

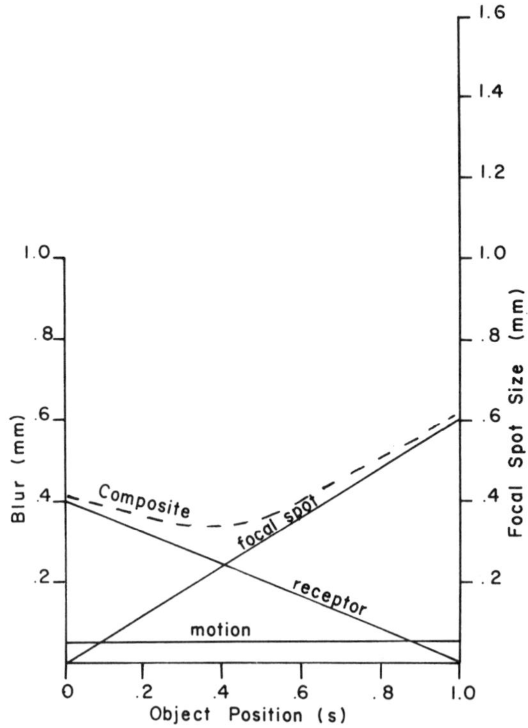

Figure 16. The relationship of blur to object position.

receptor surface. Either increasing receptor blur or decreasing focal spot size will shift the minimum blur point to higher values on the s scale. Inspection of the diagram leads to the following very significant observations:

1. When an object is located near the receptor surface (low s scale values), the total blur is essentially a function of the characteristic receptor blur.
2. As an object is moved away from the receptor surface (high s scale values), the focal spot becomes the major determining factor in overall system blur.

MODULATION TRANSFER FUNCTION

The modulation transfer function (MTF) is a graphical description of the blur or resolution characteristics of an x-ray system or its individual com-

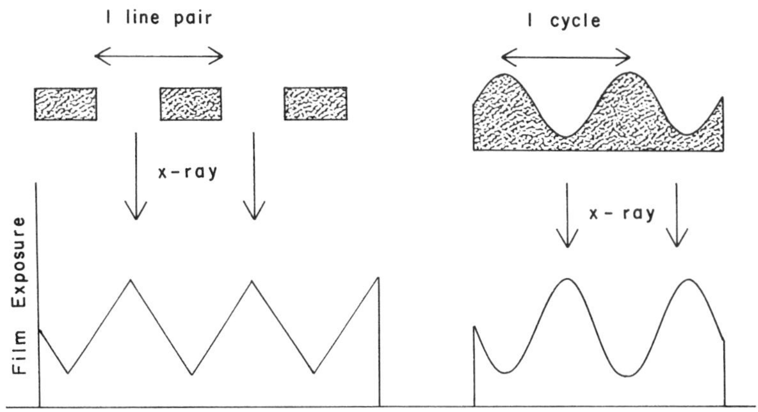

Figure 17. Comparison of test objects for determining the CTF and MTF of an imaging system.

ponents. In many respects, the MTF is similar to the contrast transfer function (CTF) shown in Figure 5. The difference is that, whereas the CTF describes a system's ability to image line pairs, the MTF describes the ability to image an object with "sine wave" shapes, as shown in Figure 17. Rather than a line and space, as in the CTF test object, a true MTF test object would have peaks and valleys, as shown. Actually, the MTF is seldom determined by using such a test object, but the idea is useful in understanding the concept of MTF. One peak and valley make up one cycle of the object. Such a test object is characterized by its spatial frequency, which is the number of cycles (peaks and valleys) per millimeter of length. In other words, an MTF test object will have a certain number of peaks and valleys (cycles) per millimeter, whereas a CTF test object has a certain number of lines and spaces (line pairs) per millimeter. The ability of a system to image the various spatial frequencies is related to the amount of blur present.

Three sections of a hypothetical MTF test object are shown in Figure 18. For low spatial frequencies, where the peaks and valleys are relatively wide, the image system blur does not spread the peaks and valleys into each other and the image has high contrast. However, as the spatial frequency is increased by packing the peaks and valleys closer together, the blurring begins to blend them and contrast is reduced. Finally, a spatial frequency is reached at which the peak and valley images are completely mixed and all contrast between the two is lost. This would generally be referred to as the resolution limit. When the relative contrast between the

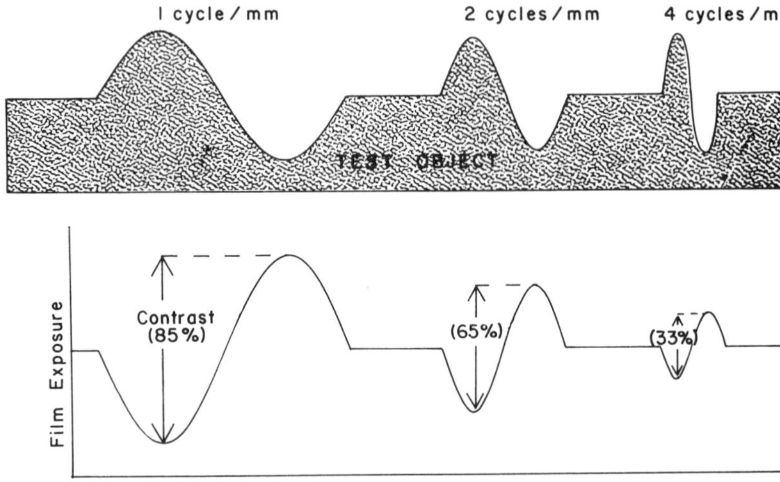

Figure 18. The contrast produced at different spatial frequencies by a hypothetical MTF test object.

peaks and valleys is plotted with respect to spatial frequency (in cycles per millimeter), as in Figure 19, the resulting curve is an MTF.

Most objects do not have just a few frequency components like the test object shown in Figure 18 but contain a continuous spectrum of spatial frequencies. It is helpful to have some concept of the general relationship between an object's size and shape and its spatial frequency components. It is the shape of an object, as seen in a cross-sectional view, which determines its spatial frequency content. Generally speaking, spatial frequency is associated with the rate with which an object's thickness changes. Attention is called once again to the test object in Figure 18. In the portion of the test object with the lower spatial frequency, the variation in thickness (along the length of the object) is not as rapid as in the higher frequency sections. A large flat object of relatively uniform thickness contains low frequency components. However, at the edge of such an object, high frequency components are created by the sudden change in thickness. Generally speaking, small objects of a given cross-sectional shape have higher frequency components than larger objects. This is illustrated in Figure 20. Two round objects, such as the cross-section of blood vessels, are shown. The exposure profile produced by x-raying these is plotted along with one cycle of a sine wave which has approximately the same shape. It is shown that the small object is best approximated by a sine wave

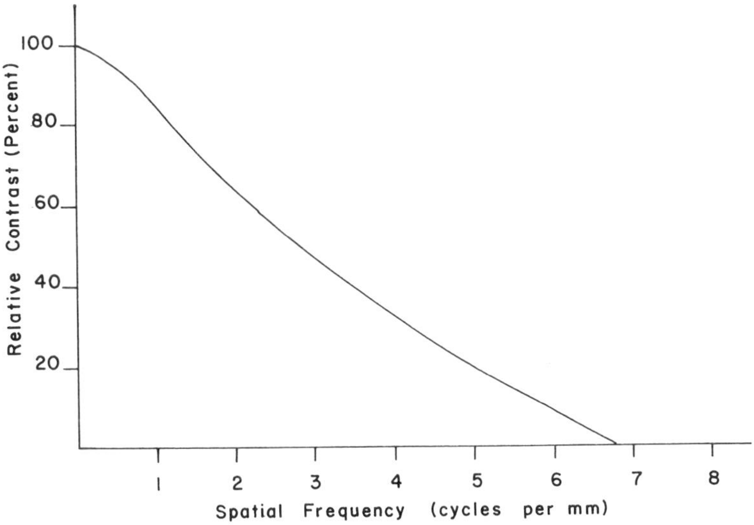

Figure 19. The modulation transfer function (MTF) from the contrast values shown in Figure 18.

which has a frequency of 0.5 cycle per mm, whereas the large object profile is close to a frequency of 0.12 cycle per mm. Shapes such as these are not described by a single frequency, but rather as a combination of many frequencies. The frequency content of such an object can be described in terms of a frequency spectrum of the object as shown in Figure

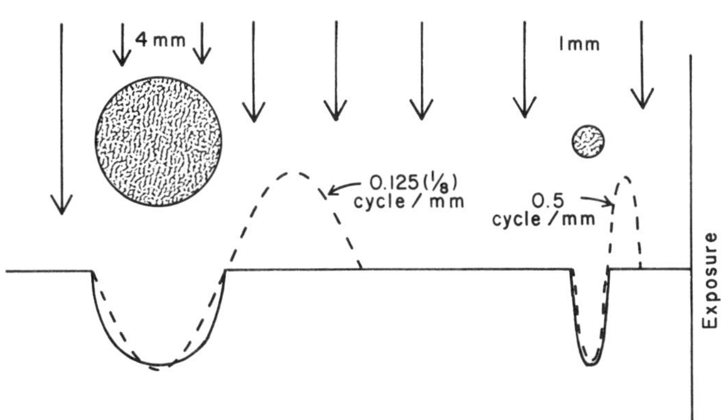

Figure 20. The relationship of spatial frequency to object size.

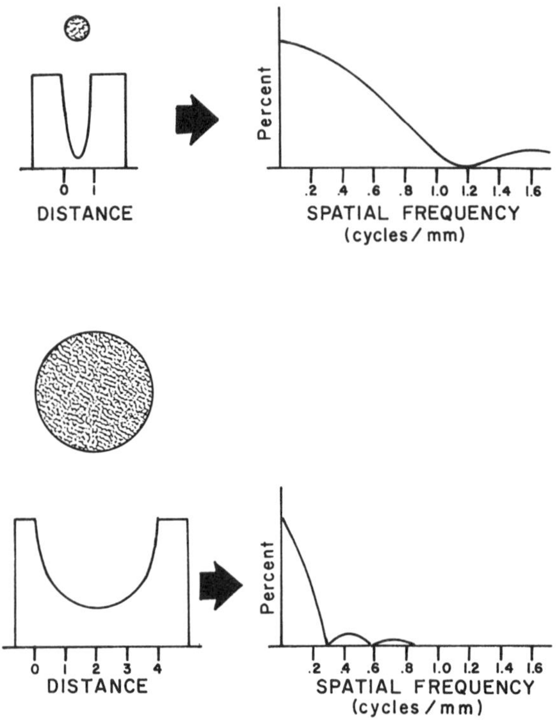

Figure 21. Exposure profiles and spatial frequency spectra for two different object sizes.

21. It indicates the relative composition of the object in terms of different frequency components. An object whose cross-sectional thickness changes rapidly will contain more high frequency components than an object whose thickness changes more gradually.

An object which is to be imaged has certain spatial frequencies which are related to the changes in thickness which produce image contrast. In order to form an unblurred image of the object, the x-ray imaging system must be able to produce sufficient contrast for all spatial frequencies contained in the object. If some of the frequency components are lost in the imaging process, the image will be distorted. For example, if the high frequency components are not present in the image, the image will be blurred. The spatial frequency content of the image which reaches the film is determined by the frequency content of the object being imaged and the MTF of the imaging system. This is illustrated in Figure 22. The image content at a specific frequency is found by multiplying the object content

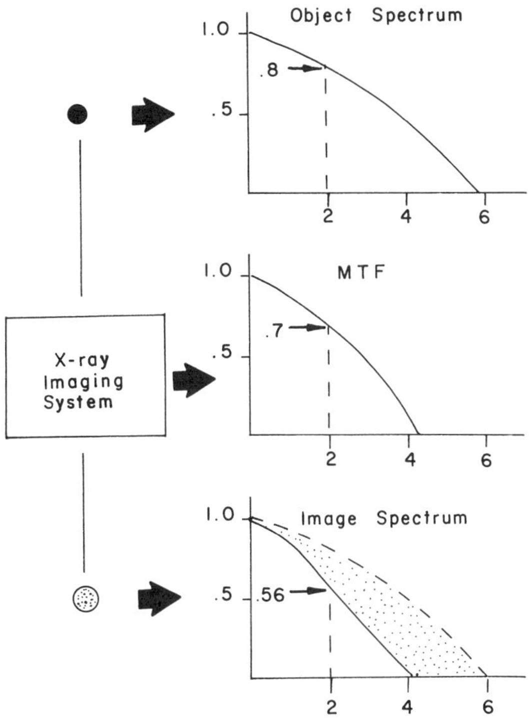

Figure 22. The relationship of an image spatial frequency spectrum to the object spectrum and the MTF of the imaging system.

by the MTF. For example, in Figure 22, the object contains 0.8 (80%) at a frequency of 2 cycles per mm. The MTF at this frequency is 0.7. Multiplying these two quantities shows that the image will contain only 0.56 (56%) at this frequency. The shaded area is the portion of the object spatial frequency spectrum that is lost because of the MTF of the imaging system. Any object frequency components above the resolution limit of the system are completely lost. In effect, the MTF of the imaging system can cut out the higher frequency components associated with an object. The image will be made up only of lower frequency components. Since low frequency components are associated with large objects with gradual changes in thickness, as opposed to sharp edges, the image will be enlarged and blurred.

A property of MTFs which is not possessed by CTFs is their ability to be cascaded. Consider an imaging system where the sources of blur are the focal spot and receptor. The blur characteristics of each of these can be

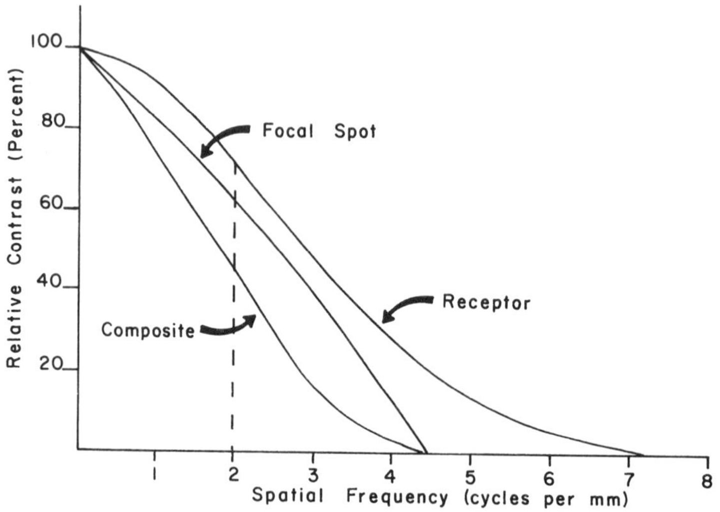

Figure 23. The composite MTF.

described by an MTF curve, as shown in Figure 23. The MTF of the total system is found by multiplying the two MTF values at each frequency. For example, the MTF at 2 cycles per mm for the focal spot is 62% and for the receptor is 72%. At this frequency, the total system will have an MTF value of 44%. It should be observed that a system cannot have frequency components which are higher than the resolution limit of either the receptor or the focal spot. This is equivalent to saying that the total system blur cannot be less than the blur from either of the two sources. If the MTFs of the different blur sources, focal spot, motion, or receptor are significantly different, the one with the lowest limiting frequency (the largest blur) will generally determine the total system MTF. In other words, if one source is producing blur which is significantly larger than from the other sources, the total system blur will be essentially equal to this larger value.

Edge Enhancement

Some imaging systems such as xeroradiography have the ability to enhance object edges. Such systems have a MTF which is quite different from that of the conventional x-ray system. The relationship of the MTF to the edge enhancement process can be seen in Figure 24. It was mentioned previously that a flat object, in principle, has low spatial-frequency regions. Most of the object is "low frequency" but the edge is made up of high

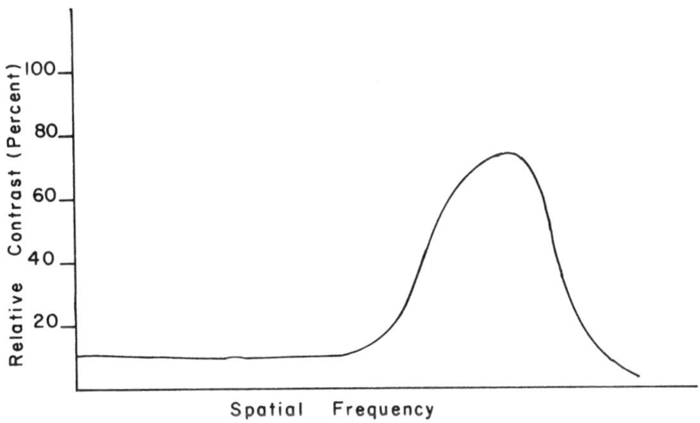

Figure 24. The MTF of an imaging system which produces edge enhancement.

frequency components. The MTF of a system which produces edge enhancement has relatively low contrast at the lower frequencies. Because of this, most of the image contrast will be in the high frequency components which are found in the edges.

Chapter XVI

The Focal Spot

One of the critical elements in an x-ray imaging system is the focal spot. The focal spot is defined as the area on the anode surface in which the bombarding electrons from the cathode produce x-radiation. The size of the focal spot is, in most cases, a compromise between two rather severe constraints. As discussed in Chapter VII, the size of the focal spot limits the operating power of a tube because of heating in the focal spot area. The heat capacity and power rating of a tube are increased by increasing the size of the focal spot. On the other hand, as discussed in Chapter XV, one source of x-ray image blur is directly proportional to the size of the focal spot. Therefore, image quality is usually improved by decreasing focal spot size.

CATHODE TYPES

The size and shape of a focal spot are determined primarily by the design and operating characteristics of the cathode. There are three basic types of cathodes used in diagnostic x-ray tubes. Each has certain characteristics which make it more or less desirable for various types of examinations.

Line Focus Cathodes

Most x-ray tubes in diagnostic equipment use line focus cathodes. A tube of this type is illustrated in Figure 1. The cathode consists of a coiled filament located in a focusing cup. The filament is heated by an electrical current to produce electron emission. The electrons emitted from the hot filament are focused onto the anode by the focusing cup. The focal spot is an approximate image of the hot cathode filament. Because of the arrangement of the cathode within the focusing cup two images are actually created. Therefore, the focal spot consists of two distinct areas from which x-ray photons are emitted. The distance between the two areas of the focal spot is determined by the position of the cathode filament within the focus-

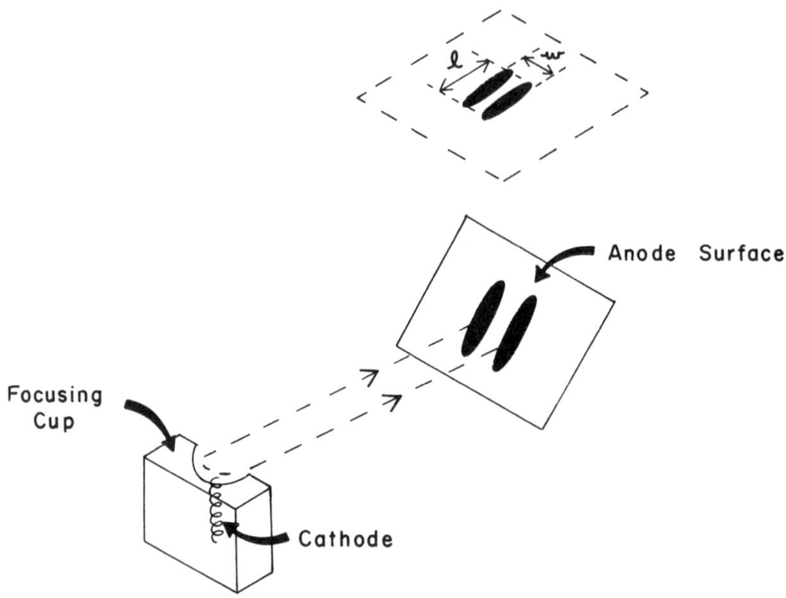

Figure 1. The focal spot shape produced by a line focus cathode.

ing cup. The size of the focal spot is related to the dimensions of the hot cathode. Most x-ray tubes contain two different filaments within the cathode assembly. One is used to form a small focal spot and the other a large spot. This allows the user to select a focal spot size in each examination which will hopefully be a reasonable compromise between blur and heat capacity. Line focus cathodes usually produce focal spots with dimensions in the range of 0.3 mm to 2.5 mm.

In some x-ray tubes a voltage is applied between the filament and the focusing cup. This causes the electrons to be focused into one area rather than the two adjacent areas as shown in Figure 1. This produces a focal spot shape which will contribute less blur than the double area spot. A tube of this type is said to have a biased cathode.

Electron Guns

One shortcoming of the line focus principle is the inability to form small focal spots which would be desirable for certain types of examinations. By using a more sophisticated design with additional electrodes within the tube it is possible to focus the electron beam onto a much smaller area of the anode. The general construction of such a tube is illustrated in Figure 2.

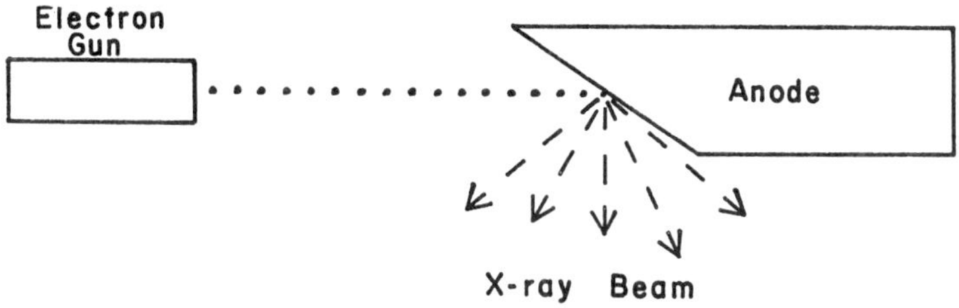

Figure 2. An electron gun x-ray tube.

The cathode and focusing electrodes form an electron gun which produces a beam of precisely controlled electrons. The focusing is adjusted by varying the voltage applied to the electrodes within the tube. A major limitation of such a tube is that it generally cannot operate at high tube currents (MA) which are required in many examinations.

Electron gun x-ray tubes can produce focal spots with a diameter of 0.2 mm or less. They generally fall into the category of tubes which are designated as microfocus devices.

Field Emission

Both line focus and electron gun x-ray tubes use a heated filament to produce electron emission. It is possible to cause electrons to be emitted from a metallic element by applying a sufficiently strong electrical field. An electrical field is created by applying a voltage between two elements such as the cathode and anode within an x-ray tube. The field is created within the space between the two elements. Electrons within the field are subjected to a force which pulls them from the negative to the positive electrode. If the field has sufficient strength it can pull electrons out of the negative element or cathode. This is called field emission. The strength of the field depends on the voltage applied between the two elements and the separation distance. The strength of this field is increased by placing the elements closer together. If the cathode has sharp points the field will be concentrated and electron emission will be enhanced. A cross-sectional view of a field emission x-ray tube is shown in Figure 3. When the high voltage is applied to the tube, electrons are emitted from the cathode points and accelerated toward the anode. The anode is generally in the shape of a cone and the x-ray photons which form the useful beam are emitted in the direction indicated. The focal spot, as viewed from the receptor direction, has an annular shape. In most field emission tubes the focal spot is relatively large. Tubes of this type also have relatively low current limits but can operate at high kilovoltage values.

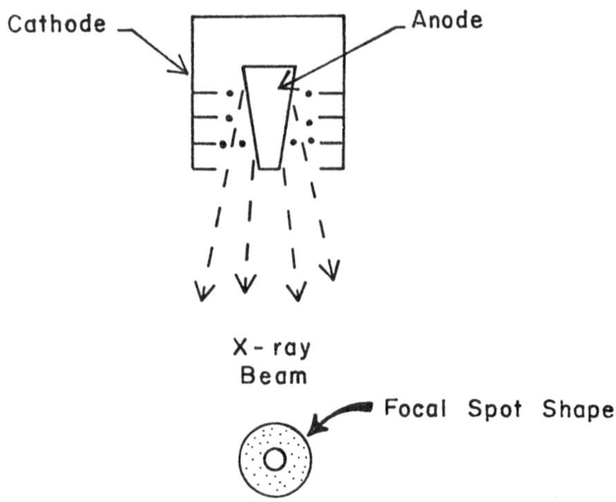

Figure 3. A field emission x-ray tube.

FOCAL SPOT SIZE

The most significant characteristic of a focal spot is its size. Most x-ray tubes have labels attached to them which specify the size of the focal spot. In most instances the labeled size of a focal spot is different from the size which determines the amount of blur. There are several factors which cause these to be different. The size specified by the manufacturer on the label is generally referred to as the nominal size. The dimension which determines the blur characteristics of the focal spot is the effective blur size. The relationship between these two sizes is illustrated in Figure 4.

Manufacturer's Tolerance

It has been a general practice to allow a discrepancy between the manufacturer's stated nominal size and the actual measured size of focal spots. In almost all cases the allowed tolerance is such that the stated nominal size is less than the measured size. The allowed tolerance generally depends on

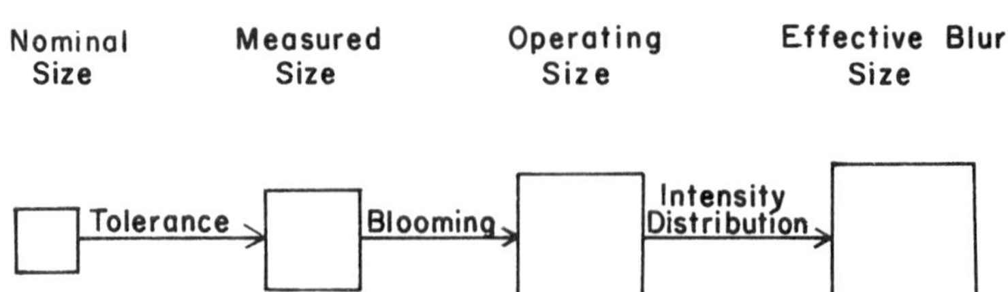

Figure 4. The different sizes of a focal spot.

the size of the focal spot but is as large as 50% for the smaller focal spot sizes. For example, a focal spot which has a measured size of 0.9 mm could be labeled as a 0.6-mm focal spot because it falls within the accepted tolerance values.

Blooming

A common characteristic of many focal spots is that they undergo a change in size with changes in tube current (MA) and voltage (KVP). This effect is known as blooming. If the size of a focal spot is measured at a relatively low tube current the size during operation at higher tube current values can be significantly larger. The amount of blooming with an increase in tube current varies from tube to tube. In some tubes the blooming of the focal spot in one direction is more than in the other. Blooming is generally greater for small focal spots.

kVp generally has less effect on focal spot size than current. Some focal spots will undergo a slight reduction in size with increased kVp.

Intensity Distribution

Most focal spots do not have a uniform distribution of radiation over their entire area. A nonuniform distribution of x-ray intensity will cause a focal spot to have an effective blur size which is different from its actual physical size. The variation in x-ray emission can be represented by an intensity profile as shown in Figure 5. The focal spot with a rectangular intensity distribution (center) will have an effective blur size which is identical to the dimensions of the spot. A focal spot with a double peak distribution (top) will have an effective blur size which is significantly larger than the actual dimension of the spot. This double peak distribution is characteristic of many focal spots produced by a line focus cathode.

The intensity distribution shown at the bottom of the illustration has a so-called Gaussian shape. A focal spot with this type of intensity distribution will have an effective blur size which is less than its actual physical size. Gaussian-shaped focal spots are highly desirable because they have a relatively low effective blur size in comparison to their heat capacity. This is the type of focal spot which is typically produced by electron gun tubes. A focal spot with an approximate Gaussian distribution can be produced in line focus tubes by applying a bias voltage between the cathode elements.

Anode Angle

The size of the focal spot is usually specified with reference to the center of the x-ray beam area or field. Because of the angle of the anode surface the

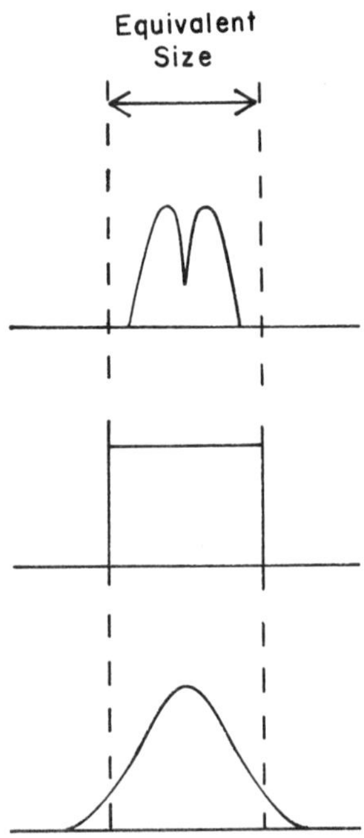

Figure 5. Three focal spot intensity distributions which have approximately the same effective blur size.

effective focal spot size changes with position in the field. It becomes smaller for points toward the anode end and larger toward the cathode end of the field. The variation in effective focal spot size with position within the field is more significant in tubes with small anode angles.

MEASUREMENT OF FOCAL SPOT SIZE

Two different methods are often used to determine the size of focal spots. The principles of the two methods are entirely different and will generally produce different dimensions for the same focal spot. The pinhole camera can be used to determine the actual dimensions of a focal spot whereas the star test pattern is used to determine the effective blur size.

Pin Hole Camera

The principle of the pinhole camera is illustrated in Figure 6. The pinhole camera consists of a very small hole in a sheet of metal such as gold or lead. The pinhole is positioned between the focal spot and a film receptor

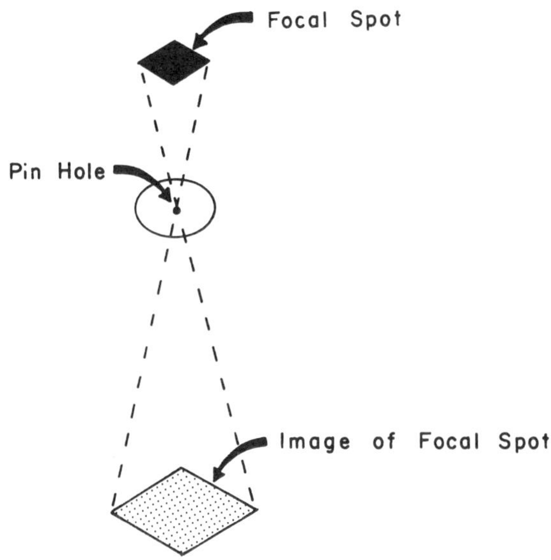

Figure 6. The pinhole method of determining focal spot size.

as shown. When the x-ray tube is energized an image of the focal spot is projected onto the film. The size of the focal spot is determined by measuring the size of the image and applying a correction factor if there is any geometric magnification present. If the pinhole is located at the midpoint between the focal spot and film the image size is equal to the focal spot size and no correction factor is required.

Star Test Pattern

The effective blur size of a focal spot can be measured by using a test object which measures blur or resolution. The most common object used for this purpose has alternating lines and spaces arranged in a star pattern as shown in Figure 7. The first step in determining focal spot size is to make a radiograph with the test object located at approximately the midpoint between the focal spot and receptor. An image is obtained in which there is a zone of blurring at some distance from the center of the object. The distance between the blur zones is measured and used to calculate the size of the focal spot by using the following formula:

$$F = \frac{\pi \theta D}{180(M-1)}$$

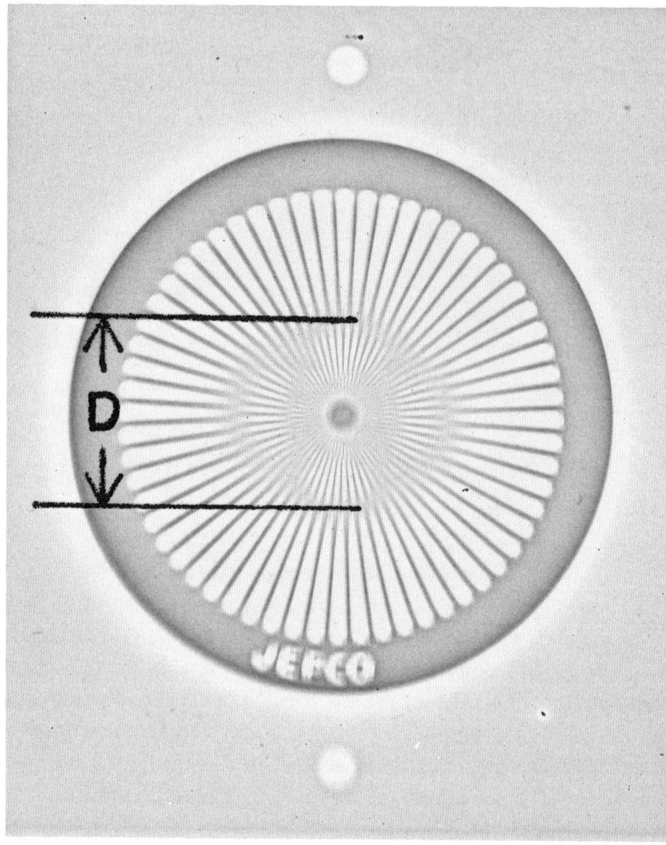

Figure 7. The image of a star test pattern used to determine focal spot size.

where F is the effective blur size, D is the diameter of the blur circle illustrated in Figure 7; M is the magnification factor; θ is the angle of one test pattern segment.

Chapter XVII

Intensifying Screens

When film is exposed by x-radiation, the sensitivity is in the range of 30 to several hundred mR, depending on the type of film and the x-ray spectrum. The receptor sensitivity can be significantly increased by using an intensifying screen. The intensifying screen is a layer of fluorescent material which is placed in contact with the film. The x-ray photons are absorbed by the material within the screen, and a portion of the energy is converted into light as shown in Figure 1. The light passes from the screen to the film and produces the exposure. The increase in film exposure results from the fact that one x-ray photon is converted into many light photons. The intensifying screen increases the number of photons by dividing high energy x-ray photons into low energy light photons. For example, one 60-keV x-ray photon has an energy equivalent to that of 20,000 light photons. However, all of the x-ray beam energy is not converted into light. This is because in most cases a significant portion of the x-ray photons are not absorbed by the screen and also much of the absorbing energy is not converted into light.

A typical intensifying screen will produce a receptor sensitivity of 0.25 to 0.5 mR. This is much more sensitive than film exposed directly by the x-ray beam.

The fluorescent material is in the form of small crystals suspended in a base material to form a layer which is approximately 0.1 to 0.2 mm thick. The screen thickness is chosen to produce a certain compromise between sensitivity and blur. The fluorescent layer is mounted on a backing support material and the front surface is covered with a transparent protective coating. A screen will typically contain a reflective surface between the fluorescent material and the back support. However, in some screens this layer is designed to absorb light. It depends on whether the screen is designed for maximum light output or for minimum blur.

In most applications the intensifying screen and film are contained in a cassette. The purpose of the cassette is to maintain good contact between

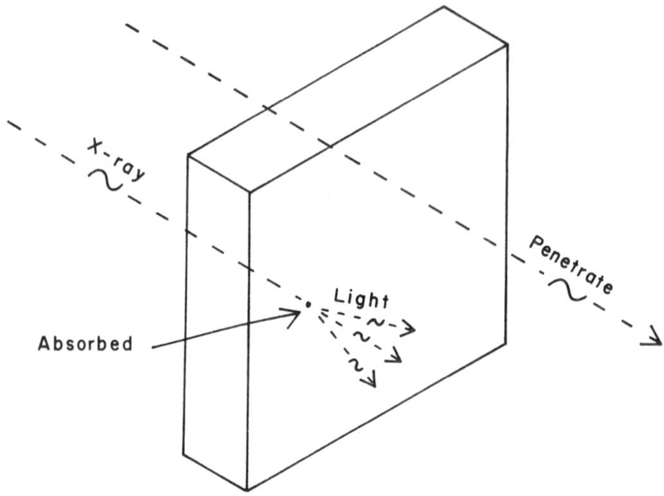

Figure 1. The interaction of x-radiation with an intensifying screen.

the intensifying screen and the film and to protect the film from unwanted light exposure. The typical cassette contains two intensifying screens and is used with a film which has sensitive emulsion on both sides. One screen is mounted on each side of the film. The use of two screens and a double emulsion film increases the overall sensitivity but also produces some increase in blur. In applications such as mammography where it is necessary to minimize blur, cassettes containing only one screen and a single emulsion film are often used. In some x-ray systems the intensifying screens are mounted in film changers rather than in individual cassettes.

SCREEN EFFICACY

The function of an intensifying screen is to absorb the x-ray energy and to convert it into light which can expose the film. One significant characteristic of a given screen is the efficacy of this conversion. Screen efficacy is defined as the ratio of light output to the x-ray exposure input. As shown in Figure 2, screen efficacy and film sensitivity are the two factors which determine the receptor sensitivity. This relationship is:

$$X_m(\text{mR}) = \frac{E_m\ (\text{ergs/cm}^2)}{E_s\ (\text{ergs/cm}^2 \cdot \text{mR})}$$

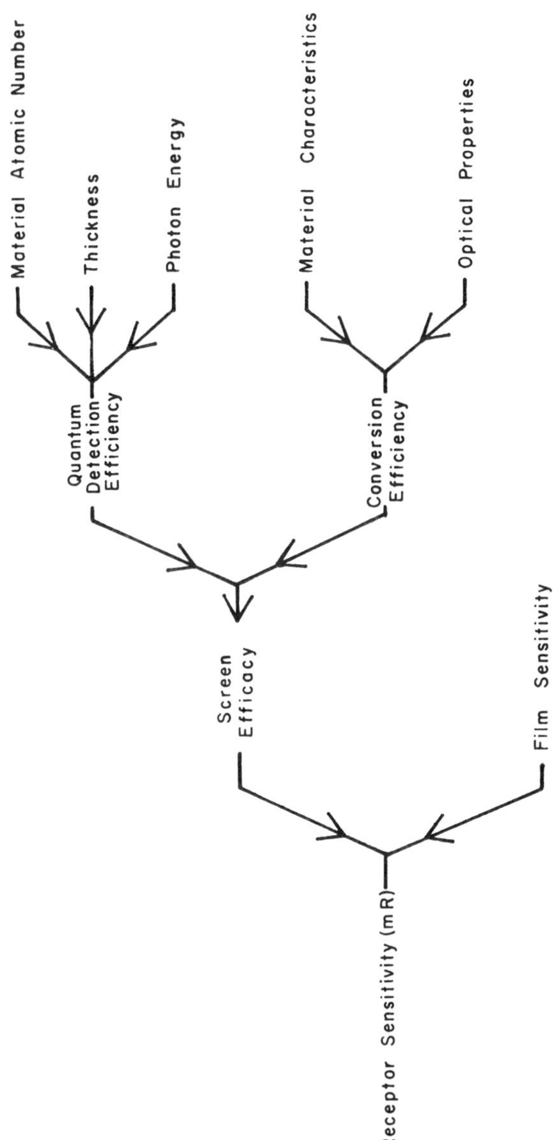

Figure 2. Relationship of receptor sensitivity to intensifying screen characteristics.

where X_m is the receptor sensitivity; E_m is the film sensitivity; E_s is the screen efficacy. For example, if a screen with an efficacy value of 0.005 is used with a film which has a sensitivity of 0.01 the receptor sensitivity would be:

$$X_m = 0.01/0.005 = 2 \text{ mR}$$

The significance of this relationship is that the x-ray exposure required to produce a given film density, X_m, is reduced by increasing the intensifying screen efficacy. The factors which affect screen efficacy are shown in Figure 2. An intensifying screen actually performs a two-step process. The first step is the absorption of the x-ray photons and the second step is the conversion of the absorbed energy into light. The efficiency of both these processes can vary from one type of screen to another and can have a significant effect on screen efficacy.

X-ray Absorption

The ideal intensifying screen would absorb all of the incident x-radiation or have a penetration of 0. Radiation which penetrates the intensifying screen does not contribute to image formation. The fraction of incident radiation which is absorbed by the screen is designated as the quantum detection efficiency (QDE). The factors which determine the value of the QDE are: 1) the material in the screen; 2) the screen's thickness; 3) the x-ray photon energy spectrum.

Most x-ray photons which are absorbed within an intensifying screen are absorbed by photoelectric interactions. Because of this the energy of the K edge has much to do with the absorption characteristics of a screen. It should be recalled that photons have the greatest chance of being absorbed if their energy is slightly above the K edge energy. Photons with energies slightly less than the K edge energy have a significantly higher chance of penetrating the screen without being absorbed.

For many years the most common fluorescent material used in intensifying screens was calcium tungstate. Tungsten, the major absorbing element in calcium tungstate screens, has a K edge at 69.5 keV. As shown in Figure 3, there is a significant change in screen absorption at the K edge energy.

In the mid-1970's a number of different screen materials began to replace calcium tungstate in many applications. Some of these screen materials are gadolinium oxysulfide and barium strontium sulfate.

Several of these contain the so-called rare earth elements. The rare earths are those elements with atomic numbers ranging from 57 to 71. Because the atomic number is lower than that of tungsten (74) the energy of

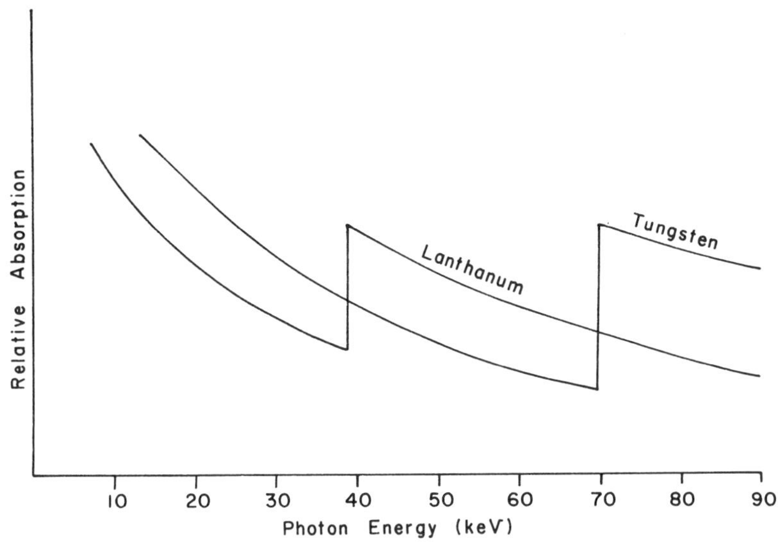

Figure 3. X-ray absorption in two different intensifying screen materials. Lanthanum is a rare earth element.

the K edge will also be lower. This is shown in Figure 3. Because of the lower K edge energy, screens containing the rare earth elements will tend to have better x-ray absorption than calcium tungstate, especially for photon energies less than 69.5 keV.

Since the quantum detection efficiency or screen absorption changes with photon energy there will also be a change in screen efficacy and receptor sensitivity. Figure 3 shows that this change is quite large, especially near the K edge energy. Since most x-ray screens are exposed to beams containing a spectrum of energies, the abrupt changes near the K edge energy are not readily apparent. The relative screen efficacy and receptor sensitivity are shown in Figure 4 for different screen materials and KVP values. It should be noticed that the relative efficacy of one screen material with respect to another changes with x-ray photon energy or KVP.

Quantum detection efficiency is also related to the thickness of the intensifying screen. A thicker screen will absorb more of the x-ray photons and increase overall receptor sensitivity. The problem is that the finite thickness of an intensifying screen produces image blur. For a given application, screens should be selected to give the most desirable compromise between sensitivity and blur.

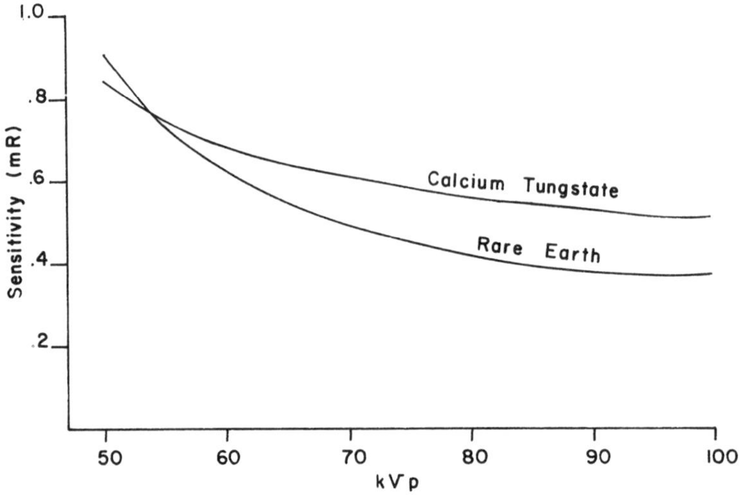

Figure 4. Relationship of sensitivity to kVp for two different intensifying screen materials.

Light Production

A relatively small fraction of the x-ray energy absorbed in intensifying screens is converted into light. The percentage of absorbed energy which is emitted as light is designated as the conversion efficiency. Values range from approximately 3% for calcium tungstate screens to approximately 10% for some of the rare earth materials. The conversion efficiency of a screen is generally a characteristic of the screen material and is not related to the x-radiation. A portion of the light which is created with any screen is absorbed and is not emitted. This can vary from one screen to another because of differences in thickness or the light transmission properties of the binding material.

Light is created in intensifying screens by the process of luminescence. The energy from the absorbed x-ray photons moves some of the screen material electrons to higher energy levels. When the electrons drop back to their normal positions, which are at lower energy levels, the excess energy is emitted as characteristic radiation. If the energy difference between the two electron energy levels is a few electron volts, the emitted energy will be in the form of light.

The energy of the light photons, which determines their color, is a characteristic of the screen material. The light emitted by intensifying screens is usually predominantly either blue or green, although some screens produce considerable light in the ultraviolet region. Figure 5 shows

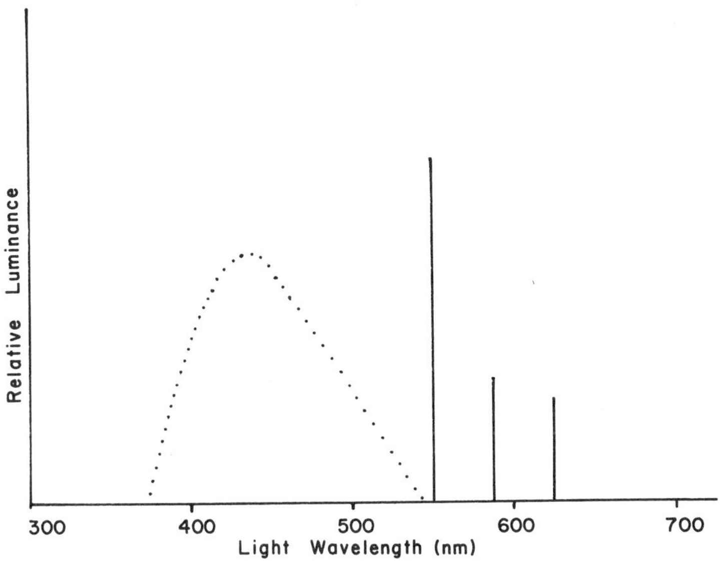

Figure 5. Light spectra for two different intensifying screen materials. Calcium tungstate (– – –) emits in the blue region. The rare earth phosphor (——) emits predominantly green light.

the typical light spectra for two different screen materials. The significance of the color of the light output is that it must be matched with the spectral response of the film in order to produce maximum film exposure.

SCREEN BLUR

X-ray photons which pass through a given object point will be absorbed and produce light along a line passing through the screen, as shown in Figure 6. The light produced along this line will spread and cover a circular area on the film. This introduces blur into an image. The amount of blurring is related to the thickness of the screen. A thick screen which has good x-ray absorption characteristics will also produce a relatively large amount of blur. In intensifying screens there is always a trade-off between sensitivity or efficacy and blur. For a given screen material, blur is approximately proportional to screen efficacy, as shown in Figure 7. This relationship must be taken into account when selecting intensifying screens for a particular application. In an examination, where blur must be kept to a minimum, the screens will have a lower efficacy value and will require more x-ray exposure.

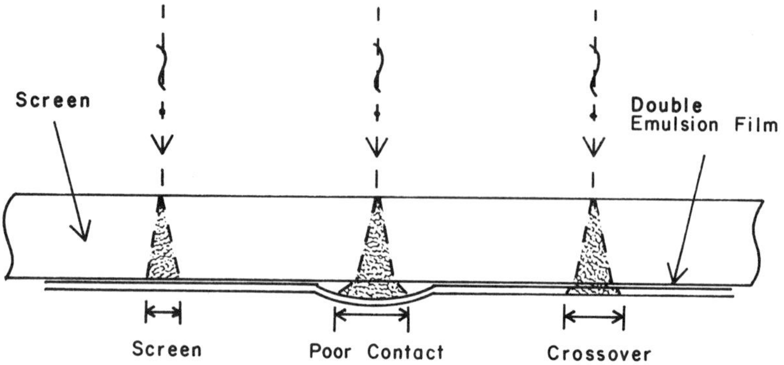

Figure 6. Sources of blur in screen-film receptors.

Most manufacturers have a selection of screens; this allows the user to select an appropriate efficacy-blur combination. Various names are used to designate the different screen types. Those which are located near the midportion of the efficacy-blur range are usually designated as par, medium speed, or as universal screens. Those which have lower efficacy

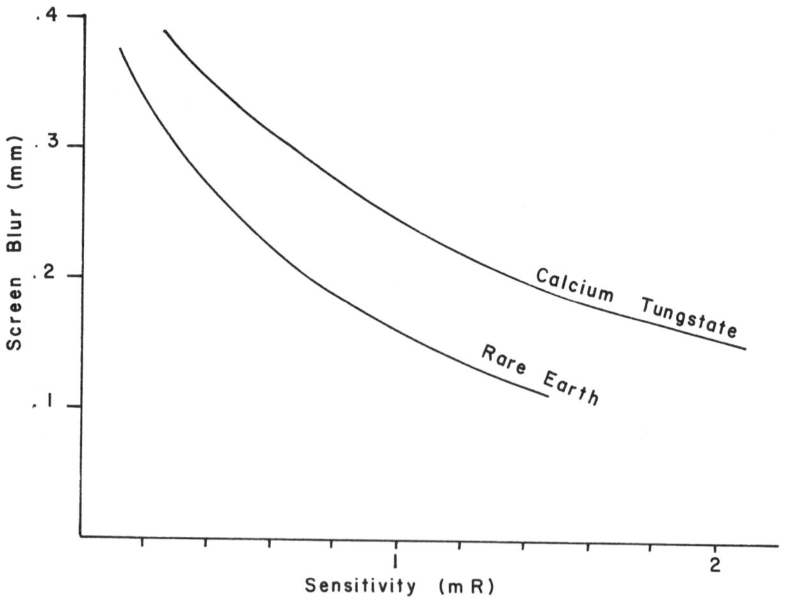

Figure 7. Approximate relationship between screen blur and sensitivity for different screen materials.

and blur values are generally designated as detail screens. Those screens which have relatively high efficacy and blur values are generally designated as high speed screens.

Another cause of blur is poor contact between the screen and film surfaces. As illustrated in Figure 6, this produces additional spreading of the light. In order to minimize blur it is necessary for the cassette or film changer to produce good screen-film contact. The usual test for adequate contact is to radiograph a wire mesh. Areas in which the film is not in direct contact with the screen surface are readily visible.

Another source of blur is ''crossover'' between the two sides of double emulsion film. This occurs when the emulsion layer and the film base do not absorb all of the light. Light from the intensifying screen enters one side of the film and spreads before it reaches the other emulsion layer. Light absorption in the film base is usually higher for ultraviolet light. Therefore, screens which emit ultraviolet light will generally have less blur because of crossover than other screens.

Chapter XVIII

Intensified Radiography

In radiography, with either direct film exposure or with intensifying screens, the energy which ultimately produces the film density is always less than the energy delivered to the receptor surface by the x-ray beam. Two factors account for this: one is that most receptors do not absorb all of the x-ray energy; the other is that the conversion from x-ray energy to film density is relatively inefficient. As indicated earlier, systems using intensifying screens require a median density exposure of approximately 0.25 to 0.5 mR. Although this type of receptor is sufficiently sensitive for many types of examinations, it is not generally appropriate when it is necessary to produce a large number of images, especially in rapid sequence. Receptor sensitivity can be increased well above that of intensifying screens by using electronic image intensifier tubes. The intensifier tube is similar to the intensifying screen in that it absorbs the x-ray beam and converts it into a light image. It differs from the intensifying screen, however, in that it can also amplify, or increase, the intensity of the image. By incorporating an image intensifier tube into the receptor system, sensitivities of 0.02 mR or more can be obtained in certain applications.

The basic system for intensified radiography contains three basic components, as shown in Figure 1. These are: 1) the intensifier tube; 2) an optical system for transferring the light image from the tube to the film; 3) the film. Actually, the optical system and film comprise a camera which is used to photograph the image which appears on the output screen, or phosphor, of the intensifier tube.

INTENSIFIER TUBE

A diagram of an image intensifier tube is shown in Figure 2. As the x-ray beam enters the larger end of the tube it encounters a layer of material which performs two functions. The first is to absorb the x-ray energy, and the second is to convert a portion of the x-ray energy into light. This part of

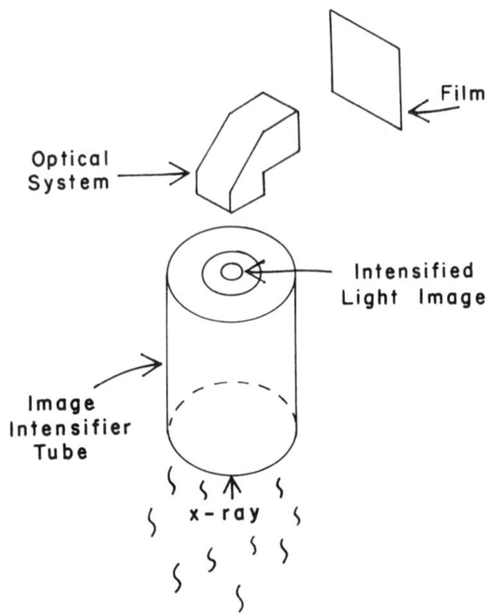

Figure 1. The basic components of a system for intensified radiography.

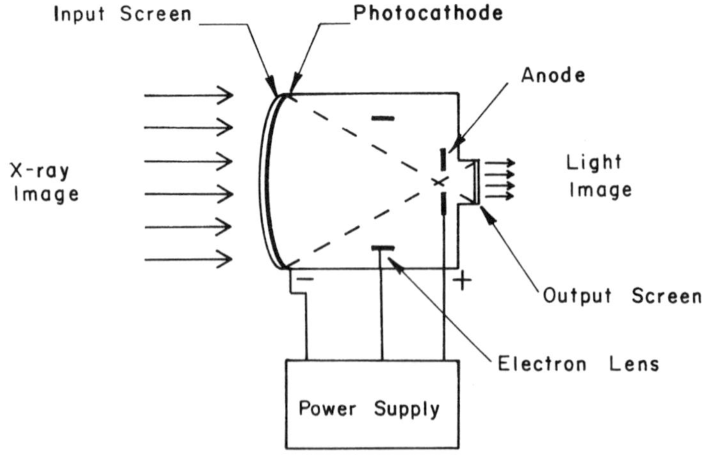

Figure 2. Cross-sectional view of image intensifier tube.

the tube is generally referred to as the input screen or phosphor. Cesium iodide is the most common input phosphor material, although other materials, such as zinc cadmium sulfide, have been used. This part of the tube is somewhat similar in function to an intensifying screen. A thickness is selected which will give a reasonable compromise between x-ray absorption (quantum detection efficiency) and blur. The input phosphor of intensifier tubes will typically absorb 50% or more of the incident radiation.

In direct contact with the input phosphor, there is a second layer of material which forms a photocathode. The function of the photocathode is to convert the light image into an image consisting of electrons. The electrons are emitted from the photocathode into the vacuum space of the tube. The number of electrons emitted at a given point is determined by the x-ray exposure to the adjacent point on the input phosphor.

The electrons leaving the photocathode come under the influence of an electrical force which is created by a relatively high voltage applied to electrodes within the tube. The electrical force accelerates the electrons toward the output screen and gives them an increase in energy. Additional electrodes are located within the tube for the purpose of focusing the electron image onto the small output screen. These electrodes form an electron lens system. The focusing of the image is controlled by varying the voltage applied to the electrodes.

The electrons strike the small output screen where they are absorbed and produce a light image.

Gain

An image intensifier tube is used to increase the intensity of the image. There are two factors which produce this increase. One is the energy gained by the electrons as they pass through the high voltage applied between the photocathode and output screen. This is generally referred to as the electronic gain, G_e. Intensification is also produced by concentrating the large image of the input to the much smaller size of the output screen. This produces the so-called "minification gain." The minification gain factor, G_m, is the ratio of the area of the total input image to that of the output. This can be expressed as:

$$G_m = \frac{\text{input area}}{\text{output area}} = \left(\frac{d_{in}}{d_{out}}\right)^2$$

where d is the diameter of the respective image areas.

A typical output screen diameter is 20 mm. Input phosphor sizes will generally range from 13 to 30 cm (5 to 12 inches). Table 1 gives values for the minification gain factors for several common input phosphor sizes. It should be noticed that a 23-cm (9-inch) tube has more than twice the gain

Table 1. Minification gain and relative exposure input for same light output

Input size	Gain	Relative exposure
13 cm (5 in)	42	1
23 cm (9 in)	132	0.3
30 cm (12 in)	225	0.19

of a 13-cm (5-inch) tube. This is because the gain is proportional to the area rather than the diameter of the input screen. The total gain in intensity produced by an image tube is the product of the electronic and minification gain values.

Some intensifier tubes are designed to operate at two or more input image sizes. The change in size is produced electronically. There are a number of applications in which it is desirable to switch from one input image size to another. The use of a large mode is indicated when it is necessary to film a relatively large area, such as the entire heart. Because of the diverging nature of the x-ray beam, the field of view within the patient is always less than the size of the image at the receptor surface. For example, a 23-cm (9-inch) intensifier input will cover an area of only 13 cm (5.3 inches) at the tabletop under normal operating conditions. The smaller modes produce image enlargement. Since the gain of the image intensifier tube is related to the size of the input image, it changes as a tube is switched from one mode to another. When used in the small mode, the tube will require a higher input exposure to produce the same output image brightness than when in the larger mode.

Up to this point, gain has been used to describe the ability of a tube to increase the intensity of an image. The amount of gain of a tube is determined by comparing the output luminance (brightness) to the luminance of a standard fluoroscopic screen with the same input exposure. This is illustrated in Figure 3. For example, if both the intensifier tube and the fluoroscopic screen are exposed to 1 mR per sec and the respective luminances are 75 and 0.014 nits, the gain of the tube would be the ratio of these two values, or 5,360. Modern intensifier tubes have gain values of 5,000 or more.

Another way of expressing the intensifying ability of a tube is in terms of the conversion factor. The conversion factor is defined as the ratio of the output phosphor luminance, in nits, to the input phosphor exposure rate in milliroentgens per sec. For the example shown in Figure 3, where the output luminance is 75 nits for an input exposure rate of 1 mR per sec, the

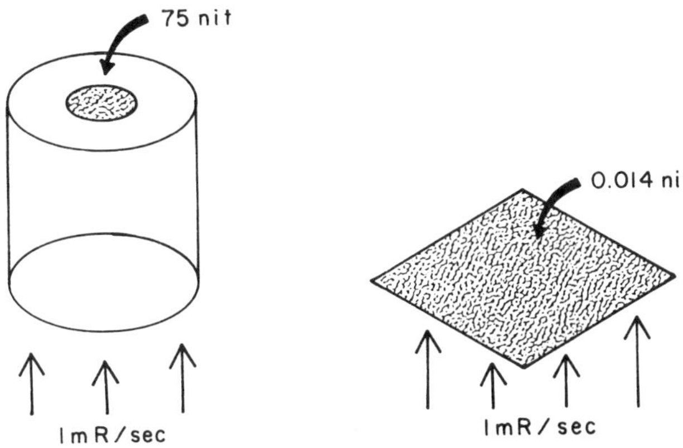

Figure 3. Comparison of the luminance produced by an image intensifier tube and a fluoroscopic screen for the same x-ray input.

conversion factor is 75. Both gain and conversion factor are used for the same purpose, that is, to express the ability of a tube to intensify an image. The use of conversion factor is becoming more common because it is relatively easy to measure and does not require the use of a reference fluoroscopic screen. An approximate relationship between gain and conversion factor is given by:

$$\text{Gain} = 70 \times \text{conversion factor}$$

For example, if a given tube has a conversion factor of 75, the approximate gain would be 5,250.

The major advantage in using an intensifier tube, rather than an intensifying screen, is that it permits films to be made with much less radiation. From that standpoint it would appear that a very high gain value is desirable. However, it will be shown later that a point is reached at which further increases in gain will significantly decrease image quality. This is because as receptor sensitivity is increased, as by increasing intensifier tube gain, the quantity of x-radiation required to produce the film exposure does not contain a sufficient number of photons to produce a smooth image. This results in image degradation because of quantum noise.

OPTICAL SYSTEM

When intensifying screens are used, the light is transferred directly to the film because the film is in direct contact with the screen. This also results in a film image which is the same size as the image from the intensifying

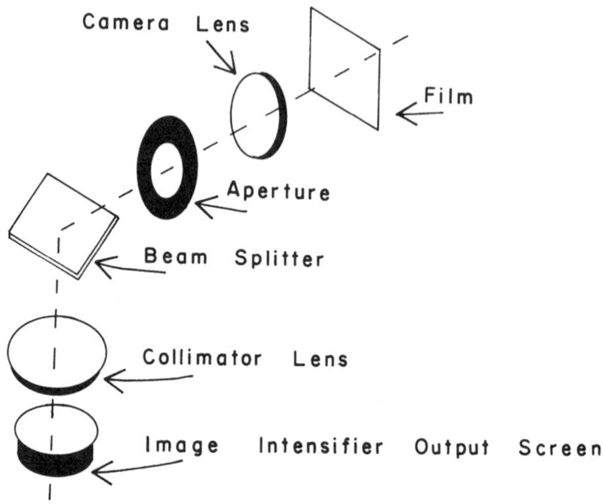

Figure 4. Components of the optical system which transfers the image from the image intensifier to the film.

screen. However, the output image from the typical intensifying tube is only about 20 mm in diameter and must be enlarged before it is applied to the film. In order to achieve enlargement, the film must be separated from the output screen. The transfer of the image from the image intensifier output to the film surface is the main function of the optical system referred to earlier. The basic components of the optical system are shown in Figure 4.

The first component of the optical system encountered by the light from the intensifier output screen is the collimator lens. The function of the collimator lens is to collect the light from the output screen and focus it into a beam of parallel light rays, as shown in Figure 5. The parallel rays are

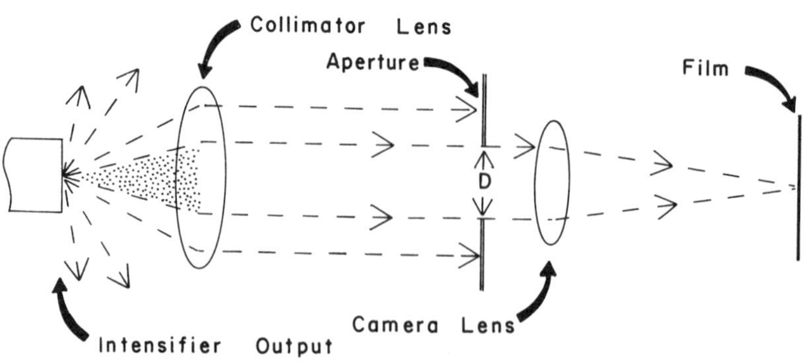

Figure 5. The transfer of light through the optical system.

produced by positioning the lens so that the image intensifier screen is located near the focal point of the lens. One of the fundamental characteristics of a converging lens is that light originating at its focal point will be formed into a beam of parallel rays after passing through the lens. Light originating from points at distances other than the focal length from the lens will be formed into either a diverging or converging beam after passing through the lens. The formation of the image into a parallel beam makes it possible to distribute the image to two or more devices, such as a spot film camera and a video camera for fluoroscopy.

The next element in the path of the light is a beam splitter. A splitter is usually a mirror which is only partially reflective. A portion of the light will be reflected by the mirror to one camera. The remaining light will pass through the mirror to a second camera. In some systems the mirror is attached to a rotating mechanism so that it can be shifted from one camera to another. The mirrors are generally designed to divide the light unevenly between two devices. For example, a 70-30 mirror may be used; this will send 70% of the light to a film camera and 30% to a video camera to form the fluoroscopic image.

After leaving the beam splitter, the light passes through a circular aperture. The aperture is usually adjustable and is used to control the quantity of light reaching the camera. The effective size of the aperture is specified in f numbers which will be discussed in more detail below.

After passing through the aperture, a second lens focuses the light onto the surface of the film to form the final image. This lens is part of the camera and serves the same function as a conventional camera lens. The most significant characteristic of this lens is its focal length. The amount of enlargement in the image between the image intensifier output and the film is given by:

Magnification (m) = focal length of camera lens/focal length of collimator lens

This lens must be selected to give the desired image size on the film as shown in Figure 6. There are five different film sizes generally used in intensified radiography. These are 16 mm, 35 mm, 70 mm, 90 mm, and 105 mm. These are the dimensions of the film. The size of the image area is somewhat less because of sprocket holes and borders. For example, 35-mm film typically has an image area of 25 mm by 18 mm. The image at the intensifier output screen is circular, but all films have either square or rectangular image areas. Because of this, it is impossible to get exact coverage on the film.

For a given film size, it is possible to obtain different degrees of coverage or framing. This is illustrated in Figure 7 for 35-mm film. With

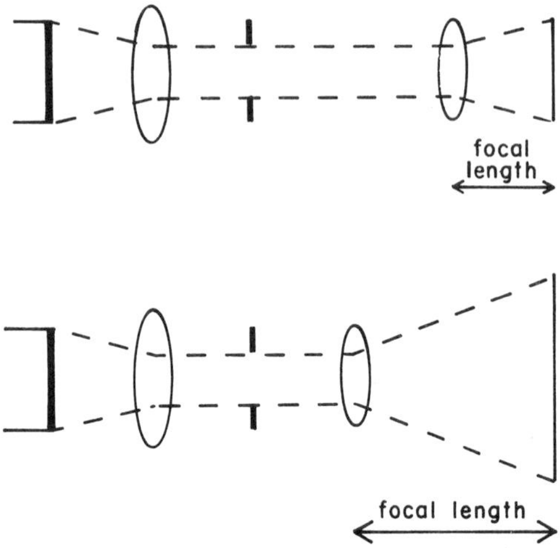

Figure 6. Relationship of image size to the focal length of the camera lens.

underframing all of the image appears on the film but will have a circular appearance. The corners of the film area are not exposed. On the other hand, overframing utilizes all of the film but some portions of the image are lost.

Optical System Efficiency

Only a fraction of the light which is emitted by the image intensifier reaches the film. The two major reasons for this are that the optical system does not capture all of the light and that a significant portion of the light is absorbed by the lens and mirrors within the system or stopped by the aperture. Figure 5 is helpful in relating these factors to the efficiency of

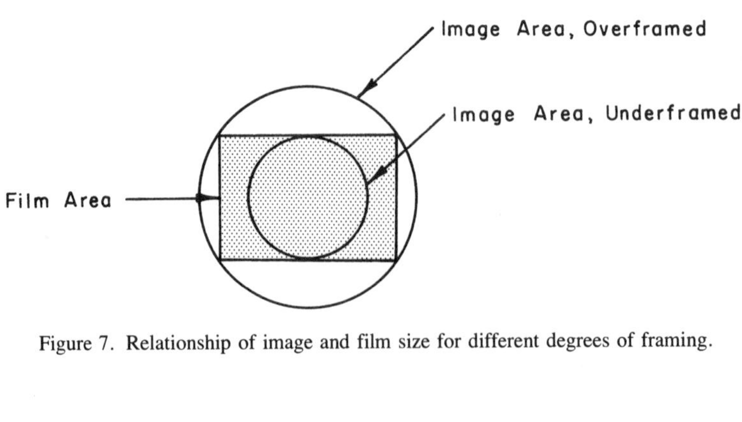

Figure 7. Relationship of image and film size for different degrees of framing.

light transfer. The fraction of the light from the intensifier which is captured by the optical system depends on the effective area of the collimator lens. The effective light-gathering area of the lens is expressed in terms of the f number. The f number is given by:

$$\text{f number} = \text{focal length of lens/diameter of aperture}$$

For a given lens, the f number is changed by adjusting the aperture. By referring to Figure 5 it can be seen that the area of the collimator lens which captures the useful light is controlled by the aperture. It should be noticed that the f number and the diameter of the aperture are inversely related. When the diameter of the aperture is increased, the f number decreases and more light will be captured. The fraction of the light captured by the optical system, or efficiency, is given by:

$$\text{Efficiency} = \frac{1}{4f^2}$$

There is a series of commonly used aperture sizes or f numbers. These are listed in Table 2 along with the relative amount of light captured by each. The difference between any two consecutive f numbers is known as one stop. Changing the aperture size by one stop changes the amount of light captured by a factor of 2. Only a fraction of the light captured by the collimator lens will reach the film because of absorption in the lens. This fraction, T, is typically about 0.8. If the light which reaches the film is spread over an area which is larger than the output screen, the intensity, but not the total number of light photons, will be reduced. By combining these various factors, it is possible to develop a relationship between the illumi-

Table 2. Standard f number values and relative lens areas

f Number	Relative area (efficiency)
16	1
11	2
8	4
5.6	8
4	16
2.8	32
2.0	64
1.4	128
1.0	256

nation on the film, E, and the luminance, L, of the output phosphor, as follows:

$$E = \frac{\pi LT}{4f^2m^2}$$

Receptor Sensitivity

The overall sensitivity of an intensified receptor system depends on three major factors. These are: 1) the gain or conversion factor of the image tube; 2) the efficiency of the optical system; 3) the sensitivity of the film. The sensitivity of film used in conjunction with image intensifiers can be specified in terms of an ASA rating which is used for conventional photographic film. The approximate light exposure, E_m, required to produce a median density is given by:

$$E_m = \frac{8}{\text{ASA number}}$$

This is not an exact relationship and will vary with the contrast characteristics of the film.

It was shown earlier that the output luminance (brightness) of the image intensifier is the product of the input exposure rate, in milliroentgens per second, and the conversion factor, G. By combining this with the relationships for film sensitivity and optical system efficiency given above, it is possible to obtain an expression for the overall receptor sensitivity which is:

$$X_m(\text{mR}) = \frac{32f^2 \cdot m^2}{\pi \cdot G \cdot T \cdot \text{ASA}}$$

In this relationship, X_m is the x-ray exposure required at the input phosphor to produce a median film density. Several aspects of this relationship should be considered. It is shown that the input exposure increases as the square of the magnification, which is, in effect, the film image size. If all other factors remain unchanged, 4 times as much x-ray exposure is required if the film size is doubled. This is because doubling the size (diameter) of the film increases the image area by a factor of 4.

A change in image size usually occurs twice in an intensified system. The image is reduced in size or minified in the image intensifier and then magnified in the optical system. Minification increases image intensity whereas magnification produces a decrease. Much of the gain in the image intensifier tube obtained from minification is lost if the image is remag-

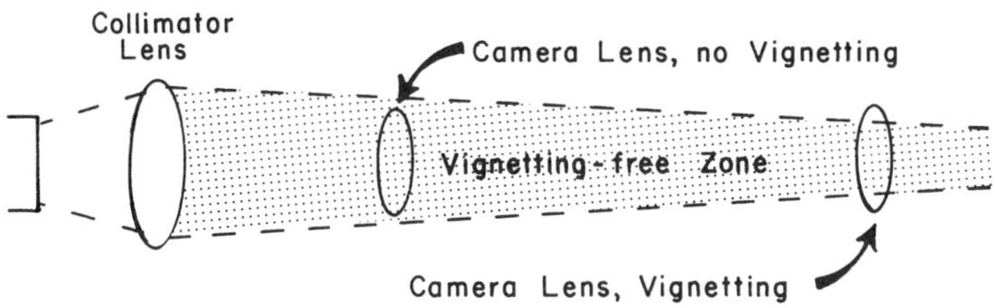

Figure 8. The vignetting-free zone.

nified on the film. In fact, if the film size is the same as the input phosphor size these two factors will cancel out.

Within a given system, the receptor sensitivity can usually be changed by adjusting the aperture. If the film is changed to one with a different sensitivity, the aperture can be used to compensate for the change and maintain the same receptor sensitivity if desired. The aperture is also used to compensate for image intensifier tubes which have different conversion factors.

The sensitivity of most intensified systems is determined either by limitations within the system, such as a tube with a low conversion factor, or by considerations for quantum noise.

Vignetting

One potential problem with a two-lens optical system is vignetting. The effect of vignetting is the loss of film exposure around the periphery of the image. The cause of vignetting is illustrated in Figure 8. Light which leaves a point near the center of the intensifier screen passes through the lens and forms a beam which is parallel to the axis running through the two lenses. Light that originates from points near the periphery of the intensifier screen also passes through the lens and forms parallel beams, but the direction is not along the axis through the lens. In order for a camera lens to capture light from the periphery of the image, it must be located in an area where the beams overlap. Vignetting usually occurs when the camera lens is mounted too far from the collimator or the camera lens is too large to be contained in the overlap area. Since the effective diameter of the camera lens is often determined by the size of the aperture, changing the aperture setting to a larger value (smaller f number) might introduce vignetting.

IMAGE QUALITY

There are a number of factors which affect the quality of images in intensified radiography systems. These should be taken into consideration when selecting an imaging system for a specific application.

There are several potential sources of blur within the system. The spreading of light in both the input and output screens of the image intensifier tube produces blur as it does in intensifying screens. In many image intensifier tubes both the input and output screens are significant sources of blur. Actually, the blur in the output screen is quite small and becomes significant only when it is referred back to the input screen. The minification of the image within the tube has the effect of magnifying the blur of most image intensifier tubes so that it increases with the size of the input image. In the use of dual mode tubes the larger field will generally produce more blur than the smaller field. In most tubes the blur varies over the image area. It is generally the smallest near the center of the field and increases toward the periphery.

In addition to blur produced in the input and output screens blur is produced by improper focusing of the electrons in the tube. Most intensifier systems have controls which can be used to adjust the electron focus. Unless the optical system is properly focused it will also be a source of image blur. It is possible for both the collimator and camera lens to be out of focus. The proper focusing of the collimator lens requires the use of special equipment and should be attempted only by qualified personnel.

Contrast

It has been shown previously that the contrast in an image delivered to the film is reduced by both object penetration and scattered radiation. When image intensifier tubes are used there is an additional loss of contrast because of events taking place within the tube. It is possible for some of the radiation which penetrates the input screen to be absorbed by the output screen and produce an effect similar to scattered radiation. Also, some of the light produced in the output screen travels back to the photocathode and causes electrons to be emitted. These electrons are accelerated to the output screen where they contribute to additional exposure to the image area and further reduce contrast. The contrast reduction in modern intensifier tubes is generally in the range of 5 to 15%.

Quantum Noise

The problem of quantum noise in intensified systems is discussed in detail in Chapter XIX. If it were not for the limitations of quantum noise, modern intensifier systems could be adjusted to operate at much lower input exposure values.

Chapter XIX
Image Noise

It is generally desirable for film density to be uniform except where it changes in order to form an image. There are factors present, however, which tend to produce variation in film density even when there is no image detail present. This variation is usually quite random and has no particular pattern. In many cases it reduces image quality. It is especially significant when the objects being imaged are small and have relatively low contrast. This random variation in film density is designated as noise or mottle.

Figure 1 shows two film areas which have the same average density. The two areas differ, however, in that the density in area A varies considerably from point to point, whereas the density in area B is quite uniform. In other words, area A contains much more noise than area B. There are generally three factors which can contribute to this undesirable nonuniformity in an x-ray image. These are shown in Figure 2.

As discussed in Chapter XIV, x-ray film is made up of a large number of individual silver grains. In films where the individual grains are relatively large they can give the image a grainy appearance which is a type of image noise. This is, however, usually a small contribution to overall image noise except in some situations, such as cineradiography, where the image is enlarged by projection. Even then film grain is usually not the major contributor to the total noise.

In both intensifying screens and image intensifier tubes the receptor surface consists of a layer of many small individual crystals. Variation in crystal size and distribution can produce some nonuniformity in the image. This is generally referred to as structure noise.

The third source of image noise is the natural fluctuation in the concentration of photons absorbed by the receptor. This is quantum noise. In most x-ray procedures this is the most significant source of image noise and will now be considered in some detail.

Figure 1. Comparison of a radiographic image which contains noise (*A*) to one that does not (*B*).

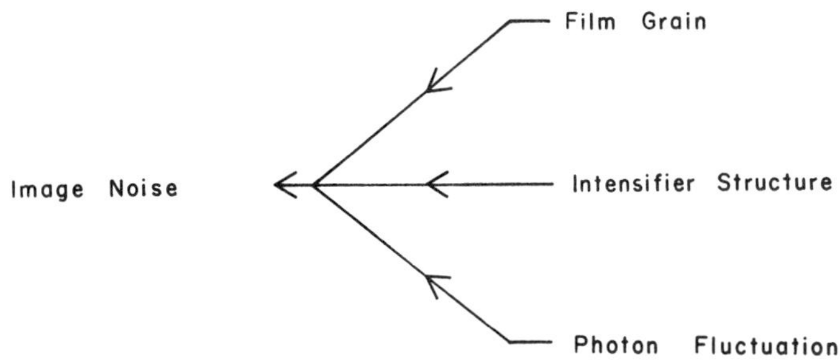

Figure 2. The three sources of radiographic image noise.

QUANTUM NOISE

X-ray photons impinging on a surface, like raindrops, will do so in a random pattern. There is no force present which will cause them to be evenly distributed over the surface. One area of the receptor surface might receive more photons than another area even when both are exposed to the same average x-ray intensity. This is illustrated in Figure 3. Several small circular areas of the same size are designated on the receptor surface. It is assumed that all of the receptor surface in this example is exposed to the same average x-ray intensity or photon fluence. However, because of the random manner in which the photons are distributed over the surface, some of the circular areas will receive more photons than others. This variation in photon fluence from point to point on the receptor surface is the source of quantum noise.

The amount of quantum noise can be expressed in terms of the variation in number of photons from one small area to another on the receptor. For example, if all of the circular areas designated in Figure 3 captured the same number of photons, the quantum noise would be 0. However, in reality they do not capture the same number of photons. Some of the areas will receive less than the average number of photons and some more. The significant factor is the amount of variation from area to area.

Figure 4 shows the relative number of areas receiving a specific number of photons. It should be noticed that most areas receive either more or less photons than the average. The statistical distribution of the number of photons falling in an area has a characteristic bell shape as shown. This is more correctly referred to as a Gaussian distribution. This type of graph shows the amount of variation in the number of photons from the average. This natural variation is the source of quantum noise. Some areas will have a larger variation or deviation from the average than others. It is therefore desirable to designate a quantity which represents an "average" variation.

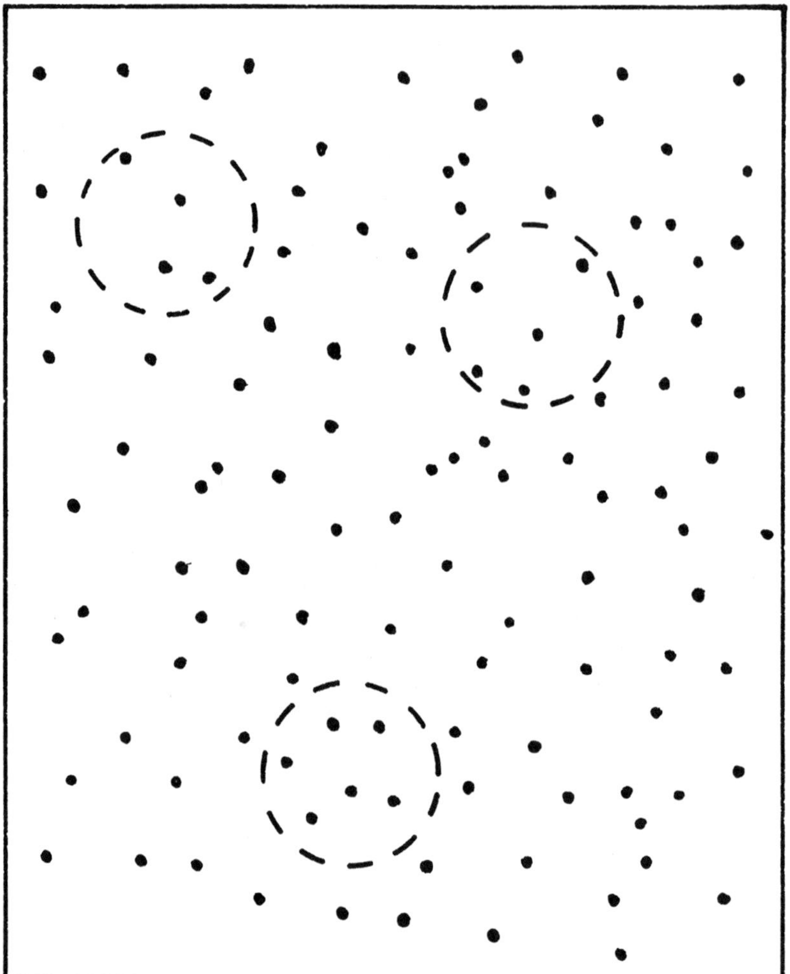

Figure 3. The random distribution of photons on a receptor surface.

This can be done in terms of the so-called standard deviation (SD). The standard deviation is a single value which can be used to express the variation in number of photons. The amount of quantum noise is proportional to the amount of variation or the value of the standard deviation.

For photon distributions the value of the standard deviation is related to the average photon fluence. Specifically, the standard deviation is equal to the square root of the average number of photons in an area. An expres-

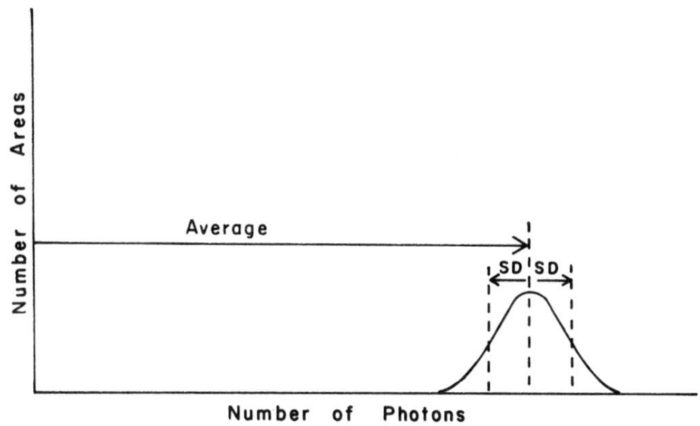

Figure 4. The natural variation in photon concentration from area to area on the receptor surface.

sion for the standard deviation as a percentage of the average can be derived as follows:

$$SD = \sqrt{N}$$

$$SD(\%) = \frac{\sqrt{N}\ 100}{N}$$

$$SD\ (\%) = \frac{100}{\sqrt{N}}$$

This relationship illustrates the basic concept of controlling quantum noise. The variation in number of photons from area to area, or relative noise, expressed in terms of the standard deviation, is inversely related to the average number of photons per area or photon fluence. Quantum noise can be decreased by increasing the average number of photons in an area.

For example, if the average number of photons per area is 100, the variation will be:

$$SD(\%) = \frac{100}{\sqrt{100}} = 10\%$$

However, if the average number of photons per area is 1,000, the variation will be:

$$SD(\%) = \frac{100}{\sqrt{1{,}000}} = 3\%$$

Assuming that the same film density is to be obtained, an increase in the number of absorbed photons is generally achieved by decreasing receptor sensitivity. This, in turn, requires more photons to produce a given film density.

A distinction must be made between the number of photons entering the receptor and the number actually absorbed. It was shown in previous chapters that most receptors have a quantum detection efficiency (QDE) of less than 100%. The photons which penetrate the receptor do not contribute to image formation or the reduction of quantum noise. For a given x-ray beam quality the average number of photons absorbed in a small area is proportional to the product of the exposure, X, and the QDE.

Up to this point it has been shown that the amount of quantum noise is related to the average number of photons absorbed in each small area of the receptor. For a given input exposure the number of photons absorbed depends on the size of the area being considered. This leads to the question of what is the size of the area which should be used to determine receptor noise characteristics. Since a receptor cannot be divided up into distinct areas, the concept of an effective area must be used. The effective area is determined by the amount of blur, B, in the receptor and is proportional to the square of the blur value. If a receptor has a relatively large amount of blur it, in effect, averages photons over a larger area and reduces the quantum noise.

Another factor which affects the appearance of quantum noise on the film is the contrast characteristics of the film. A high contrast factor, G, will produce more density variation or noise for the same photon fluctuation than a low contrast factor.

The factors discussed above can be combined as follows to indicate the relative amount of quantum noise in a given receptor system:

$$\text{Quantum noise (\%)} \propto \frac{G}{B\sqrt{X_m} \cdot \text{QDE}}$$

The previous relationship shows that quantum noise can be reduced by changing various factors within the x-ray imaging system. Unfortunately, a change which would reduce noise will generally have some adverse affect on image quality or patient exposure. For example, noise can be reduced by using a film with a lower contrast factor or an intensifying screen with more blur, both of which might reduce image quality. Within a given type of imaging system it is generally desirable to adjust the various factors to give an acceptable compromise between quantum noise and the other factors in image quality and patient exposure.

RECEPTOR SYSTEMS

Quantum noise can be a significant factor in image quality in both intensifying screen and intensifier tube receptor systems. The factors which can be used to change the quantum noise level in these two systems will now be considered.

Intensifying Screens

The purpose of an intensifying screen is to produce a given film density with a smaller quantity of radiation in comparison to direct film exposure. Because of the significantly lower exposure, films made with intensifying screens will generally have a higher level of quantum noise than film exposed directly to the x-ray beam. It should be recalled that the sensitivity (median density exposure) of an intensifying screen receptor system depends on the characteristics of both the screen and the film. It is possible to have two different screen-film systems with the same overall sensitivity but significantly different noise characteristics. The reason for this is illustrated in Figure 5.

Figure 5 shows the approximate relationship of radiation quantities in several steps of the image-forming process. The incident radiation or exposure into the intensifying screen required to produce a certain density is

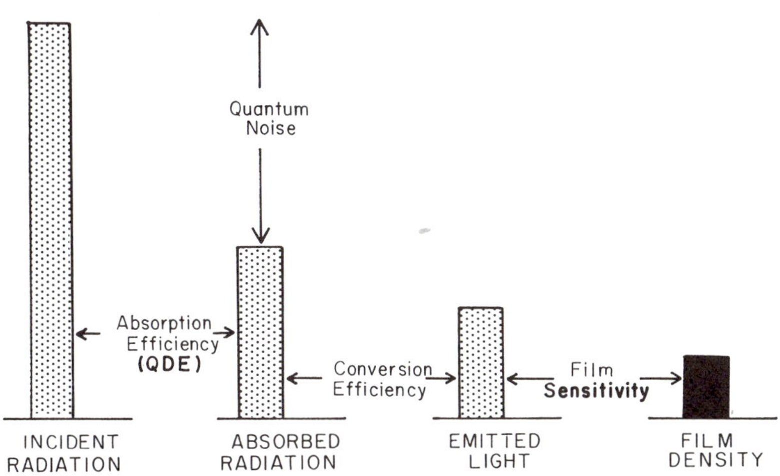

Figure 5. Relationship of radiation quantities within an intensifying screen.

determined by the receptor system sensitivity. Some fraction of this radiation is absorbed by the screens. It is the radiation absorbed which influences the quantity of quantum noise. The relationship between absorbed radiation and incident radiation is determined by the absorption efficiency (QDE) of the screen. This expresses the fraction of incident photons which will be absorbed by the screen. All of the absorbed x-ray energy is not converted into light. The fraction which is converted is the conversion efficiency of the intensifying screen material. The relationship between the quantity of light produced and the resulting film density is determined by the sensitivity of the film. With these relationships established it is now possible to consider changes which might affect quantum noise.

The goal is generally to produce a given film density with the lowest possible input exposure. The three factors which establish the relationship between input exposure and film density are QDE, conversion efficiency, and film sensitivity. Increasing any of these would allow the same film density to be produced with a lower input exposure. However, the effect on quantum noise must be considered. It will be assumed that in all cases it is desirable to obtain the same film density. Therefore, in Figure 5, that quantity will remain unchanged. If the film sensitivity is increased, less light is required. This, in turn, would allow the quantity of absorbed radiation to be reduced. Although this will allow the input exposure to be decreased it will also increase the quantum noise. The same effect would be produced by increasing conversion efficiency. That is, the input exposure is reduced at the cost of increasing quantum noise. The only way to reduce input exposure without increasing quantum noise is to increase the absorption efficiency or QDE. This is achieved by using either a thicker screen or a screen material with a higher inherent absorption efficiency. For example, some of the rare earth screen materials have larger absorption efficiencies than calcium tungstate. This permits lower exposure without a significant sacrifice in image quality or increase in quantum noise. The problem with increasing screen thickness is that it generally produces an increase in image blur.

Two screen-film combinations which have the same sensitivity are shown in Figure 6. One system uses a relatively thick "high speed" screen and a film with conventional sensitivity. The other system uses a thinner "par" speed screen and a more sensitive film. The images produced by these two systems will differ in two respects. The system using the thicker screen will have more blur but less quantum noise than the system using the more sensitive film. The reduction in noise comes from the increase in QDE and blur.

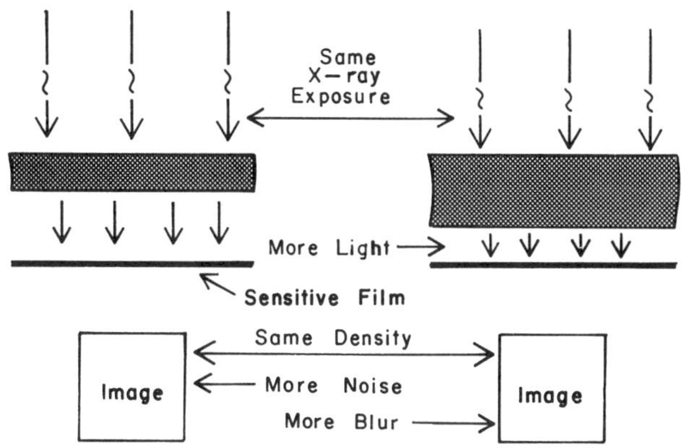

Figure 6. Comparison of image quality between two screen-film combinations.

Image Intensifiers

Quantum noise is of special concern in intensified radiography because of the potentially low receptor exposures which can produce adequate film density. Actually, it is usually possible to readjust most intensifier systems to operate at even lower exposure levels. This would, however, increase quantum noise above what is generally considered to be an acceptable level.

The amount of quantum noise in an x-ray imaging system is determined by the point within the system where the photon concentration is the lowest. This point is referred to as the quantum sink. In modern x-ray systems the quantum sink occurs at the input screen of the image intensifier. Quantum noise is therefore primarily a function of the input exposure to the image intensifier. This, in turn, is determined by the overall sensitivity of the imaging system.

The basic x-ray system illustrated in Figure 7 will be used to illustrate how it is possible to adjust the input exposure to the image intensifier for the purpose of obtaining some specified quantum noise level. All intensified radiography systems use automatic exposure control. In most systems the input to the automatic exposure control circuit is a light sensor which monitors the output of the image intensifier. The intensifier output luminance or exposure (luminance multiplied by time) is electronically compared to a pre-established reference level. The output signal from the control circuit will adjust the x-ray machine exposure factors until the desired luminance or exposure is obtained. In most spot film and some cine

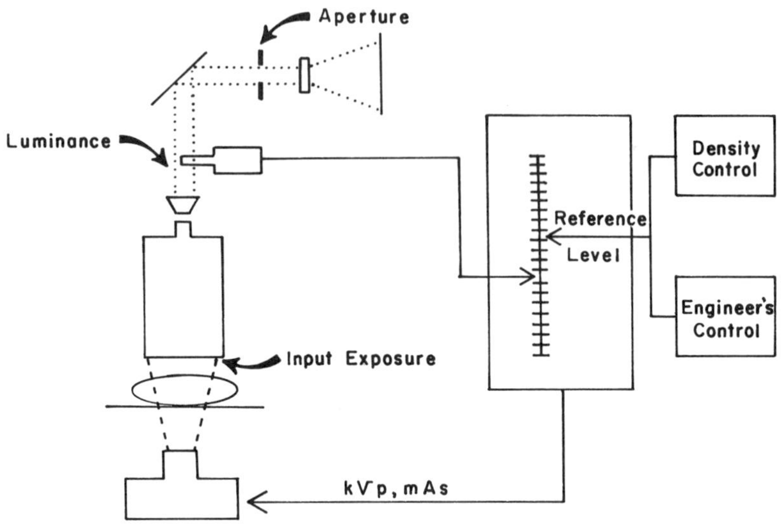

Figure 7. The factors which determine the input exposure (and quantum noise) of an intensified radiography system.

systems the KVP and MA are preset and the automatic exposure control circuit adjusts the exposure time in order to achieve proper film exposure. In some cine systems the automatic exposure control circuit adjusts the KVP, MA, or both, and the exposure time is preset. In some systems the control circuit can adjust all three exposure factors. Generally, the time will be changed within certain limits. If the desired exposure has not been obtained when time reaches a limit, either KVP or MA will be changed.

The reference level for the luminance output of the intensifier is generally adjusted by two different controls. One is the operator's control, which is used to adjust film density. The other is the engineer's control, which is used to set the approximate intensifier light output. This is usually located within the equipment and is not accessible to the equipment operator. The operator's control is essentially a fine adjustment of the engineer's control. For a given setting of the reference level the automatic exposure control circuit will produce some fixed value of intensifier input exposure. It is the readjustment of this reference level by means of the engineer's control which is used to alter the input exposure and control quantum noise.

The reference level cannot be changed without making other adjustments, or else film exposure will be incorrect. The relationship of film density to the light output from the image intensifier is determined by the film sensitivity and the size of the aperture within the optical system. The aperture and reference level are usually adjusted together to obtain the desired film exposure and image intensifier input exposure.

The adjustment of input exposure and quantum noise is illustrated in this example. Assume that a cine system is producing properly exposed films but the quantum noise is considered to be too high. A measurement of the input exposure shows that it is 10 μR per frame. It might be desirable to increase this to at least 25 μR in order to reduce the quantum noise. This can be achieved by changing the output light reference level to a higher value by means of the engineer's control. It is then necessary to reduce the size of the aperture opening to prevent the film from being overexposed.

In considering the image intensifier input exposure the relationship between the size of the image intensifier input and film must be considered. In most systems the size of the image on the film is less than the size of the image at the image intensifier input. When minification is present it is possible to form an image with a given noise level by using less radiation. The significant factor is the concentration of x-ray photons with respect to a given film area.

Many imaging systems use intensifier tubes with selectable input image sizes, as illustrated in Figure 8. Here three different image intensifier inputs or modes are compared to a 100-mm film. Intensifier input exposure values which will give approximately the same quantum noise on the film are also indicated. The relationship among the exposure values is determined by the ratio of the respective areas. In all three cases the total number of photons forming the image is the same. This is because the total

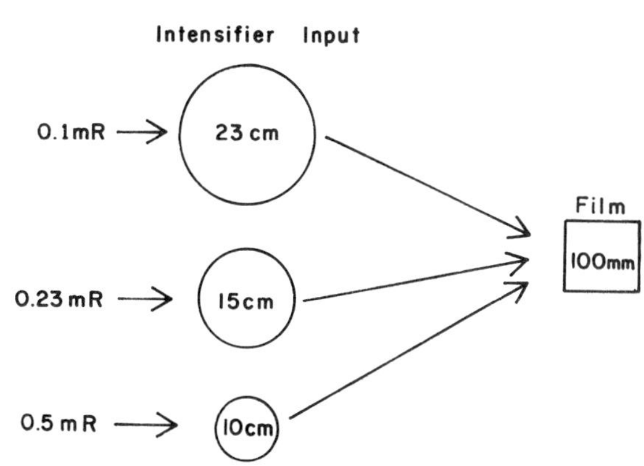

Figure 8. Relationship of intensifier tube input diameters to film size and exposure values required to produce the same image quality.

photon number is related to the product of the exposure and the image area.

When an image intensifier can be operated with different input image sizes there will be a different sensitivity value for each size. The change in sensitivity occurs because the gain of the intensifier tube is proportional to the area of the input.

In modern intensified radiography systems quantum noise is the factor that determines the maximum allowable sensitivity. Quantum noise is also a significant factor in fluoroscopic images. This will be discussed in detail in a later chapter.

Chapter XX Fluoroscopy

The fluoroscope is an x-ray imaging system that produces an immediate and continuous image for viewing by the physician. The components of a fluoroscopic system are similar to those in an intensified radiography system except that the film camera is replaced by a closed circuit video (television) system. The purpose of the video system is to transfer the image from the small output screen of the image intensifier to the larger screen of the video monitor.

The early fluoroscopes used a simple fluoroscopic screen as the image receptor and display device. The fluoroscopic screen consisted of a layer of a fluorescent material, usually zinc cadmium sulfide. It absorbed the x-ray image and converted it to light which was then viewed directly by the physician. In terms of function, the fluoroscopic screen is similar to the intensifying screen. It is generally much thicker and more efficient in absorbing the x-ray beam and converting it into light. The major shortcoming of the screen type fluoroscope was that the light output was quite low. This required that fluoroscopy be conducted in a darkened room and the physician had to dark-adapt his eyes by wearing red goggles for a period of time before conducting an examination. The quality of the images produced by the fluoroscopic screens was generally inferior to that of present day fluoroscopic images.

The first major innovation in the fluoroscopic system was to replace the fluoroscopic screen with an image intensifier tube. The light image from the intensifier tube was much brighter, by a factor of several thousand, than the image from the fluoroscopic screen. The major advantage in using the image intensifier was that it permitted fluoroscopy without the necessity of working in total darkness and without dark-adaptation of the eyes. The image from the output screen of the image intensifier was viewed through an optical system consisting of several lenses and mirrors. The major disadvantage of this type of fluoroscopy was that viewing by more than one person was difficult.

The modern fluoroscope has eliminated the major disadvantages of the early system by coupling a video system to an image intensifier tube. The result is a large, bright image of much improved quality.

VIDEO PRINCIPLES

The function of a video or television system is to transmit an image from one location to another. The two major components of this system are the camera and the monitor or receiver. Conventional broadcast television systems transmit the image from the camera to the receiver by means of radiofrequency radiation. In a closed circuit system the image is transmitted between the two devices by means of electrical conductors or cables. However, other than for the means of image transmission, the basic principles of the two types of systems are essentially the same.

A basic video system is illustrated in Figure 1. This illustration shows the major functional components which are contained in both the camera and the monitor. The ''heart'' of both the camera and monitor are two electronic tubes which convert the image into an electrical signal and vice versa.

The function of the camera tube is to convert the light image into an electronic signal. Broadcast television systems use camera tubes which are known as image orthicons. Fluoroscopic systems generally use either vidicon or plumbicon tubes. They are smaller and less complex than the image orthicons. They also require brighter input images but this is not a problem in fluoroscopy. The significant difference between the vidicon and plumbicon is one of image persistence or lag. This will be discussed later when image noise is considered. The typical camera tube has a cylindrical shape with a diameter of approximately 25 mm and a length of 15 cm. The

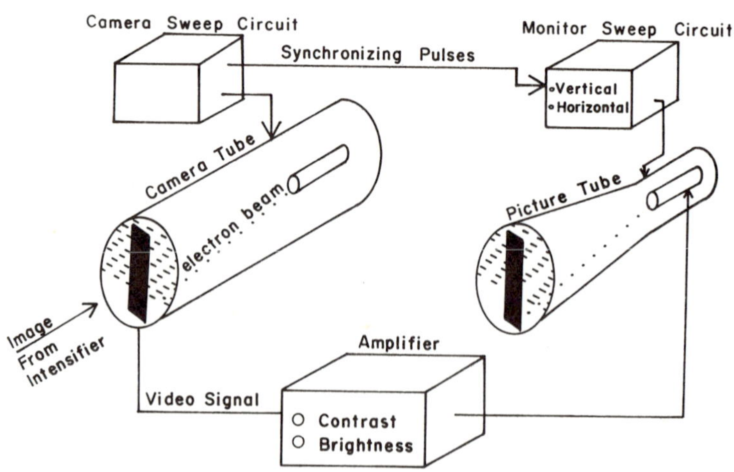

Figure 1. The major components in a video system.

image to be transmitted is projected onto the input screen of the tube. This is accomplished by using a lens like that in a conventional film camera. The other end of the tube contains a heated cathode and other electrodes which form an electron gun. The electron gun shoots a small beam of electrons down the length of the evacuated tube. The electron beam strikes the rear of the screen surface on which the input image is projected.

Electrical signals are applied to the camera tube, which causes the electron beam to be swept over the surface of the input screen. One signal moves the beam in a horizontal direction and the other signal moves it vertically. The two signals are synchronized so that they work together to move the beam in a specific pattern. Although the input screen is round, the area covered by the scanning electron beam is generally rectangular in shape. The beam begins in the upper left-hand corner and moves across the screen horizontally. In the conventional 525-line video system, lines are scanned at the rate of 15,750 per sec. When the beam reaches the right-hand side it is quickly "snapped back" to the left and deflected downward by approximately 1 beam width. It then sweeps across to form a second scan line. This process is repeated until the beam reaches the bottom of the screen. This usually requires 1/60th of a second. After reaching the bottom the beam returns to the top and resumes the scanning process. This time, however, the scan lines are slightly displaced with respect to the first set so that they fall between the lines created in the first scan. This is known as interlacing.

Interlacing is used to prevent flicker in the picture. If all of the lines were scanned consecutively it would take twice as long, that is, 1/30th of a second, for the beam to reach the bottom of the screen. This delay would be detectable by the human eye and would appear as flicker. By using interlacing, the face of the screen is actually scanned in two sets of lines. The pattern of scan lines produced in a video system is known as a raster. The conventional video system is generally set to contain 525 lines. However, the actual raster contains approximately 485 lines. The remaining lines are lost during the return of the electron beam to the left side of the screen. In a 525-line system 30 complete raster frames are formed per second.

The heart of the receiver or monitor is the picture tube. The picture tube differs from the camera tube in size and shape. One end of the tube is the screen on which the video image is displayed. Like the camera tube the picture tube has an electron gun located in the end opposite to the screen. The electron gun produces a beam of electrons which strike the rear of the screen in the picture tube. The electron beam is also scanned over the surface of the picture tube screen just as it is scanned over the camera tube screen. In fact, the scanning in the two tubes is synchronized by a signal transmitted from the camera to the monitor. If the scanning becomes unsynchronized the image will roll in the vertical direction or become distorted horizontally. The so-called horizontal and vertical controls on a video monitor are used to adjust the scan rates so that they are identical to those of the camera and can maintain synchronization.

The screen of the camera tube consists of a material which has light-sensitive electrical properties. Several different types of tubes are used but the general concept of the tube function can be described as follows.

The electrical conductivity of the screen surface depends on its illumination. When an image is projected onto the screen the conductivity from point to point will vary. A dark area will be essentially nonconductive and a brightly illuminated area will be the most conductive. As the electron beam sweeps over the surface it encounters areas with various levels of conductivity, which in turn depend on the brightness at each point. When the beam strikes a bright spot it is "conducted through" and creates a relatively high signal voltage at the output terminal of the tube. As the spot moves across the screen it creates a signal which represents the brightness of the image at each point along its path. The relationship between the video signals and image brightness is illustrated in Figure 2.

The signal from the camera tube is transmitted to the monitor, where it is applied to a control element in the electron gun. When the electron beam in the picture tube strikes the screen it produces a bright spot. The actual brightness of the spot is determined by the number of electrons in the

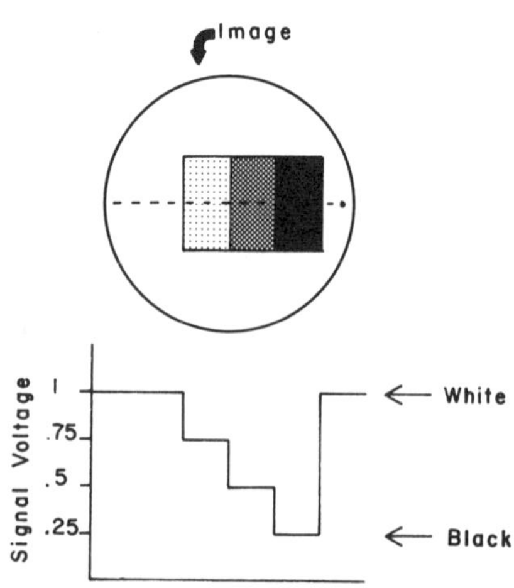

Figure 2. Relationship of video signal voltage to image brightness.

beam, which, in turn, is controlled by the signal from the camera tube. In other words, the brightness of a spot on the picture tube screen is determined by the brightness of the corresponding point on the camera tube screen. As the two electron beams scan the two screens the image is transferred from the camera tube to the picture tube. In the 525-line system complete images are transferred at the rate of 30 per sec.

VIDEO IMAGE QUALITY

The three image quality characteristics which affect fluoroscopic images are contrast, blur, and noise.

Contrast

In the typical video system image contrast can be changed by adjusting a control located in the monitor. The contrast control changes the amount of amplification of the video signal. As mentioned previously, the brightness of each point within the image on the picture tube screen is determined by the voltage of the video signal associated with the particular point. The contrast of an image on the screen is the brightness difference between two points such as a background and object area. This is determined by the voltage difference in the video signal for the two areas. When a video signal is amplified, the voltage difference between two points is increased. This, in turn, produces a larger difference in brightness or more contrast. At first it might appear that amplification of the video signals will not only increase contrast, but will also produce a brighter image. However, most circuits are designed so that changing the contrast control does not appreciably change the average signal level. The average video signal level is changed by adjusting the brightness control.

Although the contrast and brightness controls are essentially separate and independent they must generally be adjusted together for optimum image quality. The typical picture tube has a maximum brightness level which cannot be exceeded regardless of the value of the incoming video signal. If the average signal level is pushed toward this upper limit by turning up the brightness control, a decrease in contrast will generally occur. This is because the bright (white) areas have reached a limiting value and the darker areas are being increased in brightness. Since the bright areas cannot increase above the maximum limit, the contrast between the two areas is reduced.

Vertical Blur

One generally undesirable characteristic of a video imaging system is that it introduces blur into the image. One source produces blur in the vertical

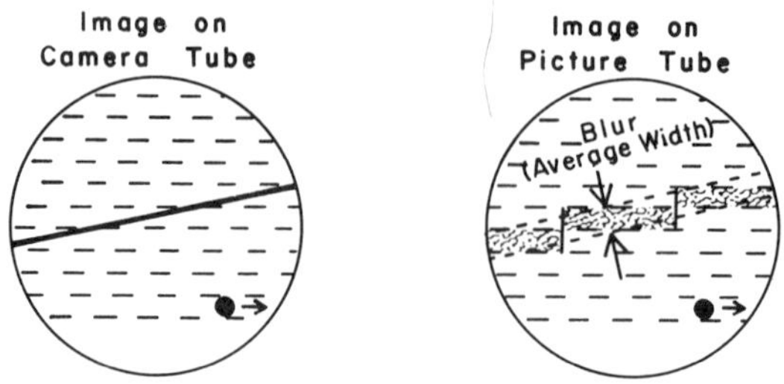

Figure 3. Vertical blur produced by scan lines.

direction and the other in the horizontal. Although it is possible for the blur values to be different for the two directions the best overall image quality is usually obtained when they are approximately equal.

Vertical blur is caused by the finite size of the electron beam and the scan lines. The effect of vertical blur is illustrated in Figure 3. If a small line-type object is oriented at a slight angle to the scan lines the image of the object will appear to be wider because of blur. At any instant the width of a line in the image cannot be less than the width of one scan line. An object will normally not be perfectly aligned with a single scan line. Therefore, the image of the line will have a width which is slightly larger than the width of a single scan line. The relationship between blur (image line width), B_v, and scan line width, w, is given by:

$$B_v = 1.4 \text{ w}$$

The width of a scan line, w, is in turn related to the vertical dimensions of the image and the number of actual scan lines. These factors can be incorporated into the above relationship to give the following:

$$B_v = \frac{1.4 \text{ V}}{\text{n}}$$

where V is the vertical dimension of the image and n is the number of useful scan lines within that dimension. It is seen that for an image containing a given number of scan lines vertical blur is directly proportional to the dimension of the image, V. The question then arises as to where within the system is the image dimension determined. Should it be on the monitor screen, at the camera tube, or at some other point? The appropriate location for determining image size is in the plane through the object being imaged as illustrated in Figure 4.

The blur value determined by using this image dimension will be properly scaled to the size of the object. It can then be easily compared to

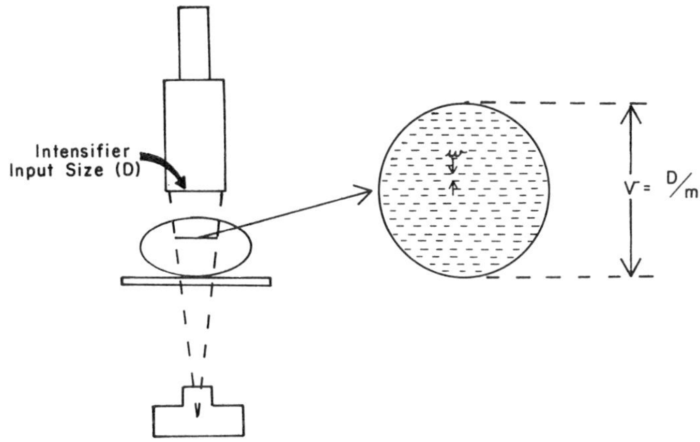

Figure 4. Video image size in the object plane.

blur values from the focal spot and receptor. In the plane of the object the image diameter, V, is equal to the diameter, D, of the image at the input to the image intensifier divided by the geometric magnification factor, m. Substitution of this expression for image size gives an expression for image blur which is related to three specific factors:

$$B_v = \frac{1.4\ D}{nm}$$

Special attention is called to the fact that video blur is directly proportional to the size of the image at the input to the image-intensifier tube. For example, assume that a system has 485 useful lines and a magnification factor, m, of 1.2. For a 15-cm (6-inch) input image size the blur will be 0.36 mm. However, if the image size is switched to 23 cm (9 inches), the blur will increase to 0.55 mm. When the size of the image at the input of the image intensifier is increased the video lines are spread over a larger object area. Since the number of lines is not changed the width of the lines must increase. Since blur is directly related to line width it is obvious that it must increase with an increase in image size. Blur can be decreased by increasing the number of lines used to form the video image.

Horizontal Blur

Blur in the horizontal direction, B_h, is determined by the response time of the electronic circuitry through which the video signal passes in going from the camera to the picture tube. The response time of a video circuit is generally specified in terms of a frequency bandwidth, f. The bandwidth is in the units of megahertz (MHz). The relationship between image blur and the response time or bandwidth of the video circuitry is illustrated in Figure 5. The best approach in developing a concept of horizontal blur is to consider the events during one scan across a very thin vertical line object. The video signal created in the camera tube will contain a narrow discrete line, as shown. However, after the video signal passes through the electronic circuit, the line will be spread over a longer time interval. This spreading of the video signal by the electronic circuitry is the source of blur in the horizontal direction. The spreading is introduced because the circuitry does not respond instantaneously to the signal. In other words, there is a lag between the time a portion of the video signal reaches the input and when it leaves the output of the circuit. The amount of blur is directly related to the amount of lag produced by the electronic circuit. A point within a video signal will generally be spread in time by an amount given by:

$$t = \frac{1}{2f}$$

where f is the bandpass of the circuit. In this relationship, t is blur expressed in units of time. The blur value expressed as a distance is obtained by multiplying the "time" blur by the velocity of the scanning electron beam spot. The spot velocity, v, is given by:

$$v = WNn_t r$$

where W is image width, N is the number of images per second (typically 30), n_t is the total number of lines, and r is a factor used to compensate for

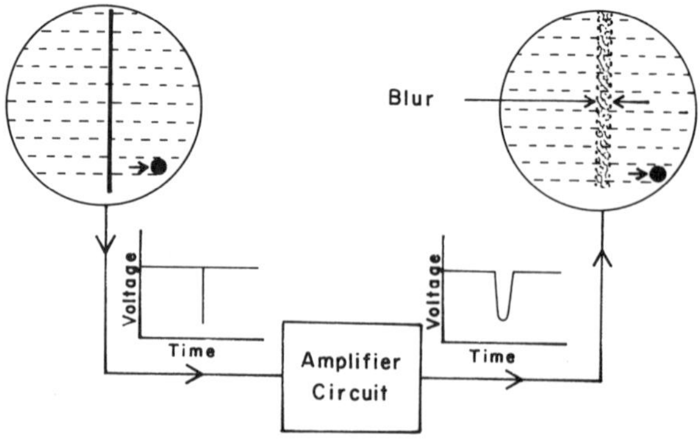

Figure 5. Horizontal blur produced by video amplifier circuit.

the time required to return the beam. It usually has a value of approximately 1.2. By combining the relationships given above an expression for horizontal blur will be:

$$B_n = \frac{WNn_t r}{2f}$$

In order for the blur value to be scaled to the object size the image width, W, must be the dimension of the image in the plane through the object. It was shown that this dimension is related to the image size at the input of the image intensifier and the geometric magnification factor. One additional factor must be added to account for the fact that a video image is generally wider (by a factor of 1.33) than it is tall. Substitution of this expression for image width in the object plane gives the following expression for horizontal blur:

$$B_n = \frac{1.33\ DNn_t r}{2fm}$$

It is seen that image blur in the horizontal direction is determined by the characteristics of the video raster such as number of lines and dimensions, and the frequency response or bandwidth of the circuitry. In most cases the bandwidth can be readily changed by the circuit designer. It is usually the factor which is used to adjust the horizontal blur value. In most systems the horizontal blur is adjusted to be approximately equal to the vertical blur. There is probably no advantage in having significantly more or less blur in one direction than the other.

Image Noise

The two types of noise in a fluoroscopic system are electronic and quantum. Electronic noise produces "snow," which is familiar to most television viewers. It is usually significant only when the video signals are extremely weak. Signal strength is not a problem in the typical closed circuit video system. Therefore, the presence of significant "snow" or electronic noise is usually an indication of problems within the video system.

In Chapter XIX it was shown that quantum noise depends on the number of photons used to form the image. The number of photons involved in image formation is directly related to the receptor input exposure. The input exposure, for a specific image brightness, can be adjusted by changing the automatic brightness control circuit reference level as discussed in Chapter XIX. An input exposure rate of approximately 0.025 mR per sec (1.5 mR per min) is usually required to reduce quantum noise to an acceptable level.

The noise level is related to the total number of photons used to form an image, not the rate. It is generally believed that the human eye has an effective ''collection'' time of approximately 0.2 sec. In video systems the time over which photons are collected to form an image is longer because of the persistence or lag inherent in the camera tube. Vidicon tubes generally have more lag than plumbicons. Because of this they average photons over a longer period of time and produce less quantum noise for the same input exposure rate.

Chapter XXI Tomography

In conventional radiography the images of all objects within the x-ray beam are superimposed. In many examinations this is undesirable because the image of one object interferes with the visualization of the object of interest. Tomography is an imaging technique that produces an image of objects located in a selection layer or slice through the body. There are two general methods used to produce tomographic images. One method is based on the movement of the x-ray tube and receptor during the exposure interval. This blurs and reduces the contrast of objects outside of the selected layer. The second method utilizes a scanning x-ray beam and a digital computer to construct the tomographic image. Computed tomography has little in common with conventional tomography except that the images are of a selected body layer.

CONVENTIONAL TOMOGRAPHY

Conventional tomography is performed by using specially designed x-ray equipment. The system consists of an x-ray tube and receptor which are linked together as shown in Figure 1. The arm is pivoted at a point that lies in a plane passing through the patient. During the exposure interval a motor moves the tube-receptor assembly. This motion produces blurring of all points within the patient except for points in the plane through the pivot point. In some examinations the motion is simple, with the tube moving in an essentially straight line. In other examinations the tube-receptor movement follows a complex path in two directions. The various motion patterns will be discussed later.

The advantage of tomography is that it can selectively blur certain object points within the body. The basic principle is illustrated in Figure 2. Object point 1 is located on the plane passing through the pivot point. Object point 2 is located some distance above this plane. When the tube and receptor are in position a the images of both points 1 and 2 are located at the same point on the receptor surface. When the tube and receptor move to position b, the images of both points also move. However, they do not move the same distance. By using simple geometric relationships it can be

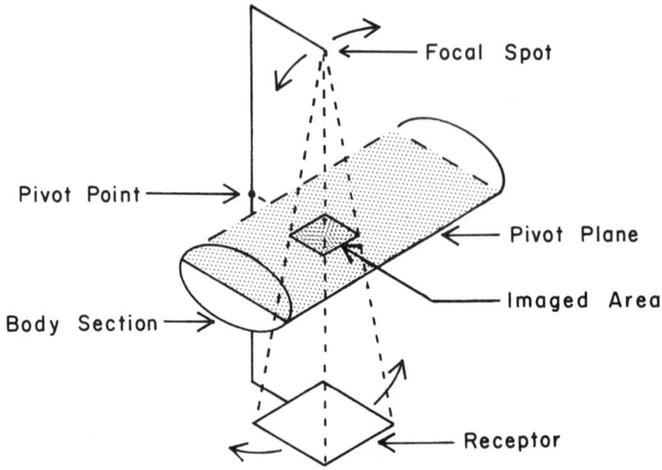

Figure 1. The basic components of a conventional tomographic imaging system shown in relationship to the image plane through the body section.

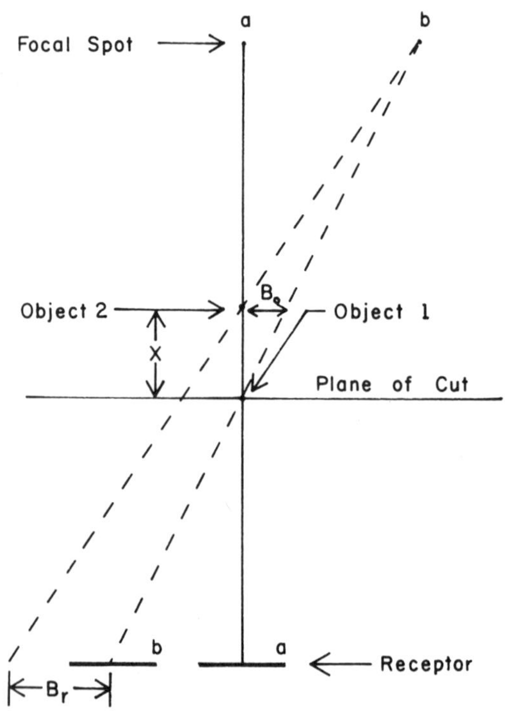

Figure 2. The relationship of object-point blur to the movement of the focal spot and receptor.

shown that the image of object 2 moves a greater distance than the image of point 1. The important factor, however, is that the receptor moves exactly the same distance as the image of object 1. Because the movement of image 1 and the receptor are the same, image 1 is not blurred. However, because the movement of image 2 is different from the movement of the receptor it is blurred. The amount of blur, B_r, at the receptor is the difference in distance moved by image 2 and the receptor. This, in turn, is determined by the distance of object point 2 from the pivot plane and the distance or angle through which the tube and receptor move. Object points located below the pivot plane will also be blurred because their images will move a shorter distance than the receptor. The blur value at the object location is the blur at the receptor divided by the magnification factor.

What actually happens in tomography is that all object points, except for those on the pivot plane, or plane of cut, appear to move during the film exposure. Perhaps this can be visualized by imagining that the x-ray tube is stationary and that the patient is moved during the exposure. This can be accomplished by rocking the patient about a pivot point located in the plane of interest. It is easy to see that the pivot point itself would not be blurred. Other points along the plane will not be blurred if the receptor surface is also rocked so that it is always parallel to the pivot plane. When viewed from this perspective, points along the pivot plane would appear not to move during the exposure interval. As shown in Figure 3, the distance "moved" by other object points and the amount of blurring of these

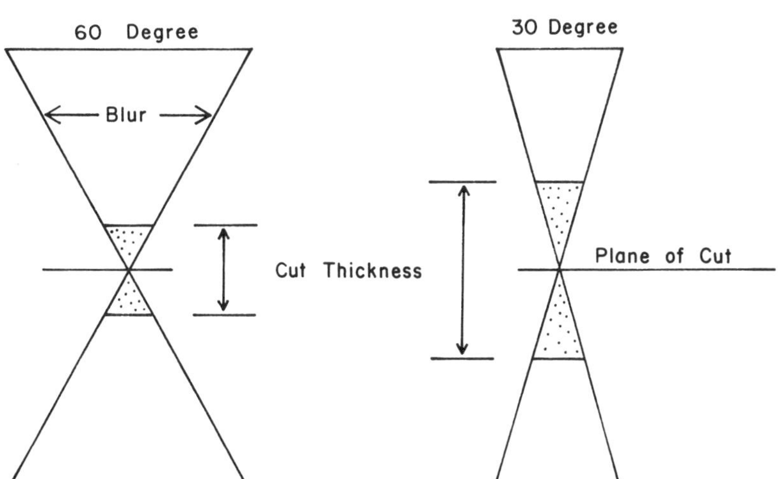

Figure 3. Relationship of object-point blur to movement angle and distance from plane of cut. The acceptable blur which establishes the cut thickness is indicated by the shaded area.

depend on two factors. These are the distance of the point from the pivot plane, x, and the angle of movement, θ, in degrees. The relationship between blur, B_0, of the object points and these two factors is given by:

$$B_0(\text{mm}) = \frac{2\pi}{360}\,\text{x(mm)}\cdot\theta(\text{degrees})$$

In tomography reference is often made to the thickness of cut. This refers to the thickness of the layer through the body in which the object points are not blurred. Actually, all points not located on the infinitely thin pivot plane are blurred to some extent. The concept of slice thickness is based on the selection of some blur value as the limits for the tomographic cut. This is usually a blur of approximately 0.5 mm. The thickness of cut, t, is 2 times the distance between the pivot plane and the object point which has a blur of 0.5 mm. When this is incorporated into the equation for blur given above, a relationship between tomographic cut thickness, t, and movement angle is obtained as follows:

$$\text{t(mm)} = \frac{360}{2\pi\theta} = \frac{57.3}{\theta(\text{degrees})}$$

The thickness of cut is controlled by adjusting the movement angle. The imaging procedure which uses a relatively small angle, producing a relatively thick cut, is called zonography.

Tomographic Motions

The blurring of object points not located on the pivot plane will be blurred in the direction of the tube motion. The simplest motion would be a linear or straight line movement of the tube and receptor as illustrated in Figure 1. This type of motion produces blur only in one direction. In many situations one-dimensional blur is not adequate for reducing the contrast of certain structures within the body. This is illustrated for a circular structure in Figure 4. A body structure is maximally blurred only when it is oriented in a direction perpendicular to the tube motion. Because of this only two sides of a circular structure will be blurred by linear motion. The other two sides, which are parallel to the tube motion, will appear to be elongated, but not blurred.

Many tomographic machines are designed to move the x-ray tube in a multidirectional pattern. The so-called polytome is a machine of this type. Several motion patterns are shown in Figure 5. The selection of a motion pattern generally depends on the shape and orientation of the body structures which are to be blurred. A disadvantage of the circular motion is that phantom images can be produced in some cases.

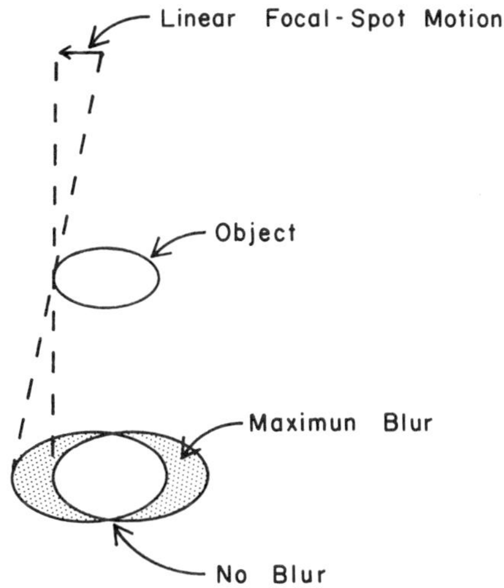

Figure 4. The blurring of a circular body structure by a linear tomographic motion.

COMPUTED TOMOGRAPHY

In the mid-1970's a method of tomographic imaging was developed which makes use of a digital computer. These systems are generally referred to as computed tomography (CT) scanners. CT imaging systems differ from conventional tomographic systems in several respects. Most CT systems produce images of body sections in the transaxial plane as shown in Figure

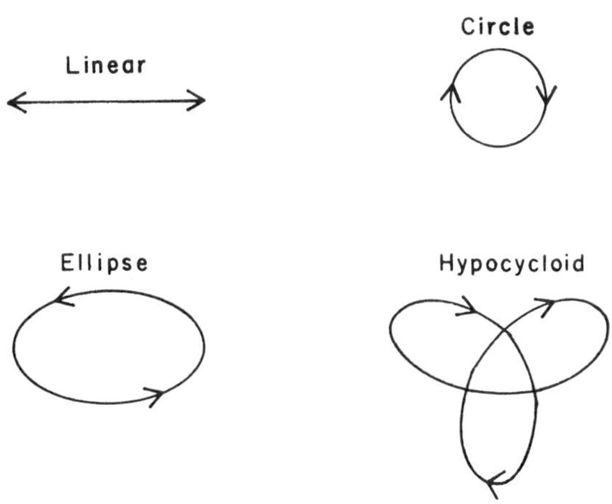

Figure 5. Various focal spot motion patterns used in tomography.

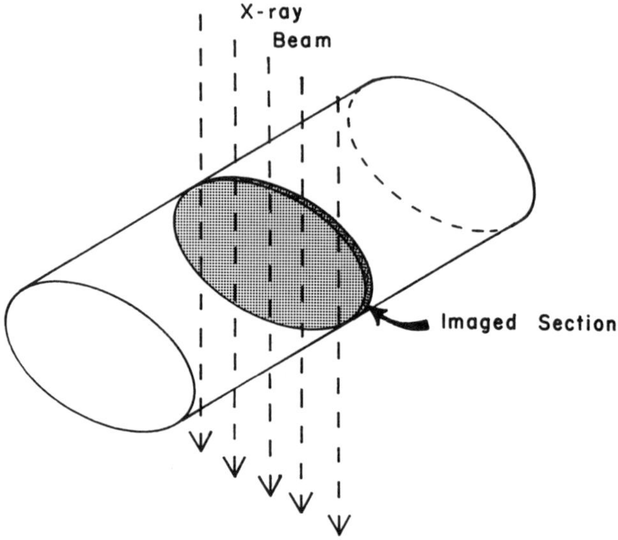

Figure 6. The relationship of the x-ray beam, imaged plane, and body section in computed tomography.

6. It was shown earlier that conventional tomographic systems produced images of axial planes through the body. In CT imaging the x-ray beam or beams pass only through the section being imaged.

In a CT system the image is not formed directly by the x-ray beam as it is in other x-ray procedures, but is a multistep process as shown in Figure 7. Most CT systems contain three functional units which are involved in the image-forming process. These are 1) the scanning unit, 2) the computer, 3) the viewing unit. In addition to these units these systems contain one or more storage devices, such as magnetic discs or tapes, which are used to store data, images, and the computer programs.

Scanning

The first step is to scan the body section with one or more small x-ray beams. The beam generally has a rectangularly shaped cross-section with a thickness on the order of 1 mm and a width which corresponds to the thickness of the body section (slice) which is being imaged. This dimension is approximately 1 cm but can be more or less depending on the design of the equipment. After passing through the body section the x-ray beam is intercepted by a radiation detector which produces an electrical signal that is proportional to the intensity of the x-ray beam. The intensity of the x-ray

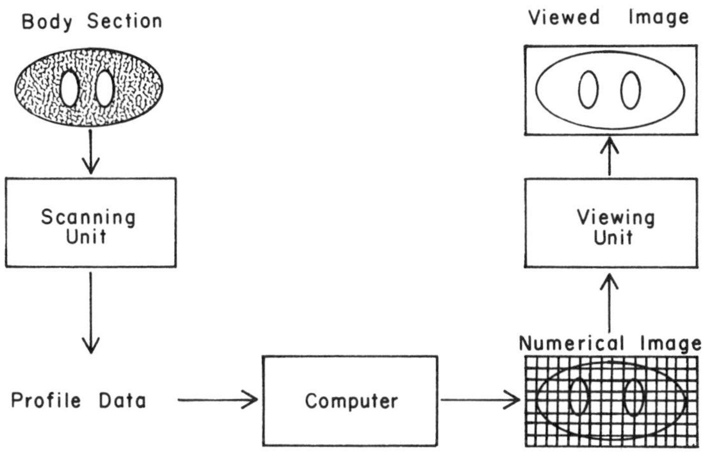

Figure 7. The steps in the formation of a CT image.

beam, in turn, is determined by the penetration of the body section. By either moving the x-ray beam or using a large number of beams a penetration profile of the body section is obtained.

The two general methods of obtaining a penetration profile are shown in Figure 8. One method is to use a small number of x-ray beams which are

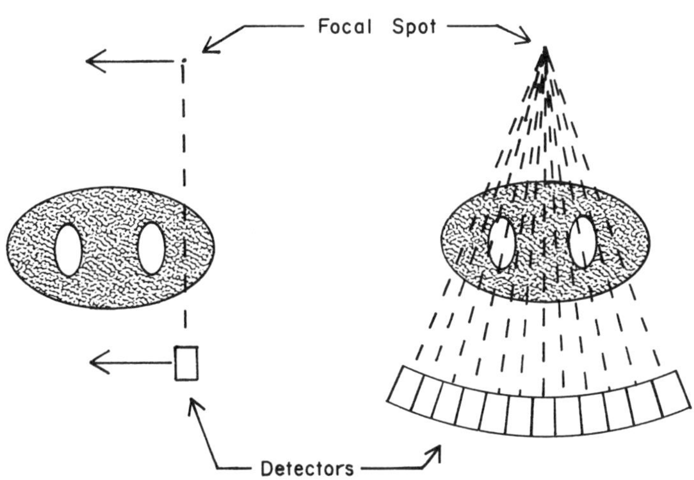

Figure 8. Two methods for obtaining a penetration profile of a body section. A single beam translate system is compared to a fan beam system.

scanned across the body section as indicated. Many of the earlier machines used a single beam. However, if multiple beams are used, it is possible to scan the body section faster. This type is usually designated as a "translate-rotate scanner."

A second method uses a so-called "fan beam." The fan beam consists of a large number of small x-ray beams coming from one x-ray tube. The individual beams are formed by a collimating device. After passing through the body section the beam is intercepted by an array of detectors. By using a fan beam it is possible to get a penetration profile without scanning across the body section. In order to form a CT image, penetration profiles taken at different angles through the body section are required. These are obtained by rotating the x-ray beam and detector assembly around the body. This is illustrated in Figure 9. In fan beam systems the rotation is continuous. In the translate-rotate systems the rotation occurs in small increments after each scan of the x-ray beam across the body section. These systems have two distinct motions of the x-ray beam with respect to the patient's body. One is the translational motion that produces data for one penetration profile, and the other is the rotation that allows penetration profiles to be obtained at different angles.

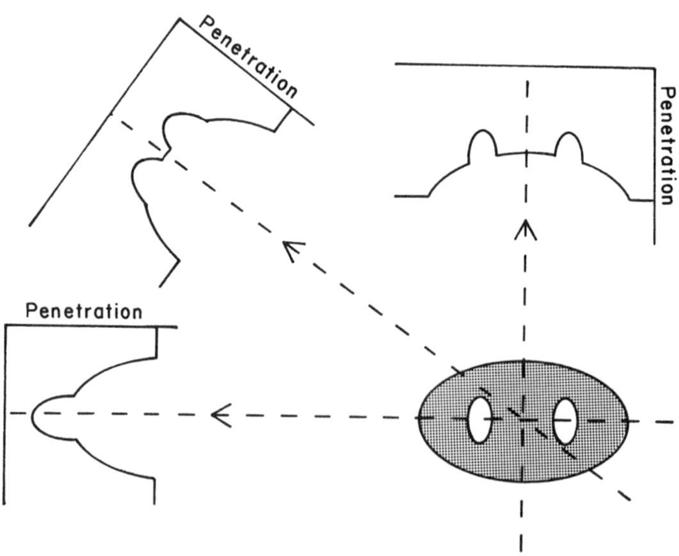

Figure 9. Penetration profiles obtained at three different angles through a body section.

Image Reconstruction

A digital computer within the system forms the CT image from the penetration profile data. This process is generally referred to as image reconstruction. It is a mathematical process and the computer actually calculates the image. The image created by the computer is a numerical image with specific values for each point within the image. The image area is divided into an array of individual miniature elements or pixels. Pixels are generally square and have dimensions in the order of 1 mm by 1 mm when referred to the body section being imaged. The specific pixel size is determined by the design of the system.

A numerical value is calculated for each pixel within the image. The pixel values are generally referred to as CT numbers. The numbers are related to the attenuation coefficient values of the materials within the body section. Most systems use water as a reference material for computing CT numbers and assign it a value of 0. Materials which have attenuation coefficient values which are larger than that of water will have positive CT numbers. Materials with lower attenuation coefficient values will have negative CT numbers. The value of the CT number, N_m, for a specific material is given by:

$$N_m = C(\mu_m - \mu_{water})$$

where C is the contrast factor for the scanner being used.

All CT systems do not use the same contrast factors. Therefore, a given material will have different CT number values when imaged with the different systems. Many systems are designed to have a contrast factor value of approximately 2,600. These systems will typically have CT numbers ranging from −500 for air to +500 for bone. A system which has a contrast factor value of 5,200 would have CT numbers ranging from −1000 to +1000 for the same materials.

It should be recalled that attenuation coefficient values are not only characteristics of the material and depend on the material's density and atomic number but are also related to the x-ray photon energy. Therefore, CT systems operated at different kVp values will generally produce different CT numbers for the same material.

There are a number of different mathematical procedures which can be used to reconstruct an image from penetration profiles. The so-called back projection method is used in many systems. The basic concept of this method is illustrated in Figures 10 and 11. Figure 10 shows a simplified body section which includes a block of high density material. The penetration profiles for two different x-ray beam directions are shown. Back

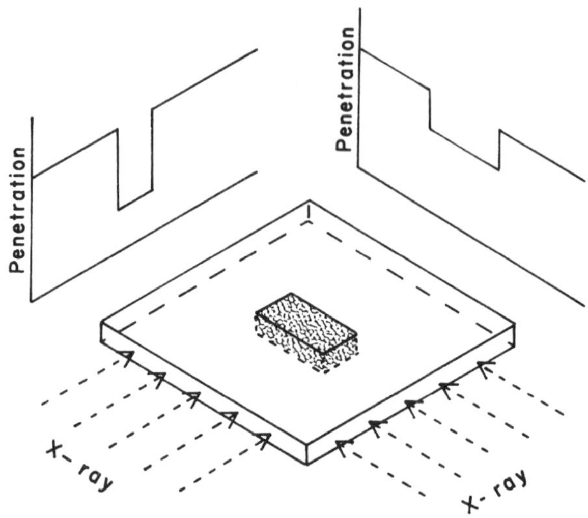

Figure 10. Penetration profiles from two directions through a simplified body section.

projection is illustrated in Figure 11. The computer takes each profile and assigns penetration values (CT numbers) to rows of pixels as shown. Different degrees of shading are used to represent different CT numbers. This is what is meant by back projection. The image is formed by the composite back projections from all of the profiles. Although Figure 11 uses only two

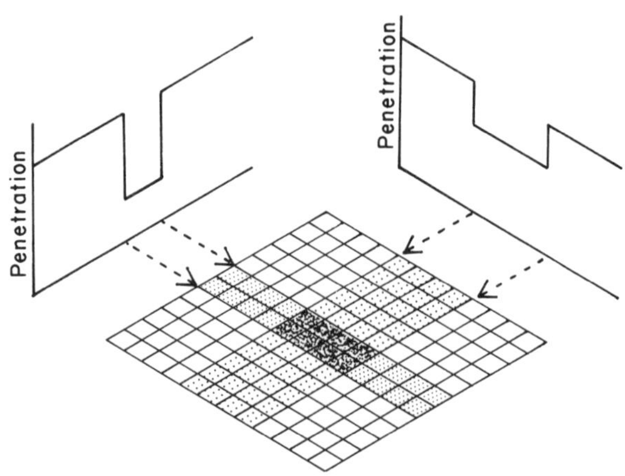

Figure 11. Back projection of penetration profiles to form a CT image.

profiles an image of the rectangular high density area can be seen. The problem with this particular image is that it contains artifacts in the form of streaks running across the image. However, if a large number of profiles, rather than just two, were used these streaks would not be present. Most CT systems use over 10 profiles to form one image.

Image Display

The numerical image must be converted into another form for viewing. Most systems use different brightness levels to represent the CT number values in each pixel. This conversion is made by the viewing unit portion of the system. The numerical image is converted into a video type signal which is displayed on a screen. Permanent images are obtained by photographing the screen.

The viewing unit contains controls; this allows the user to establish a specific relationship between pixel brightness (shades of gray) and the CT numbers. This general relationship is illustrated in Figure 12. The range of CT numbers which covers the complete gray scale or brightness range is commonly referred to as the window. Controls are available which can place the window at any position along the CT number scale and also change the window range. The window range is, in effect, a contrast control. A short window range setting will spread a smaller CT number range (subject contrast) over the entire brightness range and will therefore produce more image (radiographic) contrast.

The quality of a CT image depends on the design and operating characteristics of the imaging system. When describing CT image quality several different parameters must be considered.

Blur

The blur in most CT images is much greater than in conventional radiographs. The most significant source of blur is the division of the image into discrete pixels. Since a given pixel can have only one CT number value the image of a small object point cannot be smaller than a single pixel. The pixel size determines the minimum blur in a CT image. The image of an object point is generally not confined to a single pixel. Therefore, the actual blur is somewhat larger than the size of a single pixel. The blur produced by dividing an image into discrete pixels represents a minimum blur which will be present in all CT images. There are factors associated with the scanning and image reconstruction process which can cause the blur to be greater than this theoretical minimum value. In most systems, however, the blur is related to the pixel size.

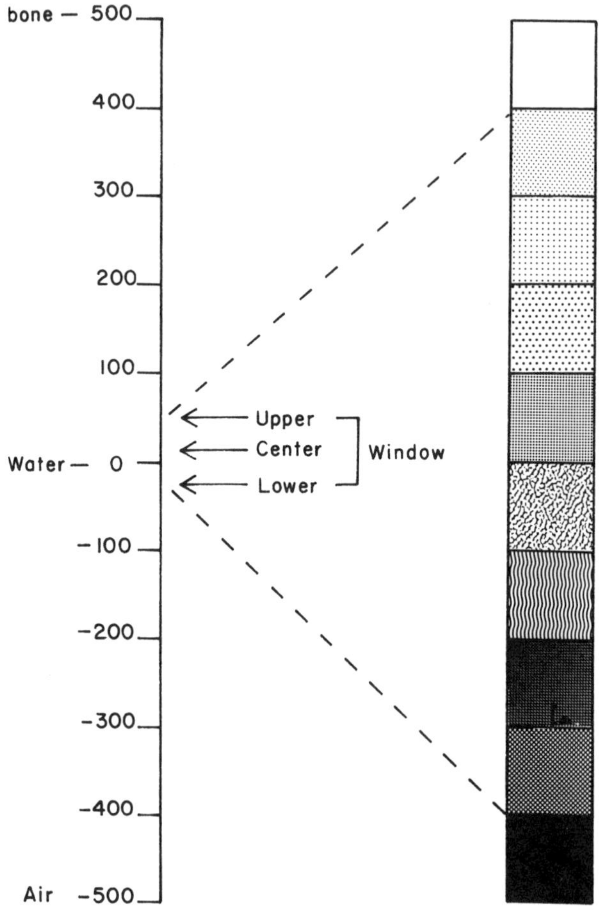

Figure 12. Relationship of image brightness or gray scale to CT numbers.

Noise

Noise in a CT image is a variation in CT number values from pixel to pixel even when all of the pixels are associated with the same material. A section of a CT image of water is shown in Figure 13. Water has an average CT number value of 0. However, because of the presence of noise individual pixel values will have a range of values as indicated. The variation in CT numbers (noise) can be expressed in terms of the standard deviation (SD) of the values. Figure 14 shows a typical distribution of CT numbers for water. The range of values represented by 1 SD below and above the

2	-2	-3	0	-6	-6	1	0
4	1	2	5	-1	1	5	3
2	-1	0	5	0	0	2	1
-1	-1	-2	0	0	1	0	0
1	1	-2	-1	1	-1	-4	-2
-2	2	-1	0	1	-1	-3	0
6	-3	2	1	-4	3	1	4
3	4	2	-4	-3	-1	-2	-5

Figure 13. Typical CT numbers in an image of a volume of water.

average value (0) is indicated. The value of the standard deviation can be expressed in CT numbers or as a percentage. Because different scanning systems have different contrast factors, it is necessary to express percentage of standard deviation in terms of attenuation coefficient values. Since different CT number scales are used a percentage standard deviation based on CT numbers alone cannot be used for comparing image quality of the different systems.

The statistical fluctuation of photon concentration is the major source of noise in CT images. As discussed in Chapter XIX, noise is reduced by increasing the number of photons used to form the image. The number of photons contributing to the CT number value for a given pixel is related to the size of the pixel and the thickness of the tomographic slice. These

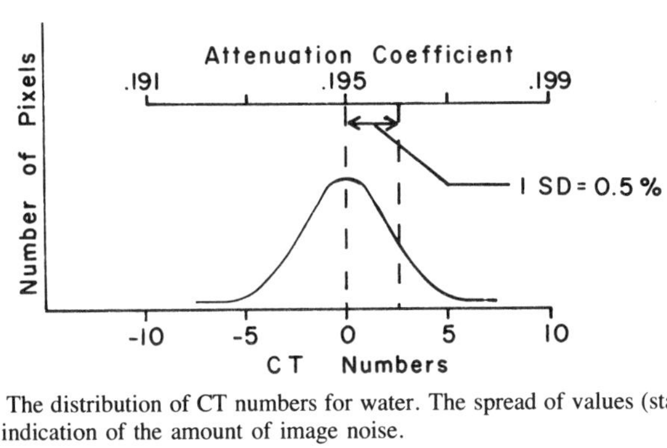

Figure 14. The distribution of CT numbers for water. The spread of values (standard deviation) is an indication of the amount of image noise.

dimensions establish the volume of tissue which is sampled to determine the CT number value.

In general, CT image noise is inversely related to pixel size, slice thickness, and patient exposure. A CT system which uses large pixels would produce an image with less noise but more blur than a system with smaller pixels operating at the same exposure levels. The relationship of noise, blur, and patient exposure should be taken into consideration when comparing various CT imaging systems.

Chapter XXII

Patient Exposure

It has been demonstrated that x-radiation can have a number of undesirable effects on the human body. The relationship between the risk of these undesirable effects and the quantity of radiation absorbed by the body is not well established. In general there are not sufficient data available that directly relate risk values to the quantities of radiation normally associated with diagnostic examinations. Much of the available data are derived from radiation quantities well above those encountered in diagnostic examinations. Also, there is not good agreement about the relationship between risk and amount of radiation. Two different proposed relationships are shown in Figure 1. The linear relationship implies that there is some risk associated with any quantity of radiation. The other relationship assumes a threshold radiation quantity below which there is no risk of undesirable effects. In the absence of evidence to the contrary it is best to assume that there is some risk associated with any radiation absorbed by the patient. Therefore, the physician must make appropriate decisions concerning the relationship of the risk to the benefits derived from the x-ray examination.

FACTORS IN PATIENT EXPOSURE

The exposure, or dose, to a specific point within a patient's body is determined by a combination of factors. One of the most significant is whether the point in question is in or out of the primary beam. Points not located in the direct beam can receive exposure from scattered radiation, but this is generally much less than the exposure to points within the beam area. The factors that determine exposure levels to points within the body will now be discussed in reference to the situation illustrated in Figure 2. It is assumed that the point of interest is the organ located near the middle of the body section.

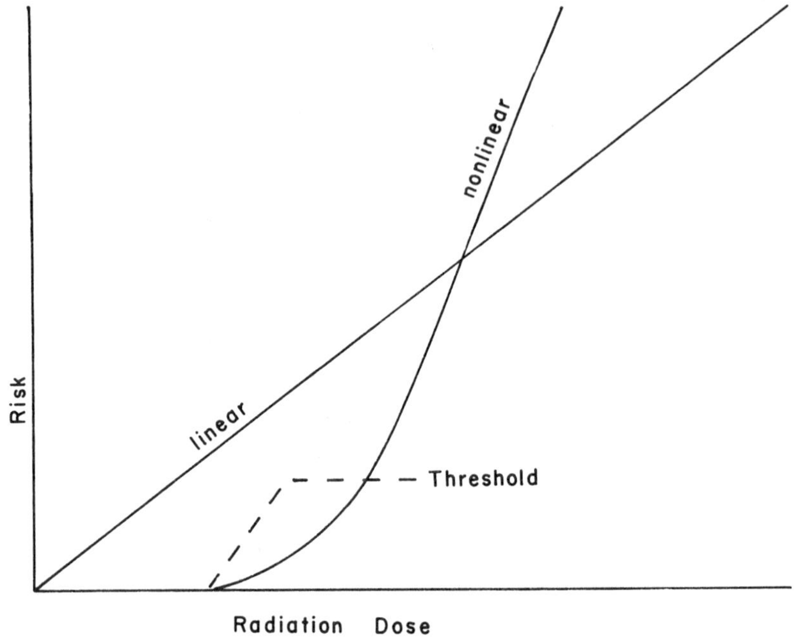

Figure 1. Two possible relationships between risk and the quantity of radiation imparted to the human body.

Receptor Sensitivity

One of the most significant factors is the amount of radiation that must be delivered to the receptor in order to form a useful image. This in turn is determined by the sensitivity of the receptor. It was shown in Table 1 of Chapter XIII that there is a rather wide range of sensitivity values, X_m, encountered in radiography. It is generally desirable to use the most sensitive receptor which will give adequate image quality. The exposure to points within the patient's body will be some multiple of the receptor exposure. The ratio of patient-to-receptor exposure is determined by the following factors.

Grids

It was shown in Chapter XII that the penetration, P_g, of grids is generally in the range of 0.17 to 0.4. This corresponds to a Bucky factor ranging from 6.0 to 2.5. The exposure to the exit surface of the patient is the product of the receptor exposure and the grid Bucky factor. This assumes that the receptor surface is not separated from the surface of the patient by a significant distance. The use of a high ratio grid, which generally has a

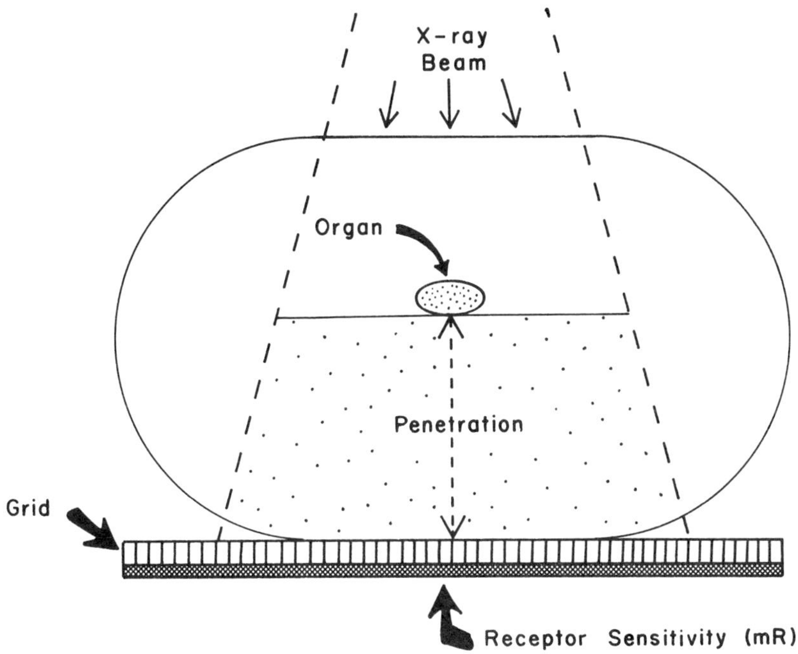

Figure 2. The elements in an x-ray system which determine the exposure to a specific organ location. The tissue located between the organ and receptor surface (shaded area) is a significant factor in organ exposure.

relatively low penetration, or a high Bucky factor will tend to increase the ratio of patient-to-receptor exposure. Low ratio grids reduce patient exposure by allowing more scattered radiation to contribute to the film exposure. In selecting grids the user should be aware of the general trade-off between patient exposure and image quality.

Table Top

In many x-ray examinations the receptor, which is typically an intensifying screen cassette, is located below the table surface which supports the patient's body. The attenuation of radiation by the table top is a factor in the ratio of patient-to-receptor exposure. It is generally recommended that the table top have a penetration, P_t, of at least 0.5 or not more than 1.0 HVL. The patient exposure with a table top which has a penetration of 0.5 will be double the exposure if no table top is located between the patient and receptor.

Tissue Penetration

If the point of interest, or organ, is not located at the exit surface of the body the attenuation in the tissue layer between the organ and exit surface will further increase the exposure. The ratio of the organ-to-exit surface exposure is determined by the penetration, P_p, of the tissue in between and the amount of scattered radiation, P_pS. The scatter factor, S, represents the scattered radiation generated in the tissue layer and scattered in the direction of the receptor. An increase in this factor would mean that more radiation contributes to exit surface exposure and reduces the organ-to-exit surface exposure ratio. However, some of the scattered radiation created in the tissue layer will be scattered back toward the organ. This radiation will increase the organ-exit surface exposure ratio. The increase in exposure due to backscatter can be represented by a backscatter factor, B. Whereas the forward scatter factor will have values ranging from 1 to approximately 5 or 6, backscatter factor values will generally range from 1 (no scatter) to approximately 1.2. The values of both factors are quite dependent on the size or area covered by the x-ray beam. A large x-ray beam area would generally produce more scattered radiation in the forward direction and would actually reduce the organ-to-exit exposure. However, a large beam area exposes more tissue and increases scatter exposure to points outside of the primary beam.

The penetration of the tissue between the point of interest and the exit surface is determined by the distance between the two points, the type of tissue (soft tissue or bone), and the effective energy of the x-ray beam. For a given patient the only factor which can be varied to alter penetration is the effective energy. This in turn depends on waveform, kVp, and filtration. Generally speaking, three-phase or constant potential waveforms produce more penetrating radiation, which reduces patient exposure. It was shown earlier that adding filters to an x-ray beam selectively removes the low energy, low penetrating photons. This in turn produces an x-ray beam with a greater penetrating ability. Filtration of an x-ray beam is especially significant in reducing the exposure to points near the entrance surface. Patient exposure is generally reduced by increasing kVp. The problem is that the higher kVp values give lower image contrast because of object penetration and more scattered radiation.

Inverse Square Effect

Because of the diverging nature of an x-ray beam the concentration of x-ray photons, or exposure, decreases with distance from the focal spot. This is the so-called inverse square effect which was discussed in Chapter IV. This effect will increase the ratio of patient-to-receptor exposure. The ratio of patient exposure, X_p, to receptor exposure, X_r, because of the inverse square effect is given by:

$$\frac{X_p}{X_r} = m^2,$$

where m is the magnification factor for the point of interest. Consider a point which is located halfway between the focal spot and receptor surface. The geometric magnification would be a factor of 2. The exposure at this point would be 4 times the receptor exposure (m^2) because of the inverse square effect. The distances which determine the magnification factor for a point on the surface of the body are shown in Figure 3. Generally the distance, t, between the surface or point of interest and receptor is fixed by the size of the patient. Therefore, the only factor which can be changed is the distance between the focal spot and point of interest, x. Since the magnification factor, m, is related to this distance by:

$$m = \frac{x + t}{x}$$

the magnification factor is increased by decreasing x. Because of this, patient exposure is reduced by using the greatest distance possible between the focal spot and body. The effect of decreasing this distance on patient exposure is illustrated in Figure 3. Here two body sections are shown with x-ray beams which cover the same receptor area. The x-ray beam with the shorter focal-to-patient distance covers a smaller area at the entrance surface. Because essentially the same radiation is concentrated into the smaller area, the exposure to the entrance surface and points within the patient will be higher than for the x-ray beam with the greater focal-patient distance.

It is generally recommended (see Reference on p. 292) that the distance between focal spot and patient surface should be at least 38 cm (15 inches) in radiographic examinations. Fluoroscopic tables should be designed so that the focal spot is at least 38 cm below the table top.

The inverse square effect increases the concentration of radiation (exposure and dose) in the patient's body. However, the total amount of radiation (surface integral exposure) is not significantly increased by decreasing the tube-to-patient distance. When this distance is decreased, the same radiation energy, or number of photons, is concentrated in a smaller area.

In procedures where the body section is separated from the receptor surface in order to achieve magnification there can be a significant increase in exposure because of the inverse square effect. Also, this introduces an

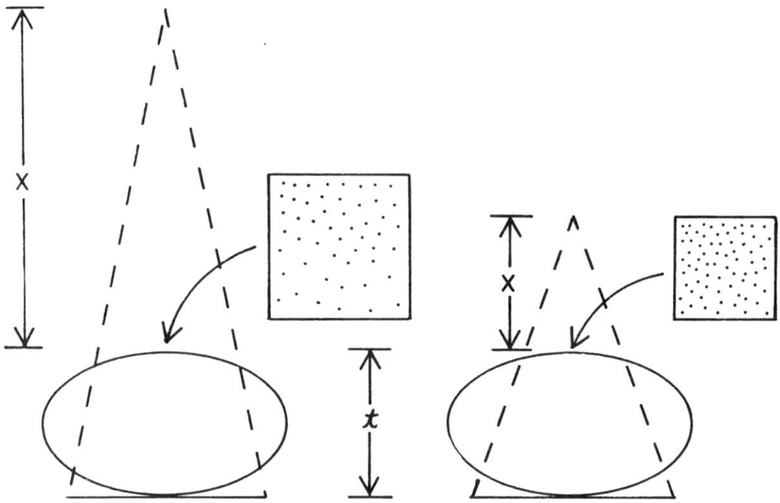

Figure 3. Decreasing the distance between the x-ray tube and patient surface increases the concentration of radiation or surface exposure.

"air gap" which reduces the amount of scattered radiation reaching the receptor. In order to compensate for this and to achieve the same film exposure it is generally necessary to increase the x-ray machine output, which increases the amount of exposure to the patient.

An approximate expression for the exposure to a point of interest which is located in the primary beam is given by:

$$X(mR) = \frac{X_m(mR) \cdot B \cdot m^2}{P_p \cdot P_g \cdot S}$$

where the various factors have been described previously. This relationship is useful in that it shows the various factors which affect patient exposure. It is not intended to be used to find exposure values for specific situations because values for penetration and the scatter factors are not generally known. A method which can be used to determine patient exposure in a specific examination will be discussed below.

DETERMINATION OF PATIENT DOSE

The previous section has identified the significant factors which affect the exposure or dose to a patient undergoing an x-ray examination. It is often desirable to determine the dose received by a patient in a specific examination. The relationships discussed above are generally not useful for this purpose because many of the factors such as receptor sensitivity, scatter factor, etc., are not precisely known. It is usually easier to determine patient exposure and dose by starting with the technical factors, KVP and MAS.

It has been shown previously that the exposure delivered to a point located 1 m from the focal spot is given by:

$$\dot{X}(mR) = E_x \cdot MAS$$

where E_x is the efficacy of the x-ray tube. In most facilities x-ray machines are calibrated periodically and the efficacy value can be obtained from the calibration reports. In the absence of a measured efficacy value for a specific machine it might be necessary to use typical values such as are found in Figure 7 of Chapter VI. It should be remembered that efficacy values depend on kVp, waveform, filtration, and the general condition of the x-ray tube anode. The exposure to points at other distances from the focal spot can be determined by adding an inverse square correction to the above relationship. This gives:

$$X(mR) = \frac{\dot{X}}{d^2} = \frac{E_x \cdot MAS}{d^2},$$

where d is the distance between the focal spot and the point of interest. The exposure value given by this relationship assumes that there is no attenuation of the x-ray beam by materials such as tissue. When the point of interest is within the body two additional factors must be considered: 1) the attenuation of the radiation as it passes through the overlying tissue; and 2) the contribution of scattered radiation to the exposure. This can be

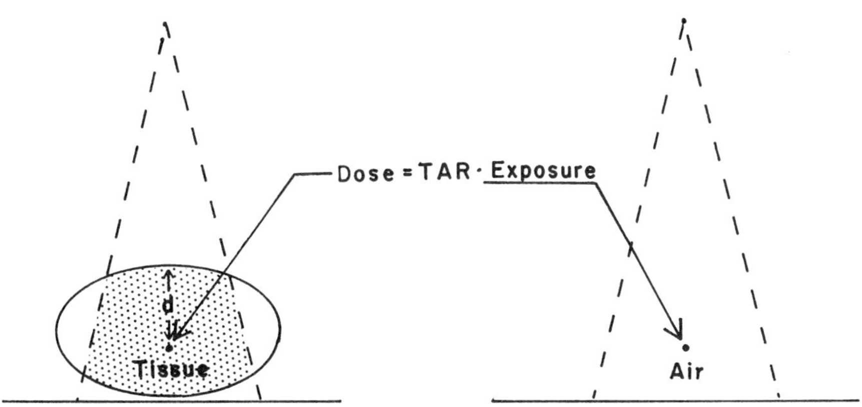

Figure 4. Relationship of tissue dose to air exposure.

Table 1. TAR values for 40-cm by 40-cm field and 2.5-mm aluminum filtration[a]

Tissue depth (cm)	kVp				
	70	80	90	100	120
0	1.07	1.10	1.12	1.14	1.15
2	1.06	1.09	1.11	1.15	1.20
4	0.791	0.845	0.904	0.955	1.09
6	0.566	0.625	0.679	0.726	0.813
8	0.406	0.461	0.510	0.552	0.630
10	0.291	0.340	0.383	0.420	0.489
12	0.208	0.250	0.288	0.320	0.379
14	0.149	0.185	0.217	0.243	0.294
16	0.107	0.136	0.163	0.185	0.228
18	0.077	0.100	0.122	0.141	0.177
20	0.055	0.074	0.092	0.107	0.137

[a]Data provided by R. J. Schulz.

done by multiplying the exposure value in air by the appropriate tissue-air ratio (TAR) as illustrated in Figure 4. Some typical TAR values for diagnostic x-ray examinations are given in Table 1. TAR values depend on the depth of the point of interest within the body, the penetrating ability of the x-ray beam (kVp, filtration, waveform), and the size of the x-ray beam field which affects the amount of scattered radiation produced.

The relationships discussed above can be combined to give:

$$\text{Dose (mrad)} = X \cdot \text{TAR} = \frac{E_x \cdot \text{MAS} \cdot \text{TAR}}{d^2}$$

The fact that both x-ray tube efficacy, E_x, and TAR increase with kVp does not mean that patients receive more radiation when the kVp is increased in an examination. An increase in kVp must be compensated for by decreasing MAS to obtain the same film exposure. This results in less radiation to the patient because of better penetration.

REFERENCES

National Council on Radiation Protection and Measurements. Medical x-ray and gamma ray protection for energies up to ten MeV. Equipment design and use, Report Number 33. Washington, D. C.

Chapter XXIII

Personnel Exposure

During the process of conducting x-ray examinations there is the possibility that persons other than the patient will receive some x-ray exposure. This chapter discusses the factors that determine the amount of exposure that such individuals might receive.

RADIATION SOURCES

Staff personnel can receive exposure from the primary x-ray beam or from stray radiation. The term 'stray radiation' as used in this discussion includes radiation scattered from the primary beam and leakage radiation. Leakage radiation is the radiation from the x-ray tube other than that contained within the beam. Regardless of the source it is useful to specify the amount of radiation from it in terms of the exposure, $\dot{X}$, at a distance of 1 m from the source.

Primary Radiation

For the primary radiation from an x-ray machine the exposure at 1 m, $\dot{X}$, is given by:

$$\dot{X}(\mathrm{mR}) = E_x \cdot \mathrm{MAS}$$

where E_x is the efficacy of the x-ray tube. Typical values of x-ray tube efficacy are shown in Figure 7 of Chapter VI.

Scattered Radiation

In most situations the most significant source of scattered radiation is the portion of the patient's body which is within the primary x-ray beam. The exposure produced by the scattered radiation at a distance of 1 m from the center of a patient's body will be some fraction, a, of the entrance surface exposure from the primary beam. The relationship of the scatter exposure at 1 m, $\dot{X}_s$, to the entrance surface exposure, X_p, depends on several

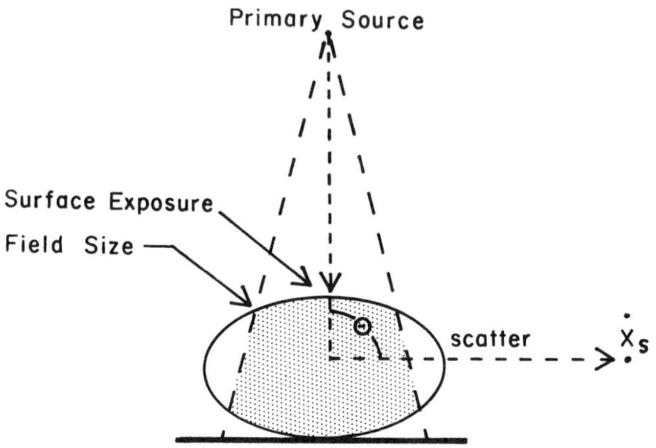

Figure 1. Factors which determine scatter radiation exposure at a point located 1 m from a patient's body.

factors, as illustrated in Figure 1. The three most significant factors are the penetrating ability of the x-ray beam, which is determined by the kVp; the size of the scatter source, which is related to the field size, F, of the primary beam; and the angle between the directions of the primary and scattered radiation. The scatter exposure at one meter from the patient is given by:

$$\dot{X}_s(\text{mR}) = a \cdot X_p \cdot \frac{F}{400}$$

Values of the fraction, a, can be obtained from published data (National Council on Radiation Protection and Measurements; Trout and Kelley, 1972). The published values are for a field size of 400 cm². This is the reason for the number 400 in the denominator of the above relationship.

In Chapter XXII it was shown that the exposure to the entrance surface of a patient, X_p, is given by:

$$X_p = \frac{E_x \cdot \text{MAS}}{d^2}$$

where d is the distance between the focal spot and the entrance surface. This expression can be substituted in the previous relationship to give:

$$\dot{X}_s = \frac{a \cdot E_x \cdot \text{MAS} \cdot F}{400\ d^2}$$

This expression can now be used to arrive at an approximate exposure value at a distance of 1 m from a patient for a specific examination condition. Although kVp does not appear in this relationship, it does have a significant effect on scatter exposure. The value of E_x and the fraction, a, increases with an increase in kVp.

Values of the fraction, a, generally increase with kVp and the angle between the primary and scattered radiation. At an angle of 90° the values range from 0.0005 at a kVp of 70 to 0.0013 at a kVp of 100.

Assume that the problem is to determine the scatter exposure from a patient for a specific examination in which a number of films were made. It is first necessary to determine the values of the various factors, as follows:

a = 0.0013 (90 degrees, 100 kVp (National Council on Radiation Protection and Measurements))

E_x = 13 mR/MAS (Figure 7, Chapter VI, 100 kVp, three phase)

F = 1,000 cm^2 (28-cm by 36-cm field size)

d = 0.8 m

MAS = 500 (total MAS for all films)

Substitution of these values in the above relationship gives:

$$X_s = \frac{(0.0013)(13)(500)(1{,}000)}{(400)(0.8)^2} = 33 \text{ mR}$$

This value would be the exposure at a distance of 1 m from the patient with no barrier.

Leakage Radiation

Diagnostic x-ray tube housings are designed so that the exposure from leakage radiation, at 1 m, does not exceed 100 mR per hour of operation. Most x-ray tubes are not operated at their maximum capacity; therefore the actual leakage radiation exposure is generally much less than 100 mR per hour.

AREA EXPOSURE

It is helpful to begin by considering the radiation exposure to an area of interest. The relationship of an area of interest to a radiation source is shown in Figure 2. The radiation source can be an x-ray tube (primary beam or leakage), a source of scattered radiation such as a patient's body, or a radioactive material.

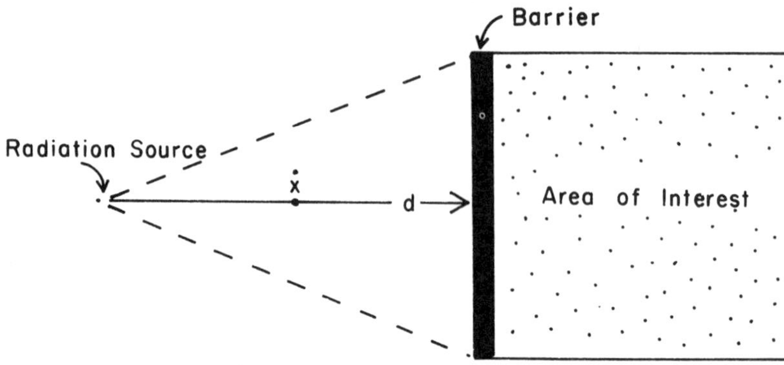

Figure 2. Exposure to an area of interest from a radiation source.

In most cases the area of interest is at a distance from the source other than 1 m and is also protected by a barrier or shield. Most protective barriers in diagnostic x-ray installations are made of lead. However, in some situations, building materials such as concrete provide adequate shielding. The exposure, X_a, to the area of interest which is located a distance, d, from the source is given by:

$$X_a = \frac{\dot{X} \cdot P_b}{d^2}$$

where P_b is the penetration of the barrier.

Several additional factors can be added to the above relationships to make them more useful for evaluating specific exposure situations. It is a common practice to consider exposure levels based on a 1-week time period. Therefore, it is necessary to know the total MAS used during a week. This quantity is generally designated as the workload, W. It is a common practice to express workload in the units of milliampere-minutes per week. Workload values are obtained from an analysis of the work performed in a specific facility, or typical values can be obtained from published reports (National Council on Radiation Protection and Measurements). In many situations the x-ray beam might not be directed at the area of interest during all of the ''on'' time. Therefore, it is necessary to introduce a factor to take this into account. The use factor, U, is the fraction of time that a particular radiation source is directed at the area of interest. By incorporating the weekly workload, W, and the use factor, U, into the relationship given above, an expression for the weekly exposure to the area of interest from primary radiation is given by:

$$X_a \text{ (mR/week)} = \frac{60\ E_x \cdot P_b \cdot W \cdot U}{d^2}$$

For scattered radiation the relationship is:

$$X_a \text{ (mR/week)} = \frac{60\ E_x \cdot P_b \cdot W \cdot U \cdot a \cdot F}{400 \cdot d_1^2 \cdot d_2^2}$$

where d_1 is the focal spot-patient distance and d_2 is the patient to area of interest distance. The value for the field size, F, is the weighted average for all of the examinations performed during a week. It is generally assumed that the scattered radiation is always directed toward the area of interest. Therefore, the use factor, U, for scattered radiation is generally assumed to have a value of 1.

DETERMINATION OF BARRIER THICKNESS

Protective barriers or shields are used to reduce the x-ray exposure in a specific area to an acceptable value. An appropriate barrier must have a penetration value, P_b, which is related to the exposure values by:

$$P_b = \frac{X_a\text{(acceptable)}}{X_a\text{(no barrier)}}$$

The exposure to the area of interest without a barrier can be determined as described above. Several factors must be considered in arriving at an acceptable exposure value for a specific area. The acceptable area exposure is determined by the permissible exposure to persons occupying the area and the degree of occupancy. Permissible personnel exposure is generally considered to be the same as the maximum permissible dose equivalent (MPD).

For the purposes of radiation protection, areas around an x-ray facility are divided into two categories, controlled and noncontrolled. The recommended MPD for a controlled area is 100 mrem per week (1). Persons occupying a controlled area (other than patients) are designated as occupationally exposed persons. Areas occupied by nonoccupationally exposed persons, such as the general public, are designated as uncontrolled areas. The recommended MPD for persons in an uncontrolled.area is 10 mrem per week. The acceptable area exposure is found by dividing the appropriate MPD value by the occupancy factor, T.

$$X_a \text{ (acceptable)} = \frac{\text{MPD}}{T}$$

The occupancy factor is related to the fraction of the total time that an area is occupied by the same person. The occupancy factor for controlled areas is generally considered to have a value of 1, which represents full time occupancy. Uncontrolled areas, such as stairways, corridors, and toilets, would generally have a lower occupancy factor.

It should be pointed out that under certain conditions both controlled and noncontrolled areas can have the same acceptable exposure. For example, a noncontrolled area (MPD of 10 mrem per week) with an occupancy factor of 0.1 would have an acceptable weekly exposure of 100 mR. This would be the same as the acceptable exposure to a controlled area (MPD of 100 mrem per week) with an occupancy factor of 1.

The appropriate relationships can be combined to give the maximum barrier penetration which would reduce the area exposure to an acceptable level.

$$P_b = \frac{MPD \cdot d^2}{T \cdot X}$$

In this equation, X is the exposure (milliroentgens per week at a distance of 1 m from the radiation source) being considered. For example, if the concern is with scattered radiation, the maximum barrier penetration which will produce the required protection is given by:

$$P_b = \frac{MPD \cdot d_1^2 \cdot d_2^2 \cdot 400}{a \cdot F \cdot T \cdot W \cdot 60\ E_x}$$

It has been a common practice in designing x-ray barriers to calculate a quantity, K, which is the product of the required barrier penetration, the x-ray tube efficacy, and the number 60. For scattered radiation the equation for K becomes:

$$K = \frac{MPD \cdot d_1^2 \cdot d_2^2 \cdot 400}{a \cdot F \cdot T \cdot W}$$

After the required barrier penetration (or K) is found, the next step is to determine the thickness of barrier material which will produce the required penetration. This is done by referring to published data (National Council on Radiation Protection and Measurements; Kelley and Trout, 1972; Trout, Kelley, and Lucas, 1959) which relates barrier penetration (K), material thickness, and kVp.

REFERENCES

Kelley, J. P., and Trout, E. D. 1972. Broad beam attenuation in lead for X-rays from 50 to 300 kVp. Radiology 104 (1):171.

National Council on Radiation Protection and Measurements. Structural shielding design and evaluation for medical use of x-rays and gamma rays of energies up to ten MeV, Report Number 49. Washington, D. C.

Trout, E. D., and Kelley, J. P. 1972. Scattered radiation from a tissue-equivalent phantom for x-rays from 50 to 300 kVp. Radiology 104(1):161.

Trout, E. D., Kelley, J. P., and Lucas, A. C. 1959. Broad beam attenuation in concrete for 50 to 300 kVp x-rays and in lead for 300-kVp x-rays. Radiology 72 (1):62.

Chapter XXIV

Measurement of X-ray Quantities

It is often desirable to measure the amount of x-radiation in order to determine patient or personnel exposure or to evaluate x-ray equipment performance. There are several types of instruments that can be used to measure radiation in the diagnostic x-ray environment. The two devices that are the most widely used are the ionization chamber and the thermoluminescence dosimeter. It will be brought out in the following discussion that each of these has certain characteristics that make it more desirable for certain applications than the other.

In addition to these two instruments, film can be used to measure x-ray exposure. The most common application of film is to measure personnel exposure within the x-ray facility. This is normally done by placing a small piece of film in a badge that is then worn on the body. Film badges can be used to monitor personnel exposure over extended periods of time, such as 1 month or longer. Film badges generally cannot measure exposure with the same accuracy as the other devices discussed below.

IONIZATION CHAMBER

It should be recalled that the radiation quantity, exposure, is defined in terms of the amount of ionization produced by the radiation. Therefore, the most direct way to measure exposure is to collect and measure the ions produced by the radiation in air. This can be done by using a device known as an ionization chamber. Ionization chambers are constructed in many different configurations, but the two most common types are shown in Figure 1. All chambers consist of a volume of air located between two electrical conductors or electrodes. One type consists of two disc-shaped electrodes. The other type consists of one cylindrical electrode and a much

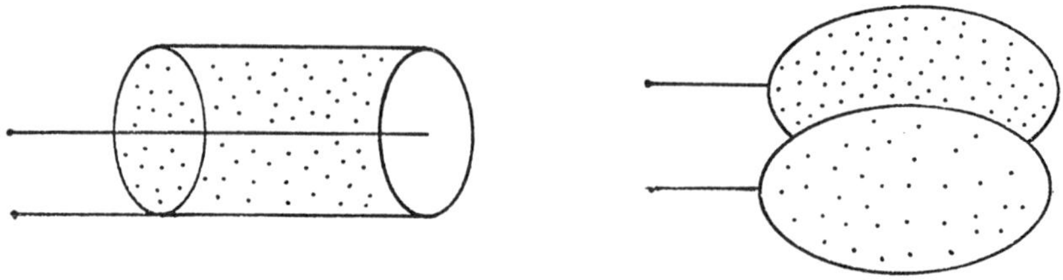

Figure 1. Two different ionization chamber electrode configurations. The sensitive volume is the air located between the electrodes.

smaller electrode rod running along the major axis of the cylinder. The electrodes are mounted on insulating material, which is not shown in the illustration. The purpose of the electrodes is to collect the ions formed within the air volume. Ionization chambers are generally used in two modes of operation. One is to measure exposure rates and the other is to measure total accumulated exposure over some period of time.

Exposure Rate Measurements

The basic system for measuring exposure rate with an ionization chamber is shown in Figure 2. In addition to the ionization chamber, a power supply and a device that will measure small electrical currents are required. The device normally used to measure the currents is the electrometer.

The three components are connected in a circuit, as shown in Figure 2. The power supply applies a voltage to the chamber, which causes one electrode to be negative and the other positive. If the air between the electrodes is not ionized it is an insulator and no electrical current can flow between the electrodes and through the circuit. However, when the air is exposed to x-radiation it becomes ionized and electrically conductive. Ionization is a process that either adds or removes electrons from an atom. This causes the atom to take on an electrical charge. Figure 2 shows how conduction takes place when an electron is removed from an atom by the radiation. The electron is attracted to the positive electrode, where it is

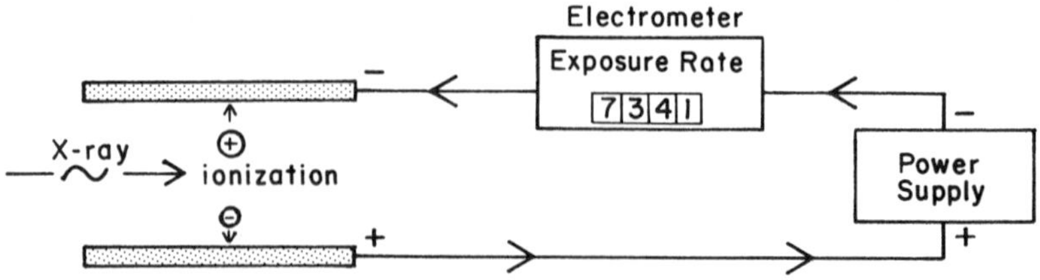

Figure 2. An ionization chamber system for measuring exposure rate.

collected and pumped through the circuit by the power supply. The arrows in Figure 2 indicate the direction of electron flow. The positive ion is attracted to the negative electrode. When it reaches the electrode it picks up an electron and becomes neutral. The electron that was absorbed from the negative electrode will be replaced by an electron from the circuit. Because electrons enter the ionization chamber at the negative terminal and leave from the positive terminal, the ionization chamber becomes, in effect, a conductor. For a given ionization chamber the amount of conduction, or current, is proportional to the exposure rate. When the system is calibrated the electrometer will indicate the exposure rate in units, such as roentgens per minute or milliroentgens per hour.

Exposure Measurements

Ionization chambers can also be used to measure accumulated exposure. One method is a three-step process, as is illustrated in Figure 3.

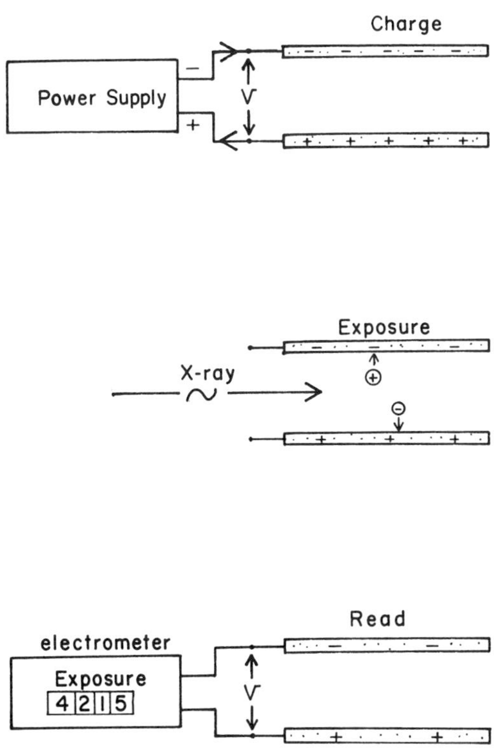

Figure 3. An ionization chamber system for measuring accumulated exposure.

The first step is to "charge" the ionization chamber by connecting it to a power supply. This is done before the chamber is exposed to the radiation. Since an ionization chamber consists of two conductors separated by an insulator (non-ionized air), it forms an electrical capacitor. The power supply pumps some of the electrons from the positive electrode to the negative. The quantity of electrons moved depends on the size of the chamber and the voltage applied by the power supply. This movement of electrons is what is generally referred to as charging the chamber. If the ionization chamber is disconnected from the power supply the charge will remain until some conductive path is formed between the two electrodes. A voltage will be present between the two electrodes even after the power supply is removed. For a given ionization chamber the voltage is proportional to the charge or number of displaced electrons.

When the charged chamber is exposed to ionizing radiation the air becomes conductive and discharges the chamber. This happens in the following way. The positively charged ions are attracted to the negative electrode, where they pick up some of the excess electrons. The electrons formed in the air by the ionization are attracted to and collected by the positive electrode. The number of electrons that are returned to their normal locations is proportional to the exposure to the air within the chamber. The third step is to determine the exposure value by reading the voltage that remains across the chamber after it is exposed to radiation. The voltage is usually read with an electrometer. By using appropriate calibration factors the drop in chamber voltage produced by the ionization can be converted into appropriate exposure units, such as roentgens or milliroentgens.

In practice, exposure measurements should be made over relatively short time intervals in order to avoid error from chamber leakage. Leakage is the discharge of the chamber from sources other than radiation, such as moisture on the insulating materials.

ERRORS IN EXPOSURE MEASUREMENT

There are several factors that must be taken into consideration when using ionization chambers to make exposure measurements. Most ionization chambers are not absolute devices and must be calibrated against some standard. A so-called "free air ionization chamber" is used as the standard in most calibration laboratories. This device is a specially designed instrument in which the sensitive air volume is not in direct contact with the electrodes but is surrounded by a buffer region of air. This prevents x-ray interactions with the electrodes from influencing the amount of ionization within the sensitive air volume. In the free air ionization chamber the ions are collected from a precisely determined volume of air. When the amount of ionization is measured with a properly calibrated electrometer an accurate exposure determination can be made. Free air ionization chambers are not used for routine exposure measurements but as a standard for calibrating other types of ionization chambers.

The response of an ionization chamber in terms of the number of ions produced and collected per unit of exposure can change with exposure conditions. Because of this, it is often necessary to use various correction factors in order to get precise exposure measurements.

Photon Energy Dependence

In most ionization chambers the amount of ionization produced per exposure unit varies with photon energy. This is usually related to the interaction of the x-ray beam with the walls of the chamber. A significant portion of the x-ray photons that contribute to the ionization are absorbed in the chamber walls. Some of the energetic electrons created by photoelectric and Compton interactions within the walls enter the air volume and produce ionization. For a given energy there is a specific wall thickness that will produce maximum ionization. This is known as the equilibrium thickness and is approximately proportional to the photon energy. At low photon energies a thick chamber wall will attenuate the x-ray beam and reduce the chamber response. At high photon energies a thin chamber wall does not provide adequate material to interact with the x-ray beam to produce maximum ionization.

An ionization chamber should be selected for the particular type of radiation that is to be measured. For example, most chambers designed for high energy therapy radiation are generally not well suited to the measurement of diagnostic x-radiation. Even when a chamber is designed for a specific photon energy range or beam quality it is often necessary to use correction factors for the different beam quality (kVp) values.

Saturation

There are conditions in which all of the ions formed by the radiation are not collected and measured. The electrons and positive ions that result from the ionization process are known as ion pairs. Unless they are quickly separated there is a good chance that they will recombine because of their opposite electrical charges. The ion pairs that recombine do not contribute to the exposure measurement. Therefore, in order to get an accurate indication of the amount of ionization produced it is necessary to separate the ion pairs before recombination can occur. This is achieved by applying a sufficient voltage between the electrodes. As the voltage across the chamber is increased the force on the ions is also increased and they are separated more quickly. When the voltage applied to the chamber is enough to prevent any recombination the chamber is said to be saturated. The voltage required to produce saturation depends on the size and shape of the chamber and the rate at which ionization is being produced. Large chambers require a higher voltage to produce saturation than small chambers. For a given chamber the voltage required to produce saturation depends on the exposure rate. When some chambers are used to make measurements at high exposure rates saturation is not achieved and it is necessary to apply a saturation correction factor in order to obtain the correct exposure value.

THERMOLUMINESCENCE DOSIMETRY

Thermoluminescence is a process in which materials emit light when they are heated. Certain thermoluminescent materials can be used as dosimeters because the amount of light emitted is proportional to the amount of radiation absorbed by the material prior to heating.

Some of the materials that are used in thermoluminescence dosimetry (TLD) are lithium fluoride and calcium fluoride. These materials consist of small crystals that can be used in a powdered form or molded into various shapes.

TLD is a two-step procedure, as is illustrated in Figure 4. The first step is to expose the TLD material to the radiation. A portion of the

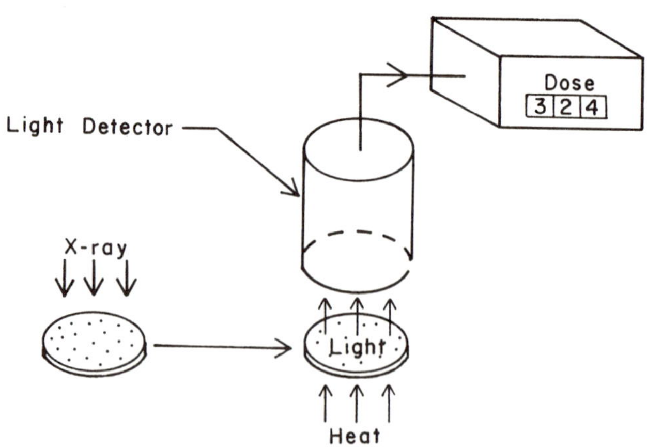

Figure 4. The two steps in radiation measurement using a thermoluminescence dosimeter.

absorbed radiation energy is used to raise electrons to higher energy levels. A characteristic of TLD material is that some of the electrons will be trapped in the higher energy locations. The number of electrons that remain in the elevated energy positions is proportional to the amount of radiation energy absorbed or the absorbed dose. The second step is to place the irradiated TLD material in a special reader unit. This unit performs two functions. It heats the TLD material and measures the amount of light emitted during the heating process. Heating causes the trapped electrons to be freed and allows them to drop back to their normal low energy positions. The energy difference between the two electron locations is given off in the form of light. By calibrating the system the light output is converted into absorbed dose values.

TLD dosimeters have several general advantages over ionization chambers. A TLD can be used to measure a much greater range of dose (or exposure) values than a single ionization chamber. They are also dose-rate independent and do not have the saturation problems that are common to ionization chambers. Another useful property is the ability of a TLD to collect radiation over a much longer period of time than is possible with ionization chambers. This makes them very useful for monitoring personnel and area exposures.

A TLD actually measures absorbed dose in the thermoluminescent material. Since most materials used as thermoluminescent dosimeters have approximately the same effective atomic number as soft tissue and air, the TLD reading will be proportional to both soft tissue absorbed dose and exposure in air. Some TLD materials will have a response that changes more with photon energy than others. Therefore, it is desirable to calibrate a TLD system for the type of radiation (photon energy) that is to be measured.

Chapter XXV Ultrasound

Sound is a physical phenomenon which transfers energy from one point to another. In this respect it is somewhat similar to x-radiation. It differs from x-rays, however, in that sound can pass only through matter and not through a vacuum. This is because the sound waves are actually vibrations passing through the material. If there is no material there is nothing to vibrate and sound cannot exist.

One of the most significant characteristics of sound is its frequency. Frequency is the rate at which the sound source and the material vibrate. The basic unit for specifying frequency is the hertz which is one vibration or cycle per second. Pitch is a term which is commonly used as a synonym for frequency.

The human ear cannot hear or respond to all sound frequencies. The range of frequencies which can be heard by a normal young adult is from approximately 20 to 20,000 Hz (20 kHz). Ultrasound is sound which has a frequency above this audible range. Frequencies in the range of 1 MHz (million cycles per second) to 15 MHz are used in diagnostic ultrasound. It is used as a diagnostic tool because it can be focused into small, well defined beams which can be used to probe the human body.

The basic components of an ultrasound imaging system are shown in Figure 1. The details of the various components will be considered later but the general principle of ultrasound imaging is as follows. The source of the ultrasound pulses is the transducer which is activated by electrical pulses from the pulse generator circuit. The ultrasound pulses, or beam, enter the body and are reflected from the various internal structures. The reflected pulses or echoes are picked up by the transducer and reconverted into electrical pulses. After appropriate amplification the electrical pulses are used to form an image on the display device.

After the following discussion of the physical characteristics of ultrasound the formation of images will be considered in more detail.

ULTRASOUND CHARACTERISTICS

Ultrasound has several physical characteristics which must be considered in order to apply it properly to diagnostic applications.

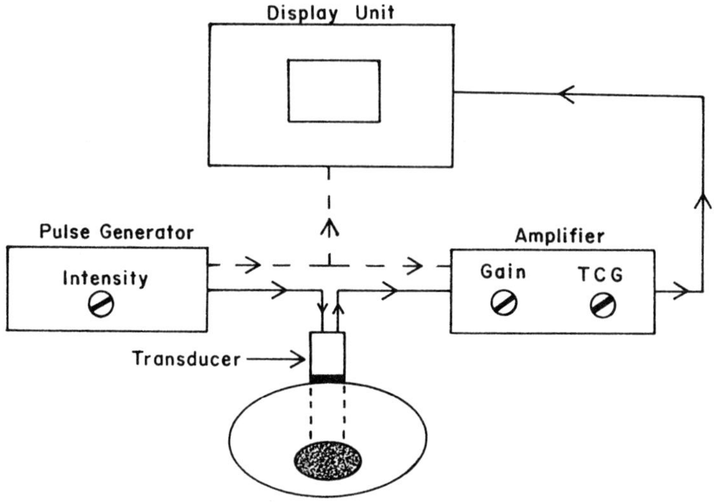

Figure 1. The basic components of an ultrasound imaging system. The solid line and arrows are the pathway of pulses. The dotted line is the pathway of synchronizing signals.

Frequency

Sound was described above as a vibration which moves through a material. The basic principle of sound transmission is illustrated in Figure 2. For simplicity the particles within the material are assumed to be arranged in rows. The source of sound is some vibrating object such as the transducer crystal. Since the vibrating source in Figure 2 is in contact with the particles in the first row, they are caused to vibrate. Because the particles in this row are in contact with those of the second row the particles in it begin to vibrate also. This process continues and the vibration, or sound, is passed along from one row of particles to another. The rate at which the particles vibrate back and forth is the frequency of the sound. The rate at which the vibrations move along from one row to another is the velocity of the sound.

Most diagnostic ultrasound systems use sound which is emitted in pulses rather than a continuous stream of vibrations. At any instant in time the vibrations are contained within a relatively small volume of the material. It is this volume of vibrating material which is referred to as the ultrasound pulse. As the vibrations are passed on from one layer of material to another the ultrasound pulse, but not the material, moves away from the source. The diameter of the pulse is determined by the characteristics of the transducer. At the transducer surface the diameter of the pulse is the same as the diameter of the vibrating crystal. As the pulse moves through the

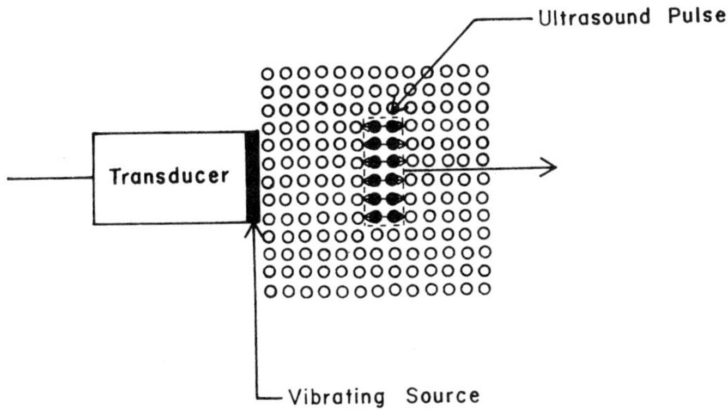

Figure 2. The movement of an ultrasound pulse through matter.

body the diameter will generally change. This is determined by the focusing characteristics of the transducer and will be discussed in detail later. As shown in Figure 3 the space through which the ultrasound pulse moves is generally referred to as the beam. In diagnostic systems pulses are emitted at a rate of approximately 1,000 per sec. The pulse rate (pulses per second) should not be confused with the frequency, which is the rate of vibration of the particles within the pulse.

The frequency of sound is determined by the source. For example, in a piano the source of sound is a string which is caused to vibrate by striking it. Each string within the piano is adjusted or tuned to vibrate with a

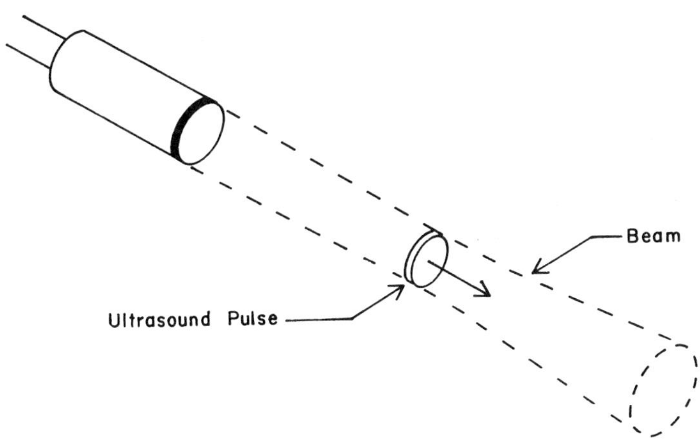

Figure 3. Relationship of the ultrasound pulse and beam to the transducer.

specific frequency. In diagnostic ultrasound equipment the sound is generated by a device called a transducer. The major element within the transducer is a special crystal which has been designed to vibrate with the desired frequency. A special property of the crystal material is that it is piezoelectrical. This means that the crystal will deform if electricity is applied to it. Therefore, if an electrical pulse is applied to the crystal it has essentially the same effect as striking a piano string: it is set into vibration. If the transducer is activated by a single electrical pulse the transducer will vibrate or "ring" for a short period of time. This creates an ultrasound pulse as opposed to a continuous ultrasound wave. Most diagnostic procedures use pulsed ultrasound. The ultrasound pulse travels through the material in contact with the transducer and moves away from the transducer surface as shown in Figure 2. A given transducer can vibrate with only one frequency, called its resonant frequency. Therefore, the only way to change ultrasound frequency is to change transducers. It will be shown later that certain frequencies are more appropriate for certain types of examination than others.

Velocity

The velocity with which sound travels through a medium is determined by the characteristics of the material and not the sound. There are several types of sound waves depending on the direction of vibration with respect to the direction of movement of the pulse. In soft tissue and fluids most of the vibration is in the same direction as that in which the sound moves. This type of vibration is designated as longitudinal waves. Shear waves exist when the vibrations are at right angles to the direction of sound movement. The velocity of longitudinal sound waves in a liquid type medium is given by:

$$\text{Velocity} = \sqrt{E/\rho}$$

where ρ is the density of the material and E is a factor related to the elastic properties of the material. The velocities of sound through several materials of interest are given in Table 1.

Some solid materials, such as bone, transmit sound by means of shear waves.

Wavelength

The distance sound travels during the period of one vibration is known as the wavelength, λ. It is related to the velocity, v, and frequency, f, by:

$$\text{Wavelength} = \frac{v}{f}$$

Table 1. Approximate velocity of sound in various materials

Material	Velocity (m/sec)
Fat	1450
Water	1480
Soft tissue (average)	1540
Bone	4100

In other words, wavelength is simply the ratio of velocity to frequency. This means that the wavelength of ultrasound is determined by the characteristics of both the transducer (frequency) and the material through which the sound is passing (velocity). Although wavelength is not a unique property of a given ultrasound pulse it is of some significance because it will be shown later that the shape of an ultrasound beam is, to some extent, determined by the wavelength of the sound.

Amplitude

The distance through which the individual particles vibrate as the ultrasound pulse passes is the amplitude of the ultrasound pulse. Generally speaking, the amplitude is related to the energy content or "loudness" of the ultrasound pulse. The amplitude of the pulse as it leaves the transducer is determined by how hard the crystal is "struck" by the electrical pulse. Most systems will have a control on the pulse generator circuit which changes the size of the electrical pulse and the ultrasound pulse amplitude. In this text this will be designated as the intensity control although different names are used by the various equipment manufacturers.

In diagnostic applications it is usually necessary to know only the relative amplitude of ultrasound pulses. For example, it is necessary to know how much the amplitude, A, of a pulse decreases as it passes through a given thickness of tissue. The relative amplitude of two ultrasound pulses, or of one pulse after it has undergone an amplitude change, can be expressed by means of a ratio as follows:

$$\text{Relative amplitude (ratio)} = \frac{A_2}{A_1}$$

There are some definite advantages in expressing relative pulse amplitude in terms of the logarithm of the amplitude ratio. When this is done the relative amplitude is specified in the units of decibels (dB). The relative pulse amplitude, in decibels, is related to the actual amplitude ratio by:

$$\text{Relative amplitude (dB)} = 20 \log \frac{A_2}{A_1}$$

When the amplitude ratio is greater than 1 (comparing a large pulse to a smaller one) the relative pulse amplitude will have a positive decibel value. However, when the ratio is less than 1 the decibel value will be negative. In other words, if the amplitude of a pulse is increased by some means it gains decibels and when the amplitude is reduced it loses decibels.

Figure 4 compares decibel values to pulse amplitude ratios. The first two pulses differ in amplitude by 1 dB. In comparing the second pulse to the first this corresponds to an amplitude ratio of 0.89 or a reduction of approximately 11%. If the pulse should be reduced in amplitude by another 11% it would be 2 dB smaller than the original pulse. If the pulse is once again reduced in amplitude by 11% (of 79%) it will now have an amplitude ratio (with respect to the first pulse) of 0.71 to 1 or is 3 dB smaller.

Perhaps the best way to establish a "feel" for the relationship between pulse amplitude expressed in decibels and in percentage is to notice that 6 dB corresponds to amplitudes which differ by a factor of 2. A reduction in amplitude of 6 dB cuts the amplitude by a factor of 2 or to 50%. The doubling of a pulse amplitude would be an increase of 6 dB.

It will be shown below that during the lifetime of an ultrasound pulse it undergoes many reductions in amplitude. If the amount of each reduction is known in decibels the total reduction can be found very simply by adding

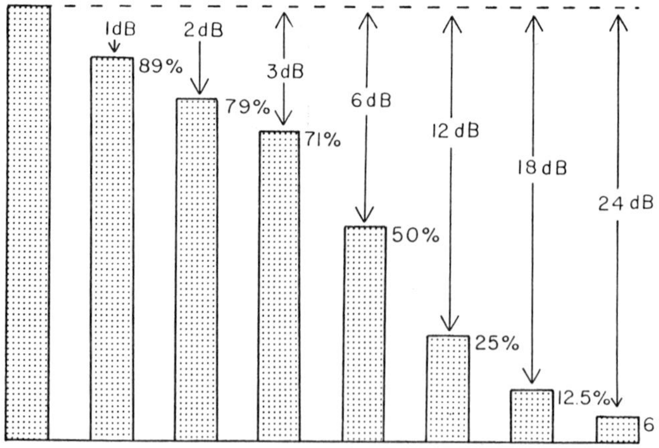

Figure 4. Pulse amplitudes expressed in decibels and percentage.

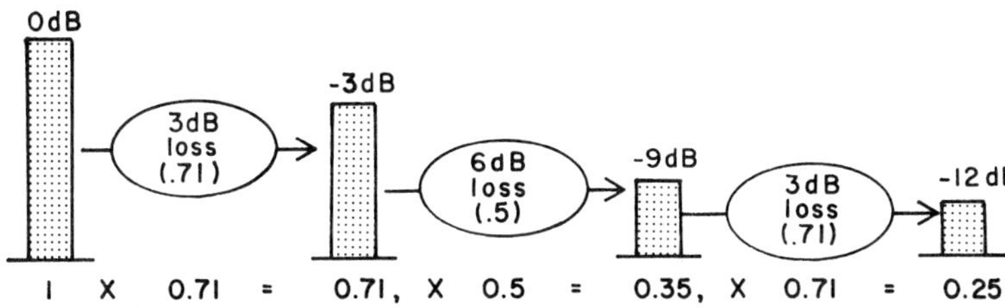

Figure 5. Final pulse amplitude is obtained by adding decibel values.

all of the decibel losses. This is much easier than having to multiply the various amplitude ratios. This is illustrated in Figure 5. Here a pulse undergoes three separate reductions in amplitude. The relative amplitude of the pulse at any point can be found by adding the decibel losses. The advantage of being able to do this rather than having to multiply the various ratios will become clear in later discussions.

In the following discussion of pulse amplitude the reader is advised to think in terms of decibels without constantly trying to convert back and forth between decibels and amplitude ratios or percentages. It is much easier to use the decibel method for computing pulse amplitude changes.

Intensity

Intensity is the amount of energy which passes through a specified area per second. Intensity is usually expressed in the units of watts per square centimeter. The intensity of most diagnostic ultrasound beams at the transducer surface is in the order of a few milliwatts per square centimeter. The intensity is related to the amplitude of the individual pulses and the pulse rate. Since the pulse rate is fixed in most systems the intensity of the beam is proportional to pulse amplitude when the amplitude is expressed in decibels.

INTERACTION OF ULTRASOUND WITH MATTER

As an ultrasound pulse passes through matter, such as the human body, it interacts with the material in several different ways. Some of these interactions are necessary in order to form an ultrasound image whereas some interactions absorb much of the ultrasound energy and are generally undesirable in diagnostic examinations. The ability to conduct and interpret the results of an ultrasound examination depends on a thorough understanding of ultrasound interactions.

Attenuation

As the ultrasound pulse moves through matter it continuously loses energy. This is generally referred to as attenuation. Several factors contribute to this reduction in energy. One of the most significant is the absorption of the ultrasound energy by the material and its conversion into heat. Ultrasound pulses lose energy continuously as they move through matter. This is unlike x-ray photons which lose energy in "one-shot" photoelectric or Compton interactions. Scattering and refraction interactions remove some of the energy from the pulse and contribute to its overall attenuation.

The rate at which an ultrasound pulse is attenuated generally depends on two factors: the material through which it is passing and the frequency of the ultrasound. The attenuation rate is specified in terms of an attenuation coefficient in the units of decibels per centimeter. Since the attenuation in tissue increases with frequency it is necessary to specify the frequency when an attenuation rate is given. The attenuation through some thickness of materials, x, is given by:

$$\text{Attenuation (dB)} = \alpha \cdot \text{f} \cdot \text{x}$$

where α is the attenuation coefficient (in decibels per centimeter at 1 MHz) and f is the ultrasound frequency in megahertz. Some approximate values of the attenuation coefficient for various materials of interest are given in Table 2.

From the attenuation coefficient values given in Table 2 it is apparent that there is a considerable variation in attenuation rate from material to material. The significance of these values will now be considered. Of all the materials listed, water produces by far the least attenuation. This means that water is a very good conductor of ultrasound. Water contained within

Table 2. Approximate attenuation coefficient values for various materials

Material	Coefficient (dB/cm MHz)
Water	0.002
Fat	0.66
Soft tissue (average)	0.9
Muscle (average)	2.0
Air	12.0
Bone	20.0
Lung	40.0

the body, such as in cysts and the bladder, forms "windows" through which underlying structures can be easily imaged. Most of the soft tissues of the body have attenuation coefficient values of approximately 1 dB per cm per MHz with the exception of fat and muscle. Muscle has a range of values depending on the direction of the ultrasound with respect to the muscle fibers. Lung has a much higher attenuation rate than either air or soft tissue. This is because the small pockets of air in the alveoli are very effective in scattering the ultrasound energy. Because of this the normal lung structure is extremely difficult to penetrate with ultrasound. Compared to the soft tissues of the body, bone has a relatively high attenuation rate. Bone, in effect, shields some parts of the body against easy access to ultrasound exploration.

Reflection

The reflection of ultrasound pulses by structures within the body is the interaction which creates the ultrasound image. The reflection of an ultrasound pulse occurs at the interface or boundary between two dissimilar materials. In order to form a reflection interface the two materials must differ in terms of a physical characteristic which is known as acoustic impedance, Z. It should be pointed out that the traditional symbol for impedance is Z, which is the same symbol used for atomic number. The two quantities are in no way related. Acoustic impedance is a characteristic of a material which is related to the density and elastic properties of a material. Since the velocity is related to the same material characteristics, a relationship exists between tissue impedance and ultrasound velocity. The relationship is such that the impedance, Z, is the product of the velocity, v, and the material density, ρ, which can be written as:

$$\text{Impedance} = \rho \cdot \text{v}$$

At most interfaces within the body only a portion of the ultrasound pulse is reflected. What happens is that the pulse is divided into two pulses. One pulse is reflected back toward the source and the other continues on into the other material as shown in Figure 6. The quality of the ultrasound image depends on the strength of the reflection or echo. This in turn depends on how much the two materials differ in terms of acoustic impedance. The amplitude ratio of the reflected to the incident pulse is related to the tissue impedance values by:

$$\text{Reflection loss (dB)} = -20 \log \frac{Z_2 - Z_1}{Z_2 + Z_1}$$

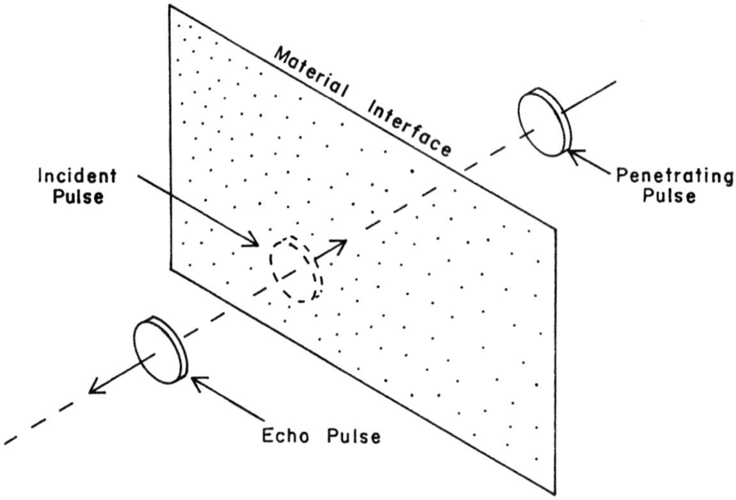

Figure 6. The creation of an echo pulse at a material interface.

At most soft tissue interfaces only a small fraction of the pulse is reflected. Therefore, the reflection process reduces the amplitude of the pulse which is reflected to the transducer. The reduction in pulse amplitude during reflection at several different interfaces is given in Table 3.

The amplitude of a pulse is reduced both by attenuation and reflection losses. Because of this an echo returning to the transducer is much smaller than the original pulse produced by the transducer.

Table 3. Pulse amplitude loss produced by a reflection

Interface	Amplitude loss (dB)
Ideal reflector	0.0
Tissue-air	−0.01
Bone-soft tissue	−3.8
Fat-muscle	−20.0
Tissue-water	−26.0
Muscle-blood	−30.0

FORMATION OF ULTRASOUND IMAGES

Most ultrasound images used for medical diagnostic purposes are formed by reflections or echoes from structural interfaces within the body. Reflected pulses, or echoes, are detected by the transducer where they are converted into electrical pulses which are then amplified and displayed in an appropriate image format. The several different types of image display will be discussed later.

When an ultrasound pulse returns to the transducer it brings with it two kinds of information as illustrated in Figure 7. Its relative amplitude provides information as to the type of interface which produced the reflection. The time interval between when a pulse leaves and when it returns to the transducer is related to the distance between the transducer and the reflecting interface. These two pulse characteristics are used to form the ultrasound image. There are some factors, however, in addition to the distance and type of interface which can alter the echo pulse. These need to be taken into consideration when performing ultrasound examinations.

In most imaging situations the ultrasound pulse will pass through several different materials on its way to a reflection site (interface) and

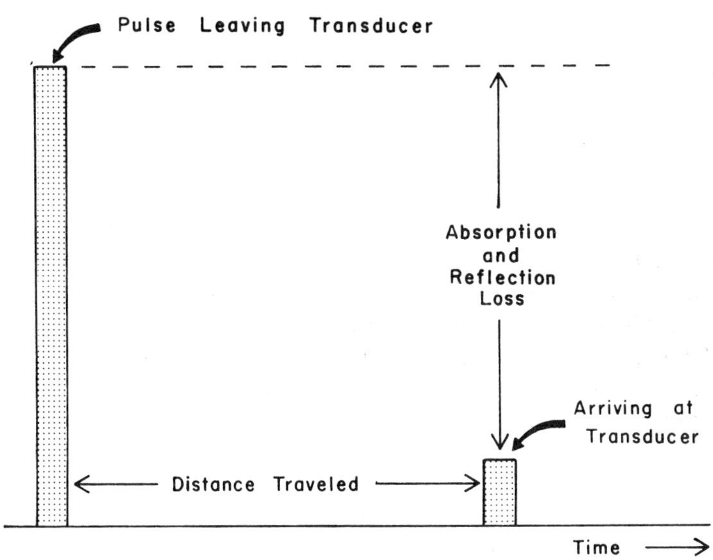

Figure 7. The relative amplitude and time of arrival of echo pulse provide the information necessary to form an ultrasound image.

back to the transducer. As discussed previously the velocity of the pulse depends on the characteristics of the material through which it is passing. Therefore, the velocity of the pulse actually changes as it passes from one material to another. The distance scale on most ultrasound equipment is calibrated for an ultrasound pulse velocity of 1540 m per sec. This is assumed to be the average velocity of a pulse passing through most soft tissues. Distance errors because of variation in ultrasound velocity are relatively small except in a material such as bone.

Echo Pulse Amplitude

When an echo pulse returns to the transducer its amplitude will be much less than when it left the transducer and began its journey into the body. It was pointed out earlier that the two factors which account for this are the attenuation of the ultrasound pulse as it passes through the various materials, and the reflection losses because of the splitting of the pulses at interface.

The body section shown in Figure 8 will be used to illustrate how both attenuation and reflection reduce the amplitude of echo pulses. This body section is not intended to represent any specific anatomical structure. The various materials have been chosen in order to demonstrate several physical phenomena which are important in ultrasound imaging. The amplitude of the pulse is plotted with respect to distance into the body in Figure 9. Reference should be made to both of these figures throughout the following discussion. It is assumed that the ultrasound frequency is 2.5 MHz.

As the pulse travels through the layer of fat it is attenuated at the rate of 1.7 dB per cm (0.66 dB per cm per MHz $\times$ 2.5 MHz). This is represented by segment a in Figure 9. After traversing the 3-cm thickness of fat the pulse amplitude will be reduced by 5 dB (1.7 dB per cm $\times$ 3 cm). At the fat-muscle interface the pulse will be split by a reflection. The reflected pulse from a fat-muscle interface is reduced in amplitude by 20 dB as indicated by segment b. The reflected pulse returns through the same layer of fat where it undergoes an additional reduction in amplitude of 5 dB as indicated by segment c. The echo which returns to the transducer is 30 dB smaller than the original pulse.

The fat-muscle interface produces a relatively weak reflection. Therefore, most of the pulse energy passes through it into the muscle. As it moves through the muscle it is attenuated at the rate of 5 dB per cm for a total loss of 15 dB in the 3-cm muscle thickness. This is represented by segment d. At the muscle-fluid interface a reflected pulse is produced which is approximately 23 dB smaller as indicated by segment e. As the reflected pulse returns to the transducer through the muscle and fat layers it

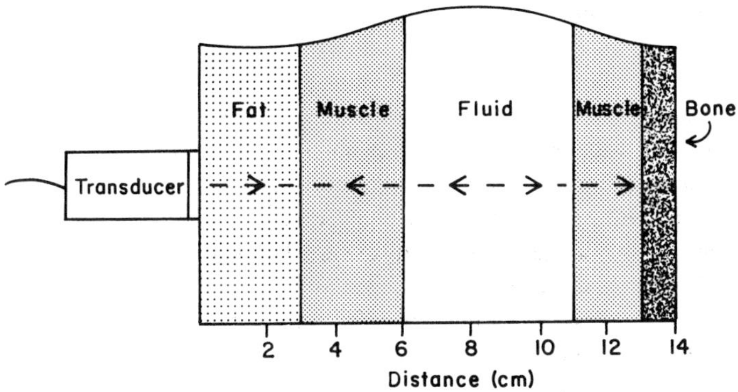

Figure 8. A body section containing different materials and interfaces.

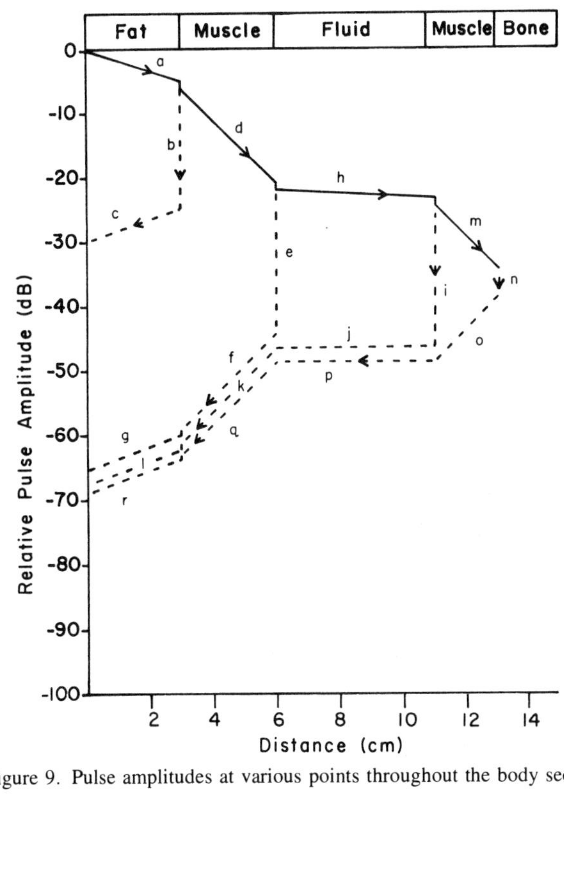

Figure 9. Pulse amplitudes at various points throughout the body section.

undergoes additional attenuation as indicated by segments f and g. The echo from the muscle-fluid interface is 65 dB smaller than the original pulse.

At the muscle-fluid interface most of the pulse energy passes on into the fluid. Since attenuation in fluid (water) is extremely small, no significant reduction in pulse amplitude occurs in the fluid as indicated by segment h. A small part of this pulse is reflected at the second fluid-muscle interface and is returned to the transducer. The loss of amplitude for this reflected pulse is represented by segments i, j, k and l.

The pulse energy which is not reflected continues on into the muscle where it undergoes additional attenuation as represented by segment m. At the muscle-bone interface a relatively strong reflection occurs and the echo is reduced by only 3.8 dB as indicated by segment n. This echo pulse returns to the transducer after undergoing the additional attenuation losses represented by segments o, p, q and r. When it reaches the transducer, its amplitude will be 69 dB smaller than the original pulse.

Amplitude Display (A-mode)

In the foregoing example each ultrasound pulse sent out by the transducer results in four echoes. The returning echo pulses are intercepted by the transducer and converted into electrical pulses. The electrical pulses are passed through an amplifier which increases their amplitude. The pulses from the amplifier go into an oscilloscope-type device which produces a visual display on a picture tube. It was pointed out earlier that the returning echo pulses picked up by the transducer differ in both amplitude and time of arrival after the initial pulse is sent out. The so-called amplitude (A) display, or mode, displays these two characteristics. The "pulses" appear on the screen of the display. The amplitude of the echo pulses is represented by the height of the pulses on the display. The position of the display pulses along the horizontal scale is proportional to echo return time which is interpreted as distance from the transducer. The purpose of an amplitude (A) mode display is to show the location and relative reflectivity of the various tissue interfaces. The relationship of the A-mode display to the structure of the body section is shown in Figure 10. In the ideal A-mode display the amplitude of the displayed pulse should indicate the strength of the reflection or echo. For example, in Figure 10 the echo pulse from the muscle-bone interface is much larger than the pulses from the fat-muscle or muscle-fluid interfaces. This relationship between pulse amplitude and type of interface can provide useful diagnostic information. It should be recalled, however, that the amplitude of the pulses returning to the transducer depends not only on the strength of the reflections but also on the

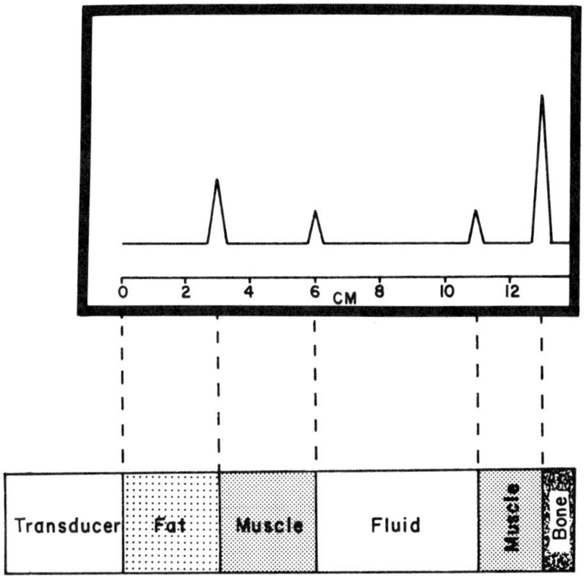

Figure 10. Relationship of A-mode display to body structure.

amount of attenuation along their path of travel. The attenuation losses can alter pulse amplitudes and make it difficult to determine the strength of a reflection from the size of a returning pulse. Attention is called once again to Figure 9. The echo from the relatively weak fat-muscle interface returns to the transducer with a reduction in amplitude of only 30 dB. However, the much stronger echo from the muscle-bone interface has been reduced in amplitude by 70 dB by the time it returns to the transducer. The reason the echo from the muscle-bone interface is smaller than the fat-muscle echo when it reaches the transducer is that it travels a much greater distance and experiences much more attenuation. The amplitude of the echo pulses reaching the transducer is shown in Figure 11 by the solid lines. The height of these should be compared to the height of the pulses in Figure 10. As stated previously the echo pulse from the fat-muscle interface is much larger than from the muscle-bone interface because it undergoes less attenuation.

In order for the pulse amplitudes to represent the strength of the various reflections it is necessary to remove the effects of attenuation on the pulse size. This can be done by amplifying the various pulses more or less in proportion to their attenuation losses. This in turn depends on the distance traveled by the ultrasound pulse and the attenuation coefficient

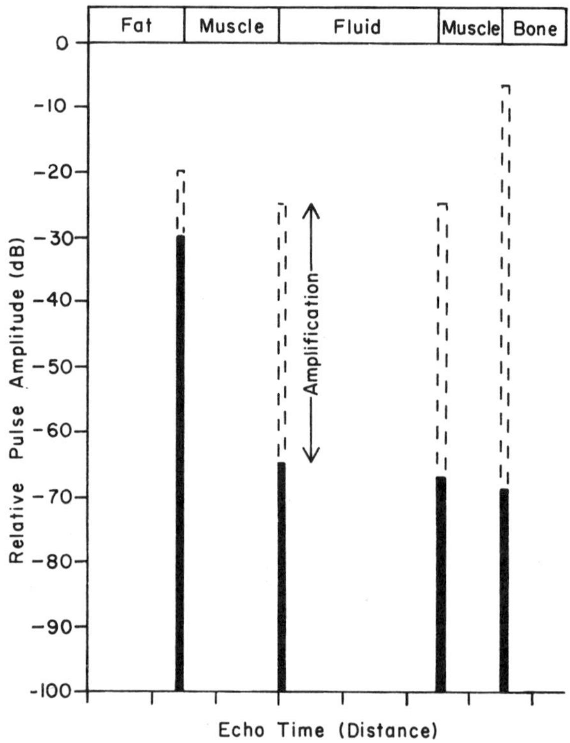

Figure 11. Amplitude of echo pulses without amplification (——) and after time-controlled amplification (- - -).

values of the material through which it passes. The attenuation loss of a 2.5-MHz pulse which is reflected from various distances within the body section is shown in the bottom of Figure 12. For example, an echo from the fat-muscle interface undergoes a 10-dB attenuation. It loses 5 dB in traveling from the transducer to the interface and another 5 dB traveling from the interface back to the transducer. As would be expected, pulses reflected from deeper within the body undergo the most attenuation. For example, echoes from the muscle-bone interface experience a 60-dB decrease in amplitude because of attenuation.

It is desirable to amplify the returning echo pulses in proportion to their attenuation losses. This is achieved by having the amplifier gain increase with time after each pulse leaves the transducer. This is generally referred to as time-controlled gain or TCG. Since the distance traveled by a pulse is proportional to its travel time, this gives a relationship between

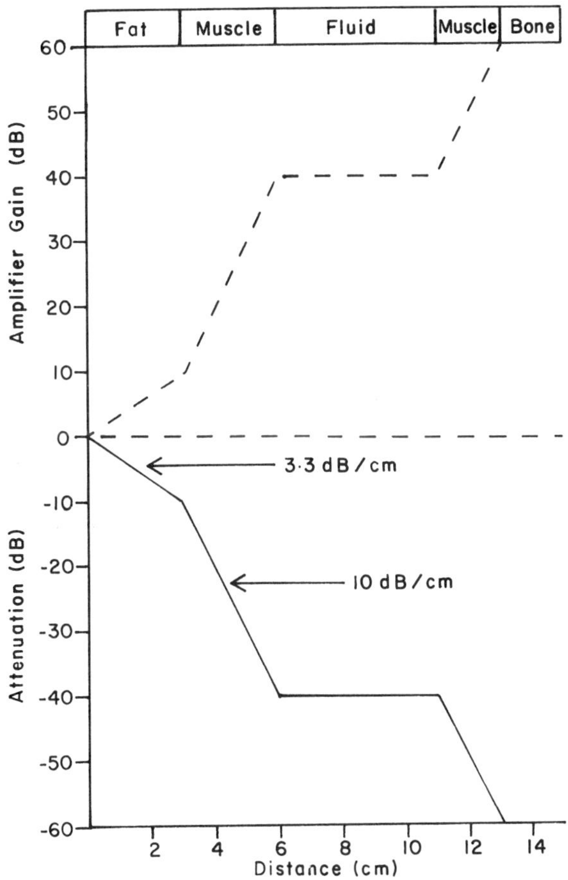

Figure 12. A TCG curve (top) which will provide compensation for the pulse attenuation described by bottom curve.

amplifier gain and distance to a reflection site. The fact that the rate of attenuation (decibels per centimeter) is not the same in all tissues must also be taken into account. When the pulse is passing through muscle the gain must increase faster than when the pulse is passing through fat. The rate at which the amplifier gain changes with time (distance) is generally expressed in units of decibels per centimeter. With most ultrasound equipment it is possible to have different TCG values over various distances within the body. The relationship between amplifier gain and the distance to an echo site is usually described by means of a TCG curve such as the one shown in the top of Figure 12. This particular TCG curve is one that would exactly compensate for the attenuation losses shown in the bottom half of the figure. In other words, the amplifier TCG curve which is a mirror image of the attenuation curve will provide complete compensation for attenuation within the tissues. When the echoes from the four interfaces are amplified in a time-controlled manner their relative amplitudes will be changed as shown in Figure 11. The echo from the fat-muscle interface will be amplified by only 10 dB. The echo from the muscle-fluid interfaces will be amplified by 40 dB and the muscle-bone echo will receive a 60-dB amplification. The increase in pulse size produced by this amplification is represented by the dotted lines in Figure 11. After passing through a properly adjusted TCG amplifier the pulse amplitudes represent the strength of the various ultrasound reflections. It should be noted that the amplified pulses in Figure 11, with respect to a −30 dB baseline, have the same relative amplitudes as the pulses in the ideal display of Figure 10.

The TCG curve is generally adjusted with respect to the particular body section being examined. Some equipment will have controls which are used to adjust the slopes (decibels per centimeter) of the various curve segments and the position of the break points. The first segment is often referred to as the near gain portion of the curve.

Brightness (B) Mode

Another useful type of ultrasound image is formed by using the amplitude of the various echo pulses to control the brightness of a spot on the display unit screen. This is a so-called B-mode display. A simple B-mode image is shown in Figure 13. This image should be compared to the A-mode image shown in Figure 10. It should be observed that the brightness (or film density) on the B-mode corresponds to the amplitude of the echo pulses shown in the A-mode display.

B-mode systems are generally classified as either bistable or gray scale. Bistable is an electronic term which means that there are only two stable states for a device. When applied to an ultrasound image it means that there are only two different brightness levels possible for any point within the image. In other words, the brightness of a point within the image can only be turned on or off by an echo. If the pulse amplitude is below some established level it does not turn the display on and nothing appears on the screen. A pulse with an amplitude above the established threshold level will cause a bright spot to appear on the screen. All pulses above the threshold level will create the same brightness on the screen regardless of their amplitudes. In a gray scale system the brightness of the spot is controlled by the amplitude of the echo pulse as shown in Figure 13. The relationship between image point brightness and the amplitude of the echo

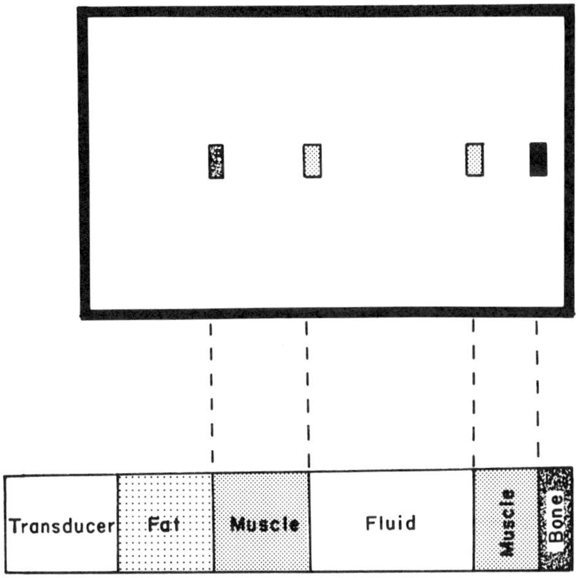

Figure 13. Relationship of a B-mode display (gray scale) to the interfaces within a body section.

pulses is determined by the characteristics and adjustment of the controls within the ultrasound system. The relationship between brightness and echo amplitude can be described by means of a graph as shown in Figure 14. An important characteristic of an ultrasound system is its dynamic range. The dynamic range is the range of pulse amplitudes corresponding to the full brightness range of the viewing unit. This is illustrated in Figure 14. The dynamic range of an ultrasound system is somewhat analogous to the latitude of an x-ray film.

If the transducer is not moved during the recording of an ultrasound image only echoes from structures within the relatively small beam area will be recorded. This is the type of image illustrated in Figure 13. A more useful B-mode image can be obtained by moving or scanning the ultrasound beam over the area of interest within the body. In order to form an image the location of the spots on the screen must be related to the position and orientation of the transducer with respect to the body section. Most transducers used for B-mode scanning are mounted on arm assemblies. Electronic sensors within the various arm joints create electrical signals which are used by the viewing unit to position the image spots on the screen. It is important for this system to be properly aligned in order to

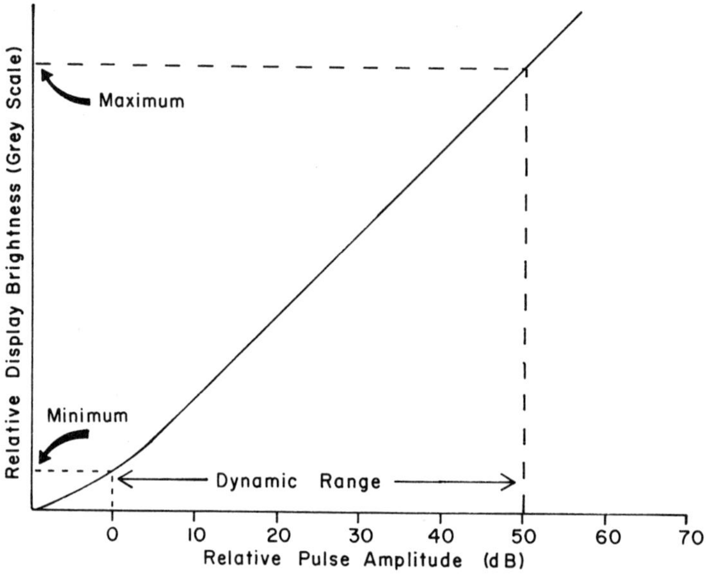

Figure 14. The relationship of dynamic range to display brightness.

establish proper registration of the image with the body section. In the absence of proper registration, object points (echo sites) within the body will appear to move when imaged with different transducer positions. This is a source of image blur which reduces the quality of the ultrasound image.

As the ultrasound beam is scanned through the area of interest the image from each beam position is stored within the viewing unit. With conventional ultrasound systems it takes several seconds to form a complete image. There are systems available, however, which can scan a body section at the rate of 10 or more times per second. These systems are generally designated as real-time devices and are useful for observing moving body structures since they give a "fluoroscopic"-type image.

Motion (M) Mode

In the M- or motion mode the ultrasound system produces a record of the motion of internal body structures. In the conventional M-mode systems the transducer is stationary with respect to the body and the echo pulses control the brightness of the display as in B-mode operation. The display of image points is moved across the screen as illustrated in Figure 15. Each echo site, in effect, leaves a track across the screen. A moving echo site will produce a curved track. By using a properly calibrated distance scale the amount of movement of the body structure can be readily determined.

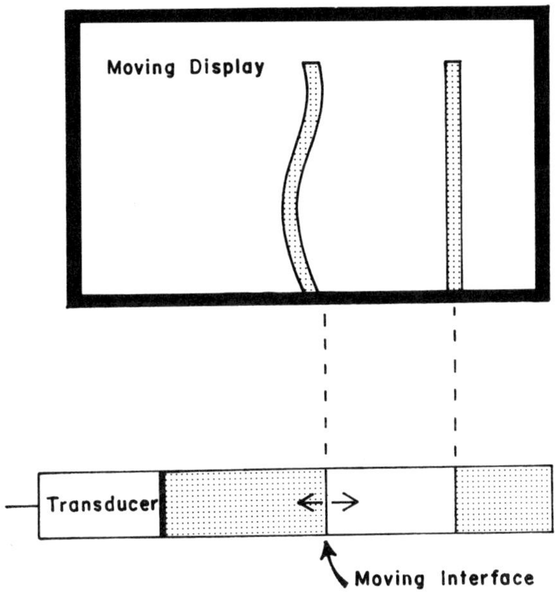

Figure 15. The recording of interface motion on an M-mode display.

BLUR AND RESOLUTION

The ultrasound image of a small object point or reflection site is usually larger than the point itself because of blur. In ultrasound imaging systems it is usually necessary to consider blur in two distinct directions as shown in Figure 16. This is because different system parameters affect blur in different directions. In some cases system blur is described in terms of resolution. In ultrasound resolution is usually defined as the minimum distance between two small echo sites which will result in a separate image of the two objects. It can be easily shown that blur and resolution, as defined above, are equivalent in value. For example, if the blur of one object point is 5 mm the separation distance between two such points (resolution) must be at least 5 mm before separate images can be created. The blur in the direction of the ultrasound beam is designated as axial blur. Blur in a direction normal to the beam axis, which is usually the direction of the scanning motion, is designated as lateral blur.

Lateral Blur

Lateral blur or resolution is determined by the diameter of the ultrasound pulse or beam at the time it interacts with the object creating the echo.

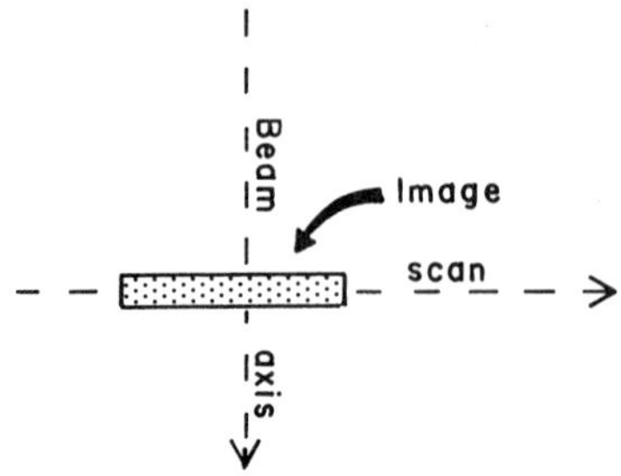

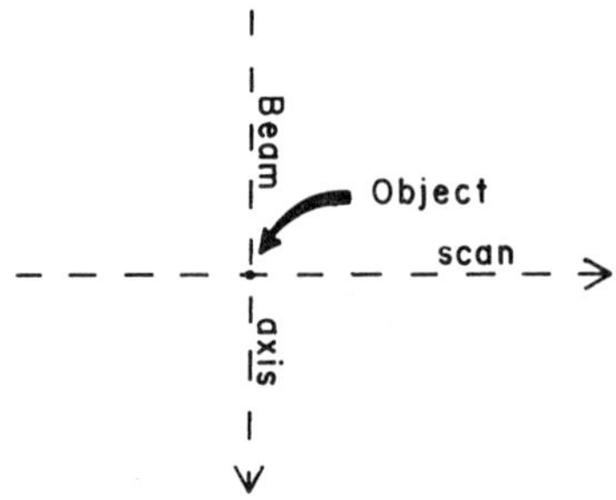

Figure 16. Relationship of image blur to the direction of the ultrasound beam and scanning motion.

Consider an ultrasound beam being scanned across an echo site as shown in Figure 17. Two beam positions during the scan are indicated. When the beam reaches position 1 during the scanning operation the edge of the beam will interact with the object and create an echo. Echoes will continue to be produced until the beam reaches position 2. This will cause an image on the B-mode display to be elongated, or blurred, in the scan direction as shown in Figure 16.

The width of the ultrasound beam is determined by certain characteristics of the transducer. The two basic types of transducers, with respect to beam shape, are the focused and unfocused.

The shape of the beam from an unfocused transducer is shown in Figure 18. The beam is divided into two rather distinct regions. The region nearest the transducer is designated as the near field or Fresnel zone. The other region is designated as the far field or Fraunhofer zone.

In the near field the beam has a constant diameter which is determined by the diameter of the transducer. The length of the near field is related to the diameter, D, of the transducer and the wavelength, λ, of the ultrasound by:

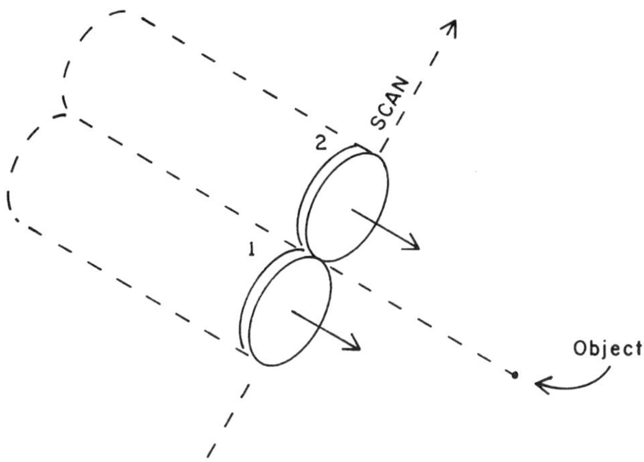

Figure 17. Two beam positions which will create echoes from a small object point. This is the source of lateral blur.

$$\text{Near field length} = \frac{D^2}{4\lambda}$$

It should be recalled that wavelength is inversely related to frequency. Therefore, for a given transducer size, the length of the near field is proportional to frequency. Another characteristic of the near field is that the intensity along the beam axis is not constant. The intensity oscillates between maximum and zero several times between the transducer surface and the boundary between the near and far field. This is because of the interference patterns created by the sound waves from the transducer surface. An intensity of zero at some point along the axis simply means that the sound vibrations are concentrated around the periphery of the beam. A picture of the ultrasound pulse in this region would look more like concentric rings or ''donuts'' than the disc which has been shown in various illustrations.

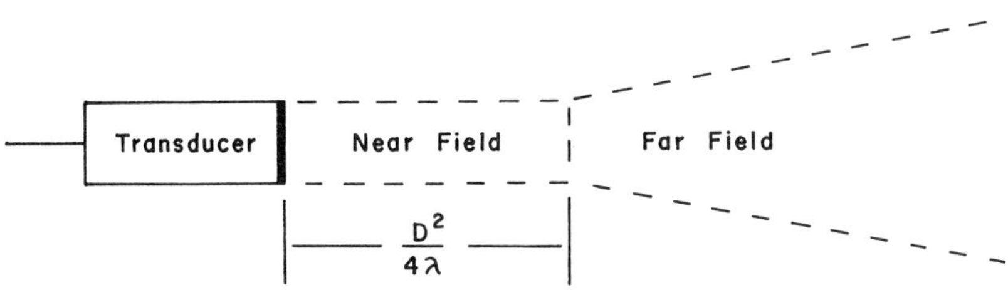

Figure 18. An unfocused ultrasound beam.

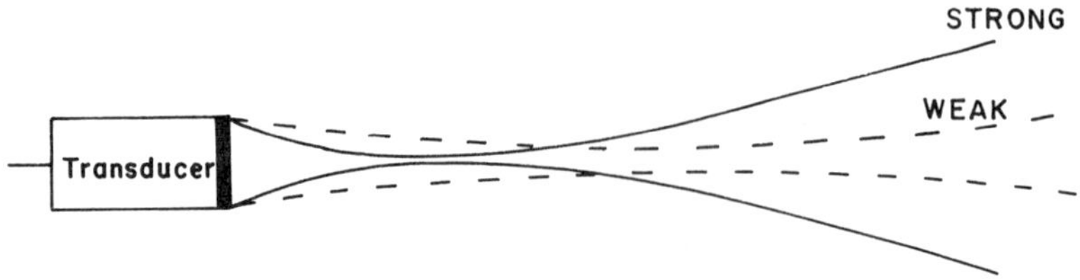

Figure 19. The variation in beam shape with degree of focusing.

The major characteristic of the far field is that the beam diverges. This causes the ultrasound pulses to be larger in diameter but to have less intensity along the central axis. The approximate angle of divergence is related to the diameter of the transducer, D, and the wavelength by:

$$\text{Divergence angle (degrees)} = \frac{70\lambda}{D}$$

Because of the inverse relationship between wavelength and frequency, divergence is decreased by increasing frequency. The major advantage of using the higher ultrasound frequencies (shorter wavelengths) is that the beams are less diverging and generally produce less blur.

An acoustical lens can be attached to the transducer to produce a focused beam as shown in Figure 19. Focusing can produce an ultrasound pulse with a diameter less than that of the transducer at some locations along the beam axis. The degree of focusing (strong or weak) is determined by the characteristics of the acoustic lens. A smaller beam can be produced by a strongly focused transducer but the small pulse size is limited to a rather short distance along the beam axis.

Axial Resolution

Axial or depth resolution is determined by the length or time duration of the ultrasound pulse. This, in turn, is determined by the characteristics of the transducer and amplifier circuit.

It has been shown that smaller beams are produced by increasing the ultrasound frequency. Therefore, it is desirable to use the higher frequencies when imaging small structures where blur might become a significant problem. The problem is that the attenuation is much greater at the higher frequencies. Therefore a transducer (frequency) must be selected which will provide a reasonable compromise between attenuation and blur.

Appendix

Mathematical Relationships in Radiology

The physics of radiology is a quantitative science. While some concepts of x-ray image formation can be discussed in a qualitative manner, an awareness of physical quantities is necessary in order to deal with the subject with any degree of completeness. For example, the formation of a simple x-ray image can be described in non-quantitative terms, but factors such as image quality and patient exposure can only be treated in a quantitative sense. The following material provides a review of the mathematical concepts that are generally encountered in radiology.

PHYSICAL QUANTITIES

In everyday life we constantly deal with such physical quantities as distance, time, weight, etc. In the field of radiology these and many more quantities are generally encountered. The basis of many radiological physics concepts is the relationship that exists between various physical quantities. After a review of the elements involved in the expression of quantities, the various types of relationships will be discussed in detail.

Symbols, Units, and Abbreviations

Every physical quantity has a name, such as weight or time. It is often desirable to use symbols as a kind of ''shorthand'' for writing the names of the various quantities. In most instances the symbols are one or more letters of the Roman (English) or Greek alphabet. Many times the chosen symbol is the first letter in the name of the quantity. Quantities are expressed in terms of a certain number of predefined units. For example, the

Table A.1. Selected unit conversion factors

From	To	Multiply by
inch	centimeter	2.54
centimeter	inch	0.394
foot	meter	0.305
meter	foot	3.28
pound	kilogram	0.456
kilogram	pound	2.20
degree F	degree C	(−32 first) 0.555
degree C	degree F	1.8 (+32)
quart	liter	0.946
liter	quart	1.06

weight of a patient might be expressed as 80 kg. In this case the unit used is the kilogram. It is possible to encounter more than one unit used for some quantities. A patient's weight can also be expressed in the units of pounds. The weight of the patient referred to above can also be specified as 176.4 pounds. The two most common systems of units are the metric and the English. A quantity expressed in one system of units can be converted to the other by multiplying by the appropriate conversion factor. A number of such conversion factors are given in Table A.1.

Standard abbreviations have been established for most units. Unit abbreviations make use of both small and capital letters of the alphabet. In most cases the small and capital letters cannot be interchanged because each has a specific meaning. For example, Mw is the abbreviation for the unit megawatt (one million watts), whereas mw is the abbreviation for milliwatt (0.001 watt).

Numbers and Scales

A given quantity can be specified by either stating the number of units, such as five roentgens, or by indicating a point on an appropriate scale. The two types of scales normally encountered in radiology are shown in Figure A.1. The scale at the top is a linear scale on which the quantity value is directly proportional to distance along the scale. A given distance between two points anywhere along the scale represents a specific difference in quantity values.

The second type of scale encountered is a logarithmic scale, as shown at the bottom. On a logarithmic scale, it is the logarithm of the quantity value that is directly proportional to distance along the scale. Logarithms will be discussed in more detail below. A logarithmic scale is in effect

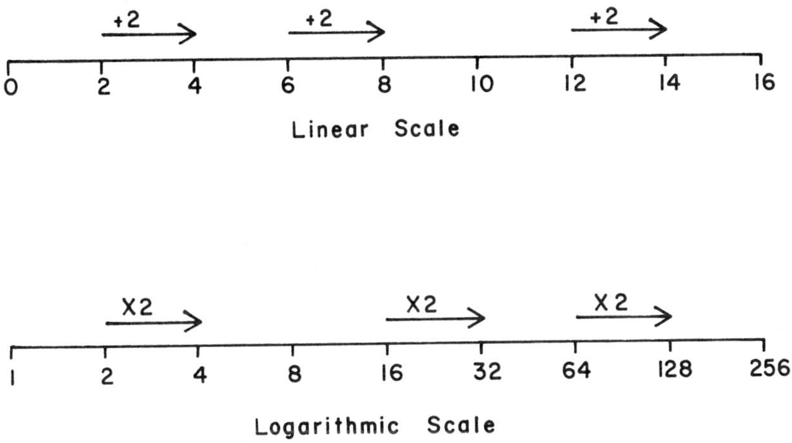

Figure A.1. Linear and logarithmic scales.

a ratio scale. The main characteristic of such a scale is that a specific distance between two points anywhere along the scale represents a certain *ratio* of quantity values rather than a *difference* in values as on the linear scale. Logarithmic scales are used either when the interest is in the ratio of quantities or when the quantity values cover a very large range.

MATHEMATICAL RELATIONSHIPS

Most of the physical principles of radiology are based on the relationship of one physical quantity to another. For example, the quantity of energy (E) delivered to an x-ray tube is directly related to the voltage (V) applied to the tube, the current (I) passing through the tube, and the duration (t) of the exposure, as is illustrated in the Figure A.2. Usually one quantity can be expressed in terms of some combination of other quantities. The energy deposited in an x-ray tube, for example, is equal to the product of tube voltage, current, and time. This relationship is usually expressed by means of an equation as follows:

$$E = V \cdot I \cdot t$$

An equation is a simple statement of a relationship among physical quantities. In many cases it is desirable to make a distinction between dependent and independent quantities involved in a relationship. In the present example energy (E) is the dependent quantity because its value depends on the values of voltage, current, and time. These quantities, in

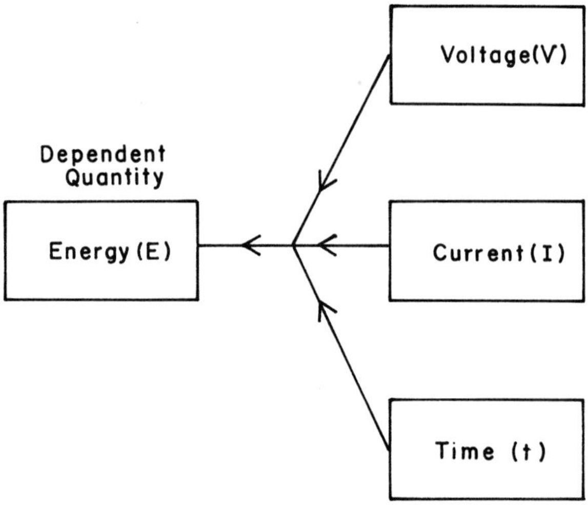

Figure A.2. The concept of a dependent physical quantity.

turn, depend on other quantities through other relationships. Equations usually express the dependent quantity in terms of the independent quantity or quantities.

In radiology equations are used for two different purposes. Equations can be used to find the value of a physical quantity that cannot be easily determined directly. The energy delivered to an x-ray tube is an example of this. Most x-ray machines do not have energy meters. They do have, however, either meters or controls that indicate the values of the voltage, current, and time. By knowing these values and the appropriate relationship it is possible to determine the energy. This is done by substituting the known values into the equation and then performing the necessary mathematical operations. Most equations encountered in radiology involve only the mathematical operations of addition, subtraction, multiplication, and division. A few relationships will involve logarithmic, exponential, and trigonometric functions. These special relationships will be discussed later.

It is not always necessary to determine the value of a specific physical quantity. However, in order to completely deal with a physical concept it is desirable to understand the nature of the relationships among the quantities involved. Usually the question is how much, and in what direction, will a dependent physical quantity change if other quantities are changed by a specified amount. This is generally determined by the type of relationship involved. The various types of relationships that are generally encountered in radiology will now be considered.

Proportional Relationships

Perhaps the most frequently encountered relationship between quantities in radiology is the proportional, or linear, type. In this type of relationship the value of the dependent quantity is proportional to the value of the independent quantities and will change accordingly. The simplest form of this type of relationship is represented by an equation such as:

$$Y = cX$$

where Y is the dependent quantity, X is the independent quantity, and c is a quantity or number that is generally considered to have a fixed or constant value. The value of c affects the value of the quantity Y. It does not, however, alter the relationship concerning changes in the quantities Y and X. When the quantity X changes, Y will change proportionally. That is, it will change by the same ratio or percentage as the change in X. For example, if the value of X is increased by 25%, the value of Y will also increase by 25% regardless of the value of c.

This type of relationship can be represented by a graph as shown in Figure A.3. When linear scales are used for the two quantities, X and Y, the relationship between the two is represented by a straight line, as is indicated. The slope of the line is determined by the value of c. The significant point, however, is that the percent change in Y is always equal to the percent change in X, regardless of the value of c.

Quite often a relationship involving more than two quantities will be encountered. An example of this is the relationship between a rectangle's area, A, and its length, L, and width, W. This relationship can be expressed as:

$$A = L \cdot W$$

In this case, the dependent quantity, A, is proportional to two quantities, L and W. Actually there are two relationships involved, one between A and L and the other between A and W. With respect to changes, each relationship can be considered separately. In a situation where the length, L, is not being changed, the relationship becomes:

$$A = cW$$

When W is changed, A will change proportionately.

Inverse Relationships

Another frequently encountered relationship is of the form:

$$Y = \frac{c}{X}$$

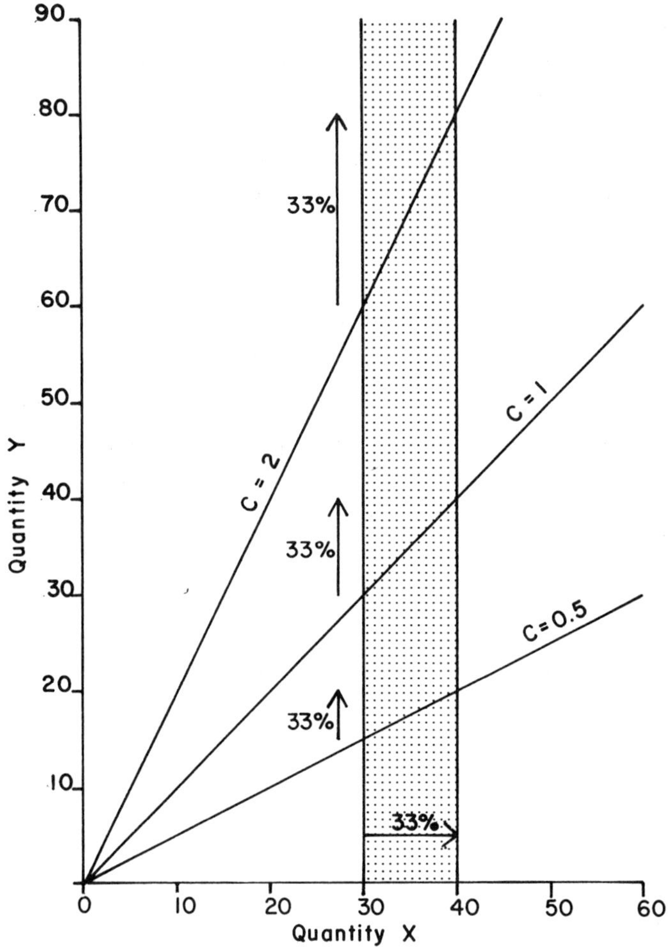

Figure A.3. A proportional relationship between quantities *Y* and *X*.

This is generally designated as an inverse, or reciprocal, relationship. When the quantity *X* increases, the dependent quantity, *Y*, decreases, and vice versa. This is actually a type of proportional relationship because the change in *Y* is proportional to the change in *X*. If *X* is increased by a factor of two, the value of the quantity *Y* is divided by two. The graph representing this relationship has a rather unique shape, as is shown in Figure A.4.

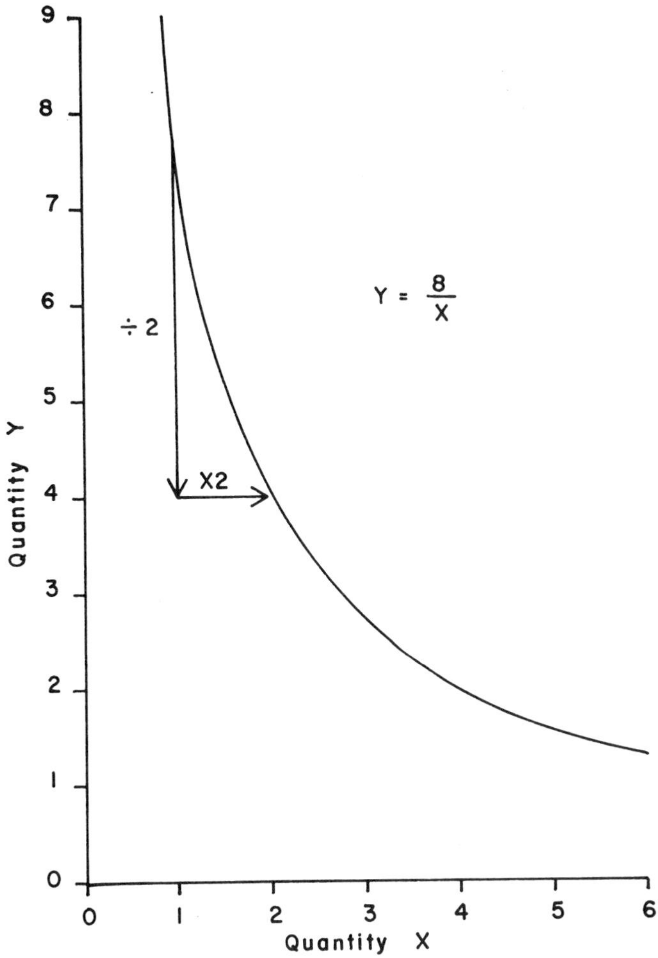

Figure A.4. An inverse relationship between quantities Y and X.

Square Relationships

In some physical situations the value of a dependent quantity is related to the product of some quantity and itself. When the relationship is of the form:

$$Y = c \cdot X \cdot X = cX^2$$

it is usually described as a square relationship because the value of Y is proportional to the square of the quantity X. When X changes, it is like two quantities undergoing a simultaneous change. This produces a change in Y that is larger than the change in X. For example, if X is increased by a factor of two, the value of Y increases by a factor of four $(2 \cdot 2)$. The significant characteristic of this relationship is that the changes in the dependent quantity, Y, are greater than the changes in X.

Another relationship encountered in radiology is a combination of the last two relationships (inverse and square) and is of the form:

$$Y = \frac{c}{X^2}$$

An increase in the quantity X produces a disproportionately larger decrease in the value of the dependent quantity, Y. If the quantity X is doubled in value, the value of Y is divided by 4 $(2 \cdot 2)$.

Logarithmic Relationships

One type of relationship often found between two quantities is the logarithmic. The concept of logarithms is related to the fact that a quantity, or number, can be expressed in terms of some multiple of another number. This is illustrated below, where several numbers are expressed as multiples of the number 10:

$$\begin{aligned} 10 &= 10 \cdot 10 = 10^2 \\ 1000 &= 10 \cdot 10 \cdot 10 = 10^3 \\ 10{,}000 &= 10 \cdot 10 \cdot 10 \cdot 10 = 10^4 \end{aligned}$$

One way of indicating the number of multiples is by using a superscript, which is known as an exponent. In the relationships shown above there are actually three different numbers involved. Each one has a special significance. It is helpful to designate each by an appropriate name, as follows:

exponent

$$10{,}000 = 10^4$$

the number — base

In this example, the number 10,000 is expressed as a multiple of the number 10. The number 10 is referred to as the base. The number 4, which designates the number of times 10 is multiplied by itself, is known as the exponent. Of special interest here is the relationship between the numbers 10,000 and 4. The number 4 (exponent) is the logarithm of the number

10,000. This is usually written as:

$$\log(10{,}000) = 4$$

In other words, the logarithm of a number is just the number of multiples of 10 that is equal to the number. For numbers that are exact multiples of 10, the value of the logarithm is obvious, such as:

$$\log(10) = 1$$
$$\log(100) = 2$$
$$\log(1000) = 3$$

The logarithm of other numbers is determined by using electronic calculators that have a logarithmic function, or by looking up the values in appropriate tables. Table A.2 gives the logarithms for some numbers encountered in radiology.

Table A.2. Logarithm values for numbers from 1 through 100[a]

X	log (X)	X	log (X)	X	log (X)	X	log (X)
1	0.000	26	1.415	51	1.708	76	1.881
2	0.301	27	1.431	52	1.716	77	1.886
3	0.477	28	1.447	53	1.724	78	1.892
4	0.602	29	1.462	54	1.732	79	1.898
5	0.699	30	1.477	55	1.740	80	1.903
6	0.778	31	1.491	56	1.748	81	1.908
7	0.845	32	1.505	57	1.756	82	1.914
8	0.903	33	1.519	58	1.763	83	1.919
9	0.954	34	1.531	59	1.771	84	1.924
10	1.000	35	1.544	60	1.778	85	1.929
11	1.041	36	1.556	61	1.785	86	1.934
12	1.079	37	1.568	62	1.792	87	1.939
13	1.114	38	1.580	63	1.799	88	1.944
14	1.146	39	1.591	64	1.806	89	1.949
15	1.176	40	1.602	65	1.813	90	1.954
16	1.204	41	1.613	66	1.820	91	1.959
17	1.230	42	1.623	67	1.826	92	1.964
18	1.255	43	1.633	68	1.833	93	1.968
19	1.279	44	1.643	69	1.839	94	1.973
20	1.301	45	1.653	70	1.845	95	1.977
21	1.322	46	1.663	71	1.851	96	1.982
22	1.342	47	1.672	72	1.857	97	1.987
23	1.362	48	1.681	73	1.863	98	1.991
24	1.380	49	1.690	74	1.869	99	1.996
25	1.398	50	1.699	75	1.875	100	2.000

[a]For larger numbers, add 1 for each multiple of 10, subtract for smaller numbers.

The general logarithmic relationship between two quantities, X and Y, can be expressed as:

$$Y = \log(X)$$

which is the same relationship as:

$$X = 10^Y$$

There are several aspects of the relationship between a number, or quantity, and its logarithm that should now be considered. One is that all numbers larger than 1 have positive logarithms, whereas all numbers smaller than 1 (fractions) have negative logarithms. The logarithm of the number 1 is 0. Another significant characteristic of the relationship is that when the number changes by some *multiple* or ratio, the logarithm changes by a *difference*. For example, if a number is multiplied by ten, the logarithm of the new number is the logarithm of the old number plus 1, regardless of the value of the original number. The relationship between numbers and their logarithms is shown graphically in Figure A.5. It should be noticed that the numbers are on a logarithmic scale. This is why the relationship can be described by a straight line.

Any number can be used as the base for logarithms but the most common base is the number ten. Logarithms using a base of ten are referred to as *common* logarithms.

Exponential Relationships

Exponential and logarithmic relationships between two quantities are essentially the same. For example, if two quantities, Y and X, have the following relationship:

$$Y = 10^X$$

it would generally be referred to as an exponential relationship. However, the same relationship can be expressed as:

$$X = \log(Y)$$

because of the definition of a logarithm. The classification of a relationship as either exponential or logarithmic depends primarily on the point of view and which is the dependent quantity. If Y is the dependent quantity and is determined by the value of the quantity X, the relationship would be stated as:

$$Y = 10^X$$

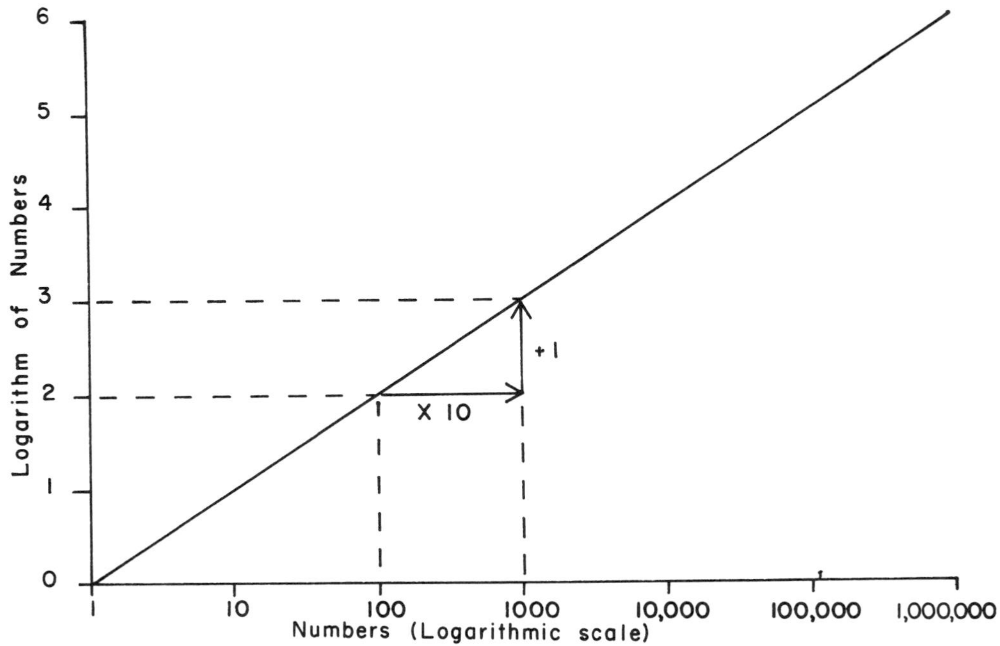

Figure A.5. The relationship between numbers and the value of their logarithms.

If, on the other hand, X is the dependent quantity the relationship is generally expressed as:

$$X = \log (Y)$$

The basic characteristic of an exponential relationship is that when the independent quantity changes by one unit the dependent quantity changes by a multiple of the base number. Consider the relationship:

$$Y = 10^X$$

when X has a value of 3. This gives Y a value of:

$$Y = 10^3 = 1000$$

If the value of X is now changed by one unit, from 3 to 4, the value of Y changes by a multiple of 10 and becomes:

$$Y = 10^4 = 10{,}000$$

The significant point is that a small change in one quantity (X) produces a large change in the other quantity.

Up to this point the discussion of exponential and logarithmic relationships have used a base number of 10. It is possible to have this type of relationship with other numbers serving as the base. There are many natural phenomena, such as x-ray penetration and radioactive decay, that can be described in terms of exponential relationships using a base number of 2.718. This is known as Euler's number, and the symbol for it is e. The general relationship involving Euler's number (e) is:

$$Y = e^X$$

Here it is assumed that Y is the quantity whose value depends on the value of X. The corresponding logarithmic relationship is:

$$X = ln\ (Y)$$

When Euler's number is used as the base the so-called *natural* logarithm is obtained. In the above relationship *ln* stands for "the natural logarithm of." It should be recalled that a base number of 10 yields *common* logarithms.

The exponential relationship most often encountered in radiology is one in which the exponent is negative, and is usually written as:

$$Y = e^{-X}$$

It should be recalled that a negative exponent indicates a reciprocal. Therefore, this particular type of relationship could also be expressed as:

$$Y = e^{-X} = \frac{1}{e^X}$$

When it is expressed in this manner, it is easy to see that as the value of X increases the quantity Y becomes smaller. More specifically, when the value of X is increased by one unit, the value of Y is divided by e (2.718), or is reduced to almost one third of its original value.

When the value of X is known, the corresponding value for the quantity Y can be found either by using an electronic calculator with exponential functions or by referring to tabulated values, such as in Table A.3.

Trigonometric Relationships

In some cases the relationship between physical quantities involves some of the so-called trigonometric functions. These functions are often involved in relationships in which one of the quantities is an angle. The

Table A.3. Values of Euler's number with negative exponents

X	e^{-X}
0.05	0.951
0.10	0.905
0.15	0.861
0.20	0.819
0.25	0.779
0.30	0.741
0.35	0.705
0.40	0.670
0.45	0.638
0.50	0.606
0.60	0.549
0.70	0.497
0.80	0.449
0.90	0.407
1.00	0.368
1.2	0.301
1.4	0.247
1.6	0.202
1.8	0.165
2.0	0.135
2.5	0.082
3.0	0.050
4.0	0.018
5.0	0.007

Table A.4. Cosine values for selected angles

X (degrees)	Cos (X)
0	1.000
10	0.985
20	0.940
30	0.866
40	0.766
50	0.643
60	0.500
70	0.342
80	0.174
90	0.000
100	−0.174
110	−0.342
120	−0.500
130	−0.643
140	−0.766
150	−0.866
160	−0.940
170	−0.985
180	−1.000

one that is encountered in radiology is the cosine function. A simple relationship involving the cosine function can be expressed as:

$$Y = \cos(X)$$

where Y is the dependent quantity and X is an angle, which is typically expressed in degrees.

The value of the cosine is related to the length of the sides of a right triangle. Specifically, the value of the cosine is the ratio of the length of the side adjacent to the angle to the length of the hypotenuse, or longest side. Cosine values range from 0 to 1 and are both positive and negative, depending on the angle. The cosine values for some selected angles are given in Table A.4.

EXERCISES

In the following problems, find the value of Y.

$$Y = W \cdot Y \cdot Z \tag{1.}$$

when, $W = 565$

$X = 2$
$Z = 27$

$$Y = \frac{X}{W \cdot Z} \tag{2.}$$

when, $W = 5$
$X = 30$
$Z = 60$

$$Y = X(W - Z) \tag{3.}$$

when, $W = 96$
$X = 3$
$Z = 64$

$$X \cdot Y \cdot Z = 400 \tag{4.}$$

when, $X = 20$
$Z = 5$

$$Y = W \cdot X^2 \tag{5.}$$

when, $W = 40$
$X = 6$

$$Y = W \cdot 10^X \tag{6.}$$

when, $W = 45$
$X = 3$

$$Y = W \cdot 10^{-X} \tag{7.}$$

when, $W = 78$
$X = 4$

$$Y = W \cdot \log X \tag{8.}$$

when, $W = 36$
$X = 27$

$$Y = W \cdot \log X \tag{9.}$$

when, $W = 25$
$X = 1500$

$$Y = W \cdot \log X \tag{10.}$$

when, $W = 65$
$X = 0.015$

$$Y = W \cdot e^{-X} \tag{11.}$$

when, $W = 50$
$X = 0.5$

$$Y = W \cdot e^{-XZ} \tag{12.}$$

when, $W = 80$
$X = 1.8$
$Z = 0.5$

$$Y = W \cdot \cos(X) \tag{13.}$$

when, $W = 98$
$X = 10$ degrees

In the following problems, describe the *change* in Y.

$$Y = W \cdot X \cdot Z \tag{14.}$$

when, X changes from 15 to 75

$$Y = W \cdot X^2 \cdot Z \tag{15.}$$

when, X changes from 75 to 150
X changes from 75 to 300
X increases by 25%

$$Y = \frac{W \cdot Z}{X} \tag{16.}$$

when, X changes from 35 to 105
X changes from 70 to 35

$$Y = \frac{W \cdot Z}{X^2} \tag{17.}$$

when, X changes from 40 to 80
X changes from 40 to 120
X changes from 40 to 20

$$Y = W \cdot Z \cdot \log X \tag{18.}$$

when, X changes from 45 to 450
X changes from 32 to 93

$$Y = W \cdot Z \cdot 10^{-X} \tag{19.}$$

when, X changes from 1 to 2
X changes from 6 to 4

$$Y = W \cdot Z \cdot e^{-X} \tag{20.}$$

when, X changes from 1 to 2
X changes from 0.2 to 0.8

Index